Fragility Fractures

Editors

SUSAN M. FRIEDMAN
DANIEL ARI MENDELSON

CLINICS IN
GERIATRIC MEDICINE

www.geriatric.theclinics.com

May 2014 • Volume 30 • Number 2

ELSEVIER

1600 John F. Kennedy Boulevard • Suite 1800 • Philadelphia, Pennsylvania, 19103-2899

http://www.theclinics.com

CLINICS IN GERIATRIC MEDICINE Volume 30, Number 2
May 2014 ISSN 0749-0690, ISBN-13: 978-0-323-26656-7

Editor: Jessica McCool
Developmental Editor: Yonah Korngold

Clinics in Geriatric Medicine (ISSN 0749-0690) is published quarterly by Elsevier Inc., 360 Park Avenue South, New York, NY 10010-1710. Months of issue are February, May, August, and November. Business and Editorial Offices: 1600 John F. Kennedy Blvd., Suite 1800, Philadelphia, PA 191023-2899. Periodicals postage paid at New York, NY, and additional mailing offices. Subscription prices are $280.00 per year (US individuals), $498.00 per year (US institutions), $145.00 per year (US student/resident), $370.00 per year (Canadian individuals), $632.00 per year (Canadian institutions), $195.00 per year (Canadian student/resident), $390.00 per year (foreign individuals), $632.00 per year (foreign institutions), and $195.00 per year (foreign student/resident). Foreign air speed delivery is included in all *Clinics* subscription prices. All prices are subject to change without notice. POSTMASTER: Send address changes to *Clinics in Geriatric Medicine,* Elsevier Health Sciences Division, Subscription Customer Service, 3251 Riverport Lane, Maryland Heights, MO 63043. Telephone: 1-800-654-2452 (U.S. and Canada); 314-447-8871 (outside U.S. and Canada). Fax: 314-447-8029. E-mail: journalscustomerservice-usa@elsevier.com (for print support) or journalsonlinesupport-usa@elsevier.com (for online support).

Reprints. For copies of 100 or more, of articles in this publication, please contact the Commercial Reprints Department, Elsevier Inc., 360 Park Avenue South, New York, New York 10010-1710. Tel.: 212-633-3874; Fax: 212-633-3820, E-mail: reprints@elsevier.com.

Clinics in Geriatric Medicine is covered in *MEDLINE/PubMed (Index Medicus), EMBASE/Excerpta Medica, Current Contents/Clinical Medicine (CC/CM),* and the *Cumulative Index to Nursing & Allied Health Literature.*

Printed and bound by CPI Group (UK) Ltd, Croydon, CR0 4YY

Contributors

EDITORS

SUSAN M. FRIEDMAN, MD, MPH, FACP, AGSF
Associate Professor of Medicine, Division of Geriatrics, University of Rochester School of Medicine and Dentistry; Department of Medicine, Highland Hospital, Rochester, New York

DANIEL ARI MENDELSON, MS, MD, FACP, AGSF, CMD
Associate Professor of Medicine, Division of Geriatrics, University of Rochester School of Medicine and Dentistry; Director, Consultative Services, Highland Hospital; Co-Director, Geriatric Fracture Center, Highland Hospital; Medical Director, Monroe Community Hospital; Medical Director, Highlands at Brighton; Department of Medicine, Highland Hospital, Rochester, New York

AUTHORS

DORCAS BEATON, BScOT, PhD
Scientist & Director, Mobility Program Clinical Research Unit, Li Ka Shing Knowledge Institute, St. Michael's Hospital; Associate Professor, Institute of Health Policy, Management & Evaluation, University of Toronto, Toronto, Ontario, Canada

MICHAEL BLAUTH, MD
Department for Trauma Surgery and Sports Medicine, Medical University of Innsbruck, Innsbruck, Austria

EARL BOGOCH, MD, MSc, FRCSC
Medical Director, Mobility Program, St. Michael's Hospital; Professor, Department of Surgery, University of Toronto, Toronto, Ontario, Canada

SUSAN BUKATA, MD
Associate Professor, Department of Orthopaedic Surgery, University of California, Los Angeles, Los Angeles, California

JEFFREY L. CARSON, MD
Vice Chair, Research, Richard C Reynolds Professor of Medicine, Chief, Division of General Internal Medicine, Rutgers Robert Wood Johnson Medical School, New Brunswick, New Jersey

ODDOM DEMONTIERO, MBBS, FRACP
Senior Staff Specialist, Department of Geriatric Medicine, Nepean Hospital; Research Fellow, Ageing Bone Research Program, Sydney Medical School Nepean, The University of Sydney, Penrith, New South Wales, Australia

GUSTAVO DUQUE, MD, PhD, FRACP
Senior Staff Specialist, Department of Geriatric Medicine, Nepean Hospital; Director, Ageing Bone Research Program, Professor, Division of Geriatric Medicine, Sydney Medical School Nepean, The University of Sydney, Penrith, New South Wales, Australia

MICHELLE ESLAMI, MD
Clinical Professor of Medicine, David Geffen School of Medicine at UCLA, Los Angeles,
California

MINDY J. FAIN, MD
Professor of Medicine, Division Chief, Geriatrics, General Internal Medicine and Palliative
Medicine, Department of Medicine, University of Arizona College of Medicine, Tucson,
Arizona

SUSAN M. FRIEDMAN, MD, MPH, FACP, AGSF
Associate Professor of Medicine, Division of Geriatrics, University of Rochester School
of Medicine and Dentistry; Department of Medicine, Highland Hospital, Rochester,
New York

LAUREN JAN GLEASON, MD
Geriatric Medicine Fellow, Department of Internal Medicine, Beth Israel Deaconess
Medical Center, Boston, Massachusetts

MARKUS GOSCH, MD
Department of Acute Geriatrics, State Hospital Hochzirl, Austria

PIUMALI GUNAWARDENE, MBBS, FRACP
Senior Staff Specialist, Department of Geriatric Medicine, Nepean Hospital; Research
Fellow, Ageing Bone Research Program, Sydney Medical School Nepean, The University
of Sydney, Penrith, New South Wales, Australia

CATHERINE A. HUMPHREY, MD
Chief, Orthopaedics, Highland Hospital, University of Rochester Medical Center;
Assistant Professor, Trauma Division, Orthopaedics, Strong Memorial Hospital, University
of Rochester Medical Center, Rochester, New York

HOUMAN JAVEDAN, MD
Instructor of Medicine, Harvard Medical School; Director Inpatient Geriatric Services,
Division of Aging, Brigham and Women's Hospital, Boston, Massachusetts

CHRISTIAN KAMMERLANDER, MD, PD
Department for Trauma Surgery and Sports Medicine, Medical University of Innsbruck,
Innsbruck, Austria

STEPHEN L. KATES, MD
Hansjörg Wyss Professor of Orthopaedic Surgery, Department of Orthopaedics and
Rehabilitation, University of Rochester, Rochester, New York

THOMAS J. LUGER, MD
Department of Anaesthesia and Intensive Care, Medical University of Innsbruck,
Innsbruck, Austria

MICHAEL A. MACEROLI, MD
Department of Orthopaedics, University of Rochester Medical Center, Rochester,
New York

SIMON C. MEARS, MD, PhD
Department of Orthopaedic Surgery, Johns Hopkins Bayview Medical Center, The Johns
Hopkins University, Baltimore, Maryland

DANIEL ARI MENDELSON, MS, MD, FACP, AGSF, CMD
Associate Professor of Medicine, Division of Geriatrics, University of Rochester School of Medicine and Dentistry; Director, Consultative Services, Highland Hospital; Co-Director, Geriatric Fracture Center, Highland Hospital; Medical Director, Monroe Community Hospital; Medical Director, Highlands at Brighton; Department of Medicine, Highland Hospital, Rochester, New York

JOSEPH A. NICHOLAS, MD, MPH
Assistant Professor of Medicine, Division of Geriatrics, Highland Hospital, University of Rochester School of Medicine, Rochester, New York

REGIS O'KEEFE, MD, PhD
Professor, Department of Orthopaedic Surgery, University of Rochester, Rochester, New York

JEAN-PIERRE P. OUANES, DO
Assistant Professor, Anesthesiology and Critical Care Medicine, Johns Hopkins University School of Medicine, The Johns Hopkins Hospital; Director, Regional Anesthesia, Johns Hopkins Bayview Medical Center, Baltimore, Maryland

JOANNA E.M. SALE, PhD
Scientist, Mobility Program Clinical Research Unit, Li Ka Shing Knowledge Institute, St. Michael's Hospital; Assistant Professor, Institute of Health Policy, Management & Evaluation, University of Toronto, Toronto, Ontario, Canada

V. ANA SANGUINETI, MD
Assistant Professor of Medicine, Division of Geriatrics, General Internal Medicine and Palliative Medicine, Department of Medicine, University of Arizona College of Medicine, Tucson, Arizona

RENE SCHMID, MD, PD
Department for Trauma Surgery and Sports Medicine, Medical University of Innsbruck, Innsbruck, Austria

FREDERICK SIEBER, MD
Professor, Chairman, Department of Anesthesiology and Critical Care Medicine, Johns Hopkins Bayview Medical Center, The Johns Hopkins Hospital, Johns Hopkins University School of Medicine, Baltimore, Maryland

VICENTE GARCIA TOMAS, MD
Assistant Professor, Department of Anesthesiology and Critical Care Medicine; Assistant Program Director, Anesthesiology Residency Program, The Johns Hopkins Hospital, Johns Hopkins University School of Medicine, Baltimore, Maryland

HONG-PHUC TRAN, MD
Assistant Clinical Professor, David Geffen School of Medicine at UCLA, Santa Monica, California

SAMIR TULEBAEV, MD
Instructor of Medicine, Harvard Medical School; Division of Aging, Brigham and Women's Hospital, Boston, Massachusetts

WAKENDA TYLER, MD, MPH
Assistant Professor, Department of Orthopaedic Surgery, University of Rochester, Rochester, New York

JOSHUA D. UY, MD
Clinical Assistant Professor, University of Pennsylvania School of Medicine, Philadelphia, Pennsylvania

JASON R. WILD, MD
Assistant Professor of Orthopaedic Surgery, Department of Orthopaedic Surgery, University of Arizona College of Medicine, Tucson, Arizona

LAURA REES WILLETT, MD, FACP
Associate Professor of Medicine, Division of Education, Rutgers Robert Wood Johnson Medical School, New Brunswick, New Jersey

MICHAEL ZEGG, MD
Department for Trauma Surgery and Sports Medicine, Medical University of Innsbruck, Innsbruck, Austria

Contents

As the world population of older adults—in particular those over age 85—increases, the incidence of fragility fractures will also increase. It is predicted that the worldwide incidence of hip fractures will grow to 6.3 million yearly by 2050. Fractures result in significant financial and personal costs. Older adults who sustain fractures are at risk for functional decline and mortality, both as a function of fractures and their complications and of the frailty of the patients who sustain fractures. Identifying individuals at high risk provides an opportunity for both primary and secondary prevention.

This article describes the principles of comanagement in an optimized geriatric fracture center. This is a collaborative model of care that uses patient-centered, protocol-driven care to standardize the care for most patient fragility fractures. This model also uses shared decision making and frequent communication to improve clinically relevant outcomes. The orthopedic and medical teams are equally responsible from admission to discharge and are responsible for daily evaluation and clinical management of the patient.

Geriatric hip fracture is a common event associated with high costs of care and often with suboptimal outcomes for the patients. Ideally, a new care model to manage geriatric hip fractures would address both quality and safety of patient care as well as the need for reduced costs of care. The geriatric fracture center model of care is one such model reported to improve both outcomes and quality of care. It is a lean business model applied to medicine. This article describes basic lean business concepts applied to geriatric fracture care and information needed to successfully implement a geriatric fracture center. It is written to assist physicians and surgeons in their efforts to implement an improved care model for their patients.

Because most older adults with hip fractures require urgent surgical intervention, the preoperative medical evaluation focuses on the exclusion of the small number of contraindications to surgery, and rapid optimization of patients for operative repair. Although many geriatric fracture patients have significant chronic medical comorbidities, most patients can be safely stabilized for surgery with medical and orthopedic comanagement by anticipating a small number of common physiologic responses and perioperative complications. In addition to estimating perioperative risk, the team should focus on intravascular volume restoration, pain control, and avoidance of perioperative hypotension.

This article describes current literature and treatment plans for managing anticoagulation and antiplatelet agents in patients presenting with hip fractures. Indications for anticoagulation and antiplatelet agents are discussed, and management techniques for when patients present with hip fractures are reviewed.

The location and type of hip fracture, and the patient's activity level, help to determine the method of surgical repair. Nondisplaced femoral neck fractures are treated with screw fixation. Displaced fractures are treated with arthroplasty. If the patient is very active, the treatment of choice should be total hip replacement, whereas if the patient is less active, the treatment of choice is hemiarthroplasty. Intertrochanteric fractures are classified as stable (treated with a sliding hip screw) or unstable (treated with an intramedullary hip screw). Subtrochanteric fractures are classified as typical or atypical. All subtrochanteric fractures are treated with intramedullary hip screws.

In this article, an overview is presented of perioperative management of the patient with a fragility fracture, including preoperative risk stratification and optimization, anesthesia risks, anesthesia options, and postoperative pain management. Issues of preoperative evaluation that are of concern for the anesthesiologist because of their direct effect on intraoperative care are discussed. A team interdisciplinary approach and good communication between specialties involved in care of elderly surgical patients is important for optimal patient outcomes and to avoid perioperative complications. Cooperation between anesthesiology and medicine is indispensable in reaching a reasonable consensus regarding preoperative evaluation and should occur on a case-by-case basis.

The goal of postoperative management is to promote early mobility and avoid postoperative complications, recognizing the potentially devastating impact of complications on elderly patients with hip fracture. The recommended approach involves early mobilization; freedom from tethers (indwelling urinary catheters and other devices); effective pain control; treating malnutrition; preventing pressure ulcers; reducing risk for pulmonary, urinary, and wound infections; and managing cognition. This carefully structured and patient-centered management provides older, vulnerable patients their best chance of returning to their previous level of functioning as quickly and safety as possible.

guidelines. Many patients can be safely and effectively managed with close attention to intravascular volume status, heart rate control, and minimization of other physiologic stresses, including pain and delirium. Many chronic cardiovascular therapies may be harmful in the immediate postoperative period, and can usually be safely omitted or attenuated until hemodynamic stability and mobility have been restored.

metaphysis. These fractures have an increased incidence in patients taking bisphosphonates for osteoporosis and develop as stress reactions in the lateral cortex of the femoral shaft. The fractures often have a distinct radiographic appearance with thickening or beaking of the lateral cortex. Treatment should be initiated immediately. There is a higher incidence of complications with atypical fractures. Early detection of these fractures can greatly reduce morbidity.

Christian Kammerlander, Michael Zegg, Rene Schmid, Markus Gosch, Thomas J. Luger, and Michael Blauth

The treatment of osteoporotic vertebral fractures is complicated because of the comorbid conditions of the elderly patient. Underlying osteoporosis leads to malalignment of the weakened bone and impedes fracture fixation. The treatment of osteoporotic vertebral fractures is widely empirical, because standardized and accepted treatment evidence-based concepts are missing for certain fracture types. As in other osteoporotic fractures in the elderly, the key for good outcome may be a combination of interdisciplinary treatment approaches and adapted surgical procedures. This article gives an overview of the underlying problems and possible treatment strategies for treatment of osteoporotic vertebral fractures in geriatric patients.

Catherine A. Humphrey and Michael A. Maceroli

Fractures of the pelvis and acetabulum in osteoporotic bone represent an important subset of fragility fractures. Pelvic fractures in the elderly patient carry a significant 1-year mortality risk, comparable to that of hip fractures. Patients often lose their ability to function independently in the community. In this group, treatment of their bone density is essential to reducing their risk of further fractures. A thorough discussion of the likely course of recovery, the prolonged need for pain medications, and the risks and benefits of intervention can help patients and their families cope with the disability.

CLINICS IN GERIATRIC MEDICINE

Preface

Fragility Fractures

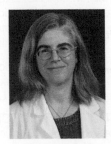 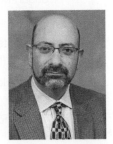

Susan M. Friedman, MD, MPH,
FACP, AGSF

Daniel Ari Mendelson, MS, MD,
FACP, AGSF, CMD

Editors

Fragility fractures are on the rise, as a function of our rapidly expanding older adult population. Fragility fractures, and particularly hip fractures, can lead to devastating consequences, including loss of mobility, institutionalization, and death. By their nature, these fractures occur in patients who are frail, who often have many comorbidities, and who may have already experienced functional decline. In addition to the personal costs of fragility fractures, they are also associated with very significant financial burdens. Because these patients are vulnerable and the consequences are substantial, it is critically important to provide thoughtful, optimized care in the perioperative setting and beyond.

A great deal of work has been done in the recent past to reduce the morbidity and mortality associated with fragility fractures. Improvement in operative techniques and implant technology, increasing appreciation of complexity and utilization of comanagement, optimized models of care through lean practices, and improved secondary prevention have all contributed to better outcomes.

This issue of *Clinics in Geriatric Medicine* will critically evaluate recent advances in the treatment of fragility fractures. As this is an interdisciplinary problem, we have asked experts from several fields, including Geriatrics, Orthopedics and Trauma Surgery, Anesthesiology, Rehabilitation Medicine, and Metabolic Bone, to participate in the writing of this issue. The focus of this discussion will be the perioperative setting, but we will also address issues related to rehabilitation and secondary prevention.

We have been extremely fortunate to work with outstanding colleagues across the globe whose driving mission is to improve the care of frail older adults. These individuals continue to inspire and motivate us to "do our part" to educate, with the goal of changing practices. Meliora!

We would like to thank our coauthors on this project, who have been our supporters, friends, and collaborators for years. We greatly appreciate the help and guidance of our editors, Yonah Korngold and Jessica McCool, and their staff. We thank the Department of Medicine and Administration at Highland Hospital for providing the resources

Clin Geriatr Med 30 (2014) xiii–xiv
http://dx.doi.org/10.1016/j.cger.2014.01.019
0749-0690/14/$ – see front matter © 2014 Elsevier Inc. All rights reserved.

geriatric.theclinics.com

to complete this project as well as the interdisciplinary team at Highland that has made our work possible. We are also grateful to our spouses and children, whose support has allowed us to do work that is so personally meaningful and rewarding.

Susan M. Friedman, MD, MPH, FACP, AGSF
Associate Professor of Medicine
Division of Geriatrics
University of Rochester School of Medicine and Dentistry

Department of Medicine
Highland Hospital, 1000 South Avenue, Box 58
Rochester, NY 14620, USA

Daniel Ari Mendelson, MS, MD, FACP, AGSF, CMD
Associate Professor of Medicine
Division of Geriatrics
University of Rochester School of Medicine and Dentistry
Director, Consultative Services, Highland Hospital
Co-Director, Geriatric Fracture Center, Highland Hospital
Medical Director, Monroe Community Hospital
Medical Director, Highlands at Brighton

Department of Medicine
Highland Hospital, 1000 South Avenue, Box 58
Rochester, NY 14620, USA

E-mail addresses:
susan_friedman@urmc.rochester.edu (S.M. Friedman)
daniel_mendelson@urmc.rochester.edu (D.A. Mendelson)

Epidemiology of Fragility Fractures

Susan M. Friedman, MD, MPH[a],*, Daniel Ari Mendelson, MD, MS[a,b]

KEYWORDS

- Frailty • Incidence • Outcomes • Predictors • Osteoporosis

KEY POINTS

- The incidence of fragility fractures is increasing rapidly, although age-adjusted rates seem to be declining.
- Poor outcomes are related both to fractures and their comorbidities and to the frailty of the patients who sustain fractures.
- Identifying individuals who are at highest risk, using a prediction tool such as the FRAX, can allow for targeted primary prevention.
- A person who sustains one fracture is at 50% to 100% higher risk of having another one; fractures, therefore, provide important opportunities for secondary prevention.
- Hip fractures cost Medicare more than $12 billion per year.

INTRODUCTION

The United States and the rest of the world are experiencing a silver tsunami. Since 2011, 10,000 American baby boomers are turning 65 daily. The older adult population in the United States is predicted to more than double, from 35 million individuals in 2000 to 72 million in 2030, and will account for approximately 20% of the population.[2]

The oldest old, those over age 85, are the fastest growing segment of the population. The baby boomers will start turning 85 in 2031, and it is predicted that the population over age 85 will increase 3-fold, from 5.5 million in 2010 to 19 million in 2050.[2] Although there is evidence that people are living healthier lives for longer,[3] and that age-adjusted fracture risk is decreasing,[4,5] these individuals remain at highest risk of sustaining fragility fractures.[6]

Fragility fracture is defined as a fracture that results from a low trauma event, such as falling from a standing height or less.[1]

[a] Division of Geriatrics, Geriatric Fracture Center, Highland Hospital, University of Rochester School of Medicine and Dentistry, 1000 South Avenue, Box 58, Rochester, NY 14620, USA;
[b] Monroe Community Hospital, 435 East Henrietta Road, Rochester, NY 14620, USA
* Corresponding author.
E-mail address: susan_friedman@URMC.rochester.edu

Clin Geriatr Med 30 (2014) 175–181
http://dx.doi.org/10.1016/j.cger.2014.01.001
0749-0690/14/$ – see front matter © 2014 Elsevier Inc. All rights reserved.

As the incidence of fragility fractures rises, it becomes more important to optimize their prevention and treatment.

PREVALENCE/INCIDENCE

For each decade after age 50, the risk of hip fracture doubles.[7] At age 50, an American white woman has a 17% lifetime risk of sustaining a hip fracture,[8,9] and a woman who lives to age 90 has a 1 in 3 chance of sustaining a hip fracture.[10] The increased risk with age combined with a rapidly expanding older adult population translates to a projected increase in worldwide hip fracture incidence, from 1.7 million in 1990 to 6.3 million in 2050.[11]

The incidence of hip fractures has been demonstrated to be increasing in many countries around the world, including Asia, North America, and Europe.[12] The risk of a hip fracture varies significantly based on gender, race, and ethnicity. The graph in **Fig. 1** shows how the expected number of hip fractures is changing over time in 8 regions around the world.[11]

When reflecting on the full burden of osteoporotic or fragility fractures, it is essential to also consider the morbidity associated with fractures other than hip fractures. The lifetime incidence of any osteoporotic fracture is estimated to be 40% to 50% in women and 13% to 22% in men.[9] At age 50, an American white woman has a 15% chance of sustaining a Colles fracture and a 32% chance of sustaining a vertebral fracture.[10]

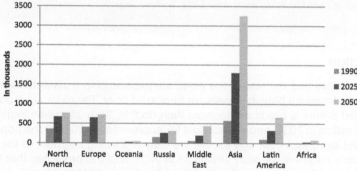

Fig. 1. The expected number of hip fractures over time in 8 regions around the world. (*Modified from* Cooper C, Campion G, Melton LJ 3rd. Hip fractures in the elderly: a world-wide projection. Osteoporos Int 1992;2(6):285–9; with permission.)

OUTCOMES

A hip fracture can be a life-changing, or life-ending, event (**Box 1**). The surgery itself carries a 4% mortality overall,[13] and within a year, approximately 20% die.[14–17] Patients with hip fracture experience a 5- to 8-fold increase in all-cause mortality in the first 3 months after the fracture, with men experiencing particularly high risk.[18] This excess risk declines over time but never resolves completely, likely reflective of the frail population who sustain the fractures in the first place. The lifetime risk of death in women from hip fractures has been noted to be comparable to that associated with breast cancer.[19]

In addition to the risk of mortality, hip fractures can lead to loss of function and mobility, which in turn can result in a loss of independence. A year after surgery, more than half of those who were previously independent are still unable to climb 5 stairs, get in and out of a shower, get on or off a toilet, walk a block, or rise from an

---

Box 1
Outcomes of hip fractures

- Increased mortality
- Loss of function
- Reduced mobility
- Need for increased health care services
- Risk of nursing home admission
- Depression
- Cognitive impairment
- Increased risk of future fracture
- High cost

---

armless chair without either equipment or human assistance.[20] Only 60% have recovered to their previous level of walking.[21] One-third of previously community-dwelling individuals require long-term nursing home care.[22] Morbidity after a hip fracture is not just physical; there is a high incidence of depression that can occur early after a hip fracture,[23] and both temporary and permanent cognitive impairment are also common.[24]

Hip fractures are costly events in the United States. The incremental direct cost to Medicare of a hip fracture has been estimated to be more than $25,000 during the period 1999–2006.[25] Although hip fractures account for only 14% of fractures, they account for 72% of costs, amounting to more than $12 billion in 2005.[26] These costs are driven by acute inpatient and postacute institutional care needs.[27]

Although fractures of the hip may be the most feared, other fragility fractures have important prognostic and functional significance. In addition to the acute and chronic pain associated with vertebral fractures, these fractures can lead to multiple outcomes that limit function. Kyphosis that occurs from vertebral collapse can lead to neck pain, reduced pulmonary function,[28] costo-iliac impingement syndrome,[29] and fear of falling.[30] The mortality after a vertebral fracture has been noted to be similar to that after a hip fracture.[31]

An individual who sustains one fracture is 50% to 100% more likely to sustain a fracture of another type.[8] Vertebral deformities from a fracture are associated with a 2.8-fold increased risk of hip fracture and 5 times the risk of another vertebral fracture in 3 years.[30] The epidemiology of fractures at different sites varies, however; the median age for sustaining a Colles fracture is 66 versus 79 for the median age of first hip fracture.[10] Identification of the fracture and understanding of future risk thereby provide an important opportunity for secondary prevention.

CLINICAL CORRELATION

As primary prevention efforts improve, the onset of first fracture is delayed. The age of hip fracture patients has increased over time,[4] and, as a concomitant phenomenon, patients have more comorbidities.[4] Fragility fractures are, therefore, not only an outcome of frailty but also a marker of frailty.

Perioperative risk is increased in the face of comorbidities, with a higher burden of chronic conditions leading to an elevated risk of postoperative complications[32,33] and mortality.[32,34] The need to optimize comorbidities in the acute setting at the time of fracture, as well as the need to manage increasingly complex individuals, is, therefore,

---

Box 2
Common comorbidities among hip fracture patients

- Chronic lung disease
- Congestive heart failure
- Diabetes
- Dementia
- Peripheral vascular disease
- Osteoporosis

---

a trend that is likely to continue over time. Common comorbidities in hip fracture patients are listed in **Box 2**.[4,33,35]

There is evidence that some outcomes are improving, with recent declines in age- and risk-adjusted short- and long-term mortality after a fracture.[4]

PREDICTORS OF FRAGILITY FRACTURE

Because fragility fractures are common and lead to significant morbidity and mortality, identifying those at risk provides opportunity for both prevention and care planning (**Box 3**).[12] The FRAX score, developed by the World Health Organization, is a tool to determine 10-year risk of hip fracture and other fragility fractures.[36] The FRAX score is available on line at http://www.shef.ac.uk/FRAX/.

FRAX uses data from cohort studies from Europe, North America, Asia, and Australia, incorporating demographic and clinical factors.

Box 3 lists common risk factors for fragility fractures.[12,35] Osteoporosis is the most important potentially treatable risk factor for fragility fractures. It is currently estimated

---

Box 3
Common risk factors for fragility fractures

Characteristics that identify high-risk individuals

- Age
- Female gender
- White race
- Cognitive impairment
- Parental history of fracture

Potentially treatable risk factors

- Osteoporosis
- Falls
- Physical inactivity
- Low body mass index
- Gait and balance disturbance
- Medications
- Alcohol
- Tobacco

---

that 10 million Americans over age 50 have osteoporosis and that this number will increase to 14 million by 2020. Additionally, 34 million have osteopenia, and this number is projected to increase to 47 million by 2020.[37]

Falls are common in older adults, with one-third of individuals over age 65 living in the community falling every year.[38] Falls increase with age, so that the risk in individuals over age 80 is 40% per year. As the oldest segment of the population increases, it is, therefore, likely that fall incidence will increase. Approximately 1% of falls result in hip fractures, and, conversely, more than 90% of hip fractures result from a fall.[39] Characteristics of falls, such as trajectory and protective reflexes, also contribute to hip fracture risk and may be associated with age and frailty.[40] A full discussion of fall risk and prevention can be found in the article by Duque and colleagues elsewhere in this issue.

Other clinical risk factors may identify individuals who are at high risk and provide opportunities to reduce that risk. Several of the risk factors listed in **Box 3** are also seen with the frailty syndrome.[41]

SUMMARY

Fragility fractures are on the rise due to the rapidly growing elderly population around the world. These fractures may be both markers of frailty as well as sentinel events leading to functional decline and other morbidity. Because of their serious consequences, efforts to prevent fragility fractures and to optimize treatment when they occur are becoming increasingly important.

REFERENCES

1. Bouxsein ML, Kaufman J, Tosi L, et al. Recommendations for optimal care of the fragility fracture patient to reduce the risk of future fracture. J Am Acad Orthop Surg 2004;12(6):385–95.
2. Statistics FIFoA-R. Older Americans 2012: key indicators of well-being. 2012. Available at: http://www.agingstats.gov/Main_Site/Data/2012_Documents/Population.aspx. Accessed June 11, 2013.
3. Tuljapurkar S, Li N, Boe C. A universal pattern of mortality decline in the G7 countries. Nature 2000;405(6788):789–92.
4. Brauer CA, Coca-Perraillon M, Cutler DM, et al. Incidence and mortality of hip fractures in the United States. JAMA 2009;302(14):1573–9.
5. Leslie WD, O'Donnell S, Jean S, et al. Trends in hip fracture rates in Canada. JAMA 2009;302(8):883–9.
6. Holt G, Smith R, Duncan K, et al. Changes in population demographics and the future incidence of hip fracture. Injury 2009;40(7):722–6.
7. Gallagher JC, Melton LJ, Riggs BL, et al. Epidemiology of fractures of the proximal femur in Rochester, Minnesota. Clin Orthop Relat Res 1980;150:163–71.
8. Cummings SR, Melton LJ. Epidemiology and outcomes of osteoporotic fractures. Lancet 2002;359(9319):1761–7.
9. Johnell O, Kanis J. Epidemiology of osteoporotic fractures. Osteoporos Int 2005; 2(Suppl 16):S3–7.
10. Cummings SR, Black DM, Rubin SM. Lifetime risks of hip, Colles', or vertebral fracture and coronary heart disease among white postmenopausal women. Arch Intern Med 1989;149(11):2445–8.
11. Cooper C, Campion G, Melton LJ 3rd. Hip fractures in the elderly: a world-wide projection. Osteoporos Int 1992;2(6):285–9.

12. Marks R. Hip fracture epidemiological trends, outcomes, and risk factors, 1970–2009. Int J Gen Med 2010;3:1–17.
13. Morris AH, Zuckerman JD. National consensus conference on improving the continuum of care for patients with hip fracture. J Bone Joint Surg Am 2002;84(4): 670–4.
14. Magaziner J, Simonsick EM, Kashner TM, et al. Survival experience of aged hip fracture patients. Am J Public Health 1989;79(3):274–8.
15. Braithwaite RS, Col NF, Wong JB. Estimating hip fracture morbidity, mortality and costs. J Am Geriatr Soc 2003;51(3):364–70.
16. Leibson CL, Tosteson AN, Gabriel SE, et al. Mortality, disability, and nursing home use for persons with and without hip fracture: a population-based study. J Am Geriatr Soc 2002;50(10):1644–50.
17. Schnell S, Friedman SM, Mendelson DA, et al. The 1-year mortality of patients treated in a hip fracture program for elders. Geriatr Orthop Surg Rehabil 2010; 1(1):6–14.
18. Haentjens P, Magaziner J, Colon-Emeric CS, et al. Meta-analysis: excess mortality after hip fracture among older women and men. Ann Intern Med 2010;152(6): 380–90.
19. Kates SL, Kates OS, Mendelson DA. Advances in the medical management of osteoporosis. Injury 2007;38(Suppl 3):S17–23.
20. Magaziner J, Hawkes W, Hebel JR, et al. Recovery from hip fracture in eight areas of function. J Gerontol A Biol Sci Med Sci 2000;55(9):M498–507.
21. Magaziner J, Simonsick EM, Kashner TM, et al. Predictors of functional recovery one year following hospital discharge for hip fracture: a prospective study. J Gerontol 1990;45(3):M101–7.
22. Bonar SK, Tinetti ME, Speechley M, et al. Factors associated with short- versus long-term skilled nursing facility placement among community-living hip fracture patients. J Am Geriatr Soc 1990;38(10):1139–44.
23. Lenze EJ, Munin MC, Skidmore ER, et al. Onset of depression in elderly persons after hip fracture: implications for prevention and early intervention of late-life depression. J Am Geriatr Soc 2007;55(1):81–6.
24. Gruber-Baldini AL, Zimmerman S, Morrison RS, et al. Cognitive impairment in hip fracture patients: timing of detection and longitudinal follow-up. J Am Geriatr Soc 2003;51(9):1227–36.
25. Pike C, Birnbaum HG, Schiller M, et al. Direct and indirect costs of non-vertebral fracture patients with osteoporosis in the US. Pharmacoeconomics 2010;28(5): 395–409.
26. Burge R, Dawson-Hughes B, Solomon DH, et al. Incidence and economic burden of osteoporosis-related fractures in the United States, 2005–2025. J Bone Miner Res 2007;22(3):465–75.
27. Nikitovic M, Wodchis WP, Krahn MD, et al. Direct health-care costs attributed to hip fractures among seniors: a matched cohort study. Osteoporos Int 2013;24(2): 659–69.
28. Schlaich C, Minne HW, Bruckner T, et al. Reduced pulmonary function in patients with spinal osteoporotic fractures. Osteoporos Int 1998;8(3):261–7.
29. Wynne AT, Nelson MA, Nordin BE. Costo-iliac impingement syndrome. J Bone Joint Surg Br 1985;67(1):124–5.
30. Papaioannou A, Watts NB, Kendler DL, et al. Diagnosis and management of vertebral fractures in elderly adults. Am J Med 2002;113(3):220–8.
31. Cauley JA, Thompson DE, Ensrud KC, et al. Risk of mortality following clinical fractures. Osteoporos Int 2000;11(7):556–61.

32. Roche JJ, Wenn RT, Sahota O, et al. Effect of comorbidities and postoperative complications on mortality after hip fracture in elderly people: prospective observational cohort study. BMJ 2005;331(7529):1374.
33. Menzies IB, Mendelson DA, Kates SL, et al. The impact of comorbidity on perioperative outcomes of hip fractures in a geriatric fracture model. Geriatr Orthop Surg Rehabil 2012;3(3):129–34.
34. Radley DC, Gottlieb DJ, Fisher ES, et al. Comorbidity risk-adjustment strategies are comparable among persons with hip fracture. J Clin Epidemiol 2008;61(6): 580–7.
35. Friedman SM, Menzies IB, Bukata SV, et al. Dementia and hip fractures: development of a pathogenic framework for understanding and studying risk. Geriatr Orthop Surg Rehabil 2010;1(2):52–62.
36. Kanis J. FRAX: WHO Fracture risk assessment tool. 2009. Accessed October 6, 2009. Available at: http://www.shef.ac.uk/FRAX/.
37. U.S. Department of Health and Human Services, Office of the Surgeon General. Bone health and osteoporosis: a report of the surgeon general. Rockville (MD): 2004.
38. Tinetti ME, Speechley M, Ginter SF. Risk factors for falls among elderly persons living in the community. N Engl J Med 1988;319(26):1701–7.
39. Hayes WC, Myers ER, Robinovitch SN, et al. Etiology and prevention of age-related hip fractures. Bone 1996;18(Suppl 1):77S–86S.
40. Cummings SR, Nevitt MC. A hypothesis: the causes of hip fractures. J Gerontol 1989;44(4):M107–11.
41. Fried LP, Tangen CM, Walston J, et al. Frailty in older adults: evidence for a phenotype. J Gerontol A Biol Sci Med Sci 2001;56(3):M146–56.

Principles of Comanagement and the Geriatric Fracture Center

Daniel Ari Mendelson, MS, MD*, Susan M. Friedman, MD, MPH

KEYWORDS

- Hip fracture • Geriatric fracture center • Hip fracture protocol • Interdisciplinary care
- Comanagement

KEY POINTS

- The 5 principles of the geriatric fracture center
  - Most patients benefit from surgical stabilization of their fracture.
  - The sooner patients have surgery, the less time they have to develop iatrogenic illness.
  - Comanagement with frequent communication avoids common medical and functional complications.
  - Standardized protocols decrease unwarranted variability.
  - Discharge planning begins at admission.
- Interdisciplinary care is multidisciplinary care that is integrated in a patient-centered fashion.
- Interdisciplinary care requires communication and shared decision making.
- Comanagement is true interdisciplinary care that results in a collaborative care environment in which all team members maximize their contributions resulting in improved outcomes.

INTRODUCTION

Fragility fractures are a common event for elders that often lead to substantial morbidity and mortality. These types of injuries have typically been classified as an orthopedic disorder rather than a geriatric syndrome; however, patients with fragility fractures have a high prevalence of comorbidity and a high risk of complications, and for these reasons, including a medical team with understanding of geriatrics principles is vital. Comanagement of osteoporotic fractures by orthopedic surgeons and

Funding Sources: None.
Conflicts of Interest: None.
Highland Hospital, Department of Medicine, 1000 South Avenue, Box 58, Rochester, NY 14620, USA
* Corresponding author.
E-mail address: daniel_mendelson@urmc.rochester.edu

geriatricians has led to better, clinically relevant outcomes.[1] This article describes the principles of a comanaged geriatric fracture center (GFC) program that results in lower-than-predicted length of stay and readmission rates, with short time to surgery, low complication rates, low mortality, and reduced cost.[1-7] This program is based on the principles of early evaluation and optimization of the patient, ongoing comanagement, protocol-driven, patient-centered care, and early discharge planning. The article by Stephen L. Kates details the development and implementation of this model.

PRINCIPLES OF COMANAGEMENT

The GFC was founded with the 5 following principles in mind[1]:

- Most patients benefit from surgical stabilization of their fracture.
- The sooner patients have surgery, the less time they have to develop iatrogenic illness.
- Comanagement with frequent communication avoids common medical and functional complications.
- Standardized protocols decrease unwarranted variability.
- Discharge planning begins at admission.

Each of these principles will be discussed in detail.

Most Patients Benefit from Surgical Stabilization of Their Fracture

The standard of care for most fragility fractures is internal fixation or partial or total joint replacement when appropriate. The article by Simon C. Mears describes surgical details. Failure to stabilize a fracture usually results in prolonged or increased pain, higher mortality, functional loss, and increased institutionalization. Timely fixation may reduce blood loss. Fixation is aimed at restoring function and reducing pain. Nonambulatory patients, who may not have functional improvement, often benefit from the pain relief that results from surgical fracture management. A nonoperative approach may be appropriate for patients who are truly moribund or give informed refusal.[8,9]

Benefits of surgical stabilization include pain relief, improved mobility and function, reduced blood loss, reduced mortality, and decreased institutionalization.

The Sooner Patients Have Surgery, the Less Time They Have to Develop Iatrogenic Illness

Unnecessary delays in surgery result in the increased risk of many negative outcomes, including

- Delirium
- Pain
- Pneumonia
- Pressure ulcers
- Malnutrition
- Urinary tract infections
- Thromboembolism
- Deconditioning
- Falls and additional injuries
- Patient, family, and staff dissatisfaction
- Higher cost
- Increased mortality

Although there are studies showing no or few sustained adverse outcomes from completing surgeries within about 48 to 72 hours, no study has shown improved outcomes by delays. There is no advantage to unnecessary delay other than provider convenience for medically optimized patients.[10] Except for cases in which further medical management is necessary, the authors recommend achieving surgical fixation within about 24 hours when appropriate resources are available.[1–3,6,7,9–12]

Comanagement with Frequent Communication Avoids Common Medical and Functional Complications

There are 4 typical models of fragility fracture care that have been recently been described (Table 1)[12–14]:

A. Orthopedics attends; geriatrics or medicine consults as requested
B. Orthopedics attends; geriatrics or medicine automatically consults
C. Geriatrics or medicine attends; orthopedics automatically consults
D. GFC; true, interdisciplinary comanagement

The first (A) model is historically the most common and simplest, in which an elder with an osteoporotic fracture is admitted to the orthopedics service, and geriatrics or medicine is consulted as needed to manage specific medical problems; usually orthopedic surgeons write orders and make most decisions. The consultant may simply clear for surgery (indicating that there is no significant medical contraindications to proceeding as planned) and then sign-off, or may be consulted postoperatively once a complication arises. In this model, the medical team does not actively manage medical conditions until asked, and medical problems may not be recognized early.

In the second (B) and third (C) models, it is agreed that the patient will be admitted to 1 service, with the other service automatically consulting. Generally the primary service writes most orders and makes most decisions. The consulting service may sign-off if there is perceived stability. Issues are usually found earlier than in the first model. Delays or errors may occur because of a lack of active, thoughtful coordination. The choice of primary service may have more to do with hospital issues and resources rather than necessarily what is best for a particular patient.

Table 1
Common models of fragility fracture care

Model	Attending Service	Consultation Type	Automatic Consultation	Who Writes Orders?	Comments
A	Orthopedics	Medicine/ geriatrics	No	Orthopedics	Simplest, most common, often single consult visit, minimal comanagement
B	Orthopedics	Medicine/ geriatrics	Yes	Usually orthopedics	Common, basic comanagement, consultant may sign off
C	Medicine/ geriatrics	Orthopedics	Yes	Usually medicine/ geriatrics	Common, basic comanagement, consultant may sign off
D	Combined	Not applicable	Not applicable	Each service writes own	Most sophisticated, true interdisciplinary care, neither service may sign off

Data from Refs.[12,13,15]

True, interdisciplinary, fully coordinated comanagement is the hallmark of the GFC model (D). Comanagement and interdisciplinary care will be further discussed.[1,15–17]

Comanagement means shared ownership, shared decision making, equal responsibility, and daily communication; each discipline writes orders, write notes, and communicates with the patient and care team. In this model, care is continuously coordinated among team members. If the geriatrics or medical team becomes aware of a surgical problem, the issue can be resolved with the orthopedics team; similarly, if the orthopedics group becomes aware of a medical problem, it is the group's responsibility to coordinate with the geriatrics or medical team to resolve the issue. Other staff is not put in the middle. In the authors' GFC, all hemodynamically stable patients are automatically officially admitted to orthopedics, with geriatrics technically consulting; this is done for documentation and system reasons, but in fact, each case is wholly and jointly the responsibility of both services at all times. Both services agree when a patient is ready for discharge and manage discharge needs together. Decisions that cross both disciplines must be shared; for example, orthopedics weighs in on whether to use heparin bridging for a patient who is usually on chronic anticoagulation with warfarin for atrial fibrillation. Care is also coordinated with other consultants and service providers, including anesthesia, nursing, therapies, and discharge planners, as well as the family.

The GFC utilizes an interdisciplinary approach rather than multidisciplinary care. Every accredited hospital uses multidisciplinary care, meaning that all appropriate services are present and available to care for the patient. In a true interdisciplinary model, not only are all appropriate services available, but they are also integrated with the common, patient-centered goal of the best outcomes. Interdisciplinary care implies a shared vision, collaboration, and coordination. In the GFC, a geriatrician attends orthopedics morbidity and mortality rounds, thereby providing additional educational opportunities and integration; this also ensures interdisciplinary review of any adverse outcomes. In an ideal system of interdisciplinary care, the whole becomes greater than the sum of the individual parts.

Standardized Protocols Decrease Unwarranted Variability

A search of Google Scholar (scholar.google.com; January 2014) for "unwarranted variations in health care delivery" revealed more than 20,000 articles. The Dartmouth Atlas of Health Care has been documenting variations in American health care for more than 20 years (http://www.dartmouthatlas.org; January 2014). The authors have shown significant local[3] and national[5] variability in the management of hip fractures.

Employing geriatrics principles to standardized order sets, protocols, and nursing care plans allows for highly standardized and evidence-based care for each patient and thus reduces inappropriate variability.[1] In the GFC model, variability is patient specific and justified rather than random or based on provider preferences or system factors. Standards are developed collaboratively between the vested services as part of the comanagement model. Compromises may be appropriate to adapt to local practices in order to gain acceptance; compromise may also be appropriate based on available resources. Not every community will be able to fully implement an optimal GFC program,[18] but the authors recommend at least adopting standard protocols.

Some of the standardized elements of the GFC include

- Emergency department order set
- Preoperative admission order set

- Postoperative order set
- Operative consent forms
- Discharge instructions
- Nursing care plan
- Geriatrics perioperative consultation
- Pain management
- Thromboembolism prophylaxis
- Delirium prevention
- Weight-bearing status, activity, physical therapy
- Implant selection algorithm
- Urinary catheter utilization
- Antibiotic prophylaxis
- Data collection form
- Osteoporosis assessment and treatment
- Transfer protocol (from outlying hospitals)
- Direct admission protocol (from partner facilities)
- Comorbidity scoring

Protocols require revision as evidence and best practices change. At the GFC, a quality improvement database is kept so that internal and published data can be used to adapt standard order sets and care plans. The service quality committee reviews outcomes at least quarterly as part of a comprehensive quality assurance and performance improvement process. A senior geriatrician attends an orthopedics morbidity and mortality conference in order to ensure interdisciplinary review of any adverse outcomes.

Protocol-driven care through a comanaged fragility fracture program has proven to improve patient centered outcomes including mortality, readmission, and complications.[2,3,5–7,16,19–22] Standardization affords better quality and cost containment by employing lower-cost, generic medications and favorable agreements among vendors for implants; additionally, length of stay is decreased, and utilization of additional services is reduced due to avoided complications and readmissions.[6,15,23]

DISCHARGE PLANNING BEGINS AT ADMISSION

In-hospital mortality rates are quite low at the GFC (less than about 2%).[7] Most patients, therefore require a discharge plan. The GFC length of stay (LOS) is quite short (<5 days average LOS).[1,3,6,7] Therefore there is little time to develop a comprehensive discharge plan. Assessing discharge needs and communicating and coordinating with the patient's family or social supports at admission can avoid delays in discharge and decrease their apprehension.

The proportion of patients who return home after hip fracture surgery varies throughout the country. Factors that affect discharge planning include availability of home health care services, family and social supports, skilled nursing facility rehabilitation beds, patient functional status and comorbidity, and local culture. At the authors' center, more than 90% of patients are discharged to a nursing facility; for many, this is a skilled admission for rehabilitation in preparation for returning to a lower level of care, but some are likely to need long-term care. Social workers are the authors' discharge planners and are involved from the time of admission in working with patients and their families for discharge planning. The relationships developed by the hospital over the past decade with outside facilities help to facilitate discharge planning. In the authors' community, there is competition to place patients in rehabilitation centers. The article by Michelle Eslami discusses transitions and rehabilitation in detail.

DISCUSSION

The evidence for this model of care continues to grow. Randomized controlled trials of this model are probably impossible to perform at this point. There is sufficient evidence that comanagement is beneficial, so that if a center is able to offer comanaged care, it would not be ethical to deny comanagement through randomization. Any center that is employing comanagement would also have contamination between randomized patients as well, since it would be impossible to fully shelter staff from the various elements. Comparison studies before and after implementation (historical control studies) will be somewhat biased by lack of blinding and participants' interest in outcomes. Case control studies and studies between centers may be revealing. There are studies indicating that comanagement can be successfully applied to other surgical programs.

The GFC model was originally developed using geriatrics hospitalists. These physicians were all internal medicine and geriatrics trained and board certified with a significant interest and experience in acute care and hospital-based care. Over the years, family medicine-trained geriatricians and internal medicine-trained hospitalists have been incorporated in to the system with continued excellent outcomes. Knowledge of geriatrics principles and perioperative medicine as well as commitment to continuous quality improvement is more important than specific credentials.

Additional study is necessary to learn which elements of the model are most important and most easily replicated. It is especially important to determine which elements are most easily translated to centers with less experience and fewer resources in order to make optimal care more readily available to more patients.

SUMMARY

The GFC is a collaborative model of care for the fragility fracture patient that employs the 5 principles discussed previously. Comanagement is the key principle. Comanagement requires true interdisciplinary care. The GFC uses patient-centered, protocol-driven care to standardize the care for most patients with fragility fractures. Quality outcomes are assessed regularly, and protocols and standards are adjusted to improve care. This model also uses shared decision making and frequent communication to improve clinically relevant and systems outcomes. Both the orthopedic and medical teams are fully responsible for the fragility fracture patient throughout the hospitalization.

REFERENCES

1. Friedman SM, Mendelson DA, Kates SL, et al. Geriatric co-management of proximal femur fractures: total quality management and protocol-driven care result in better outcomes for a frail patient population. J Am Geriatr Soc 2008;56(7):1349–56.
2. Bukata SV, Digiovanni BF, Friedman SM, et al. A guide to improving the care of patients with fragility fractures. Geriatr Orthop Surg Rehabil 2011;2(1):5–37.
3. Friedman SM, Mendelson DA, Bingham KW, et al. Impact of a comanaged geriatric fracture center on short-term hip fracture outcomes. Arch Intern Med 2009; 169(18):1712–7.
4. Kates SL, Mendelson DA, Friedman SM. Co-managed care for fragility hip fractures (Rochester model). Osteoporos Int 2010;21(Suppl 4):S621–5.
5. Kates SL, Blake D, Bingham KW, et al. Comparison of an organized geriatric fracture program to United States government data. Geriatr Orthop Surg Rehabil 2010;1(1):15–21.

6. Kates SL, Mendelson DA, Friedman SM. The value of an organized fracture program for the elderly: early results. J Orthop Trauma 2011;25(4):233–7.
7. Schnell S, Friedman SM, Mendelson DA, et al. The 1-year mortality of patients treated in a hip fracture program for elders. Geriatr Orthop Surg Rehabil 2010; 1(1):6–14.
8. Neuman MD, Fleisher LA, Even-Shoshan O, et al. Nonoperative care for hip fracture in the elderly: the influence of race, income, and comorbidities. Med Care 2010;48(4):314–20.
9. Hip Fracture Accelerated Surgical Treatment and Care Track (HIP ATTACK) Investigators. Accelerated care versus standard care among patients with hip fracture: the HIP ATTACK pilot trial. CMAJ 2014;186(1):E52–60.
10. Khan SK, Kalra S, Khanna A, et al. Timing of surgery for hip fractures: a systematic review of 52 published studies involving 291,413 patients. Injury 2009;40(7): 692–7.
11. Gleason LJ, Mendelson DA, Kates SL, et al. Anticoagulation management in individuals with hip fracture. J Am Geriatr Soc 2014;62(1):159–64.
12. Kammerlander C, Roth T, Friedman SM, et al. Ortho-geriatric service–a literature review comparing different models. Osteoporos Int 2010;21(Suppl 4):S637–46.
13. Pioli G, Giusti A, Barone A. Orthogeriatric care for the elderly with hip fractures: where are we? Aging Clin Exp Res 2008;20(2):113–22.
14. Della Rocca GJ, Crist BD. Hip fracture protocols: what have we changed? Orthop Clin North Am 2013;44(2):163–82.
15. Della Rocca GJ, Moylan KC, Crist BD, et al. Comanagement of geriatric patients with hip fractures: a retrospective, controlled, cohort study. Geriatr Orthop Surg Rehabil 2013;4(1):10–5.
16. O'Malley NT, Kates SL. Co-managed care: the gold standard for geriatric fracture care. Curr Osteoporos Rep 2012;10(4):312–6.
17. Friedman SM, Mendelson DA, Bingham KW, et al. Comanagement of elderly patients admitted to a hospital for hip fracture—reply. Arch Intern Med 2010; 170(4):392.
18. Kates SL, O'Malley N, Friedman SM, et al. Barriers to implementation of an organized geriatric fracture program. Geriatr Orthop Surg Rehabil 2012;3(1):8–16.
19. Dy CJ, Dossous PM, Ton QV, et al. Does a multidisciplinary team decrease complications in male patients with hip fractures? Clin Orthop Relat Res 2011;469(7): 1919–24.
20. Martinez-Reig M, Ahmad L, Duque G. The orthogeriatrics model of care: systematic review of predictors of institutionalization and mortality in post-hip fracture patients and evidence for interventions. J Am Med Dir Assoc 2012;13(9):770–7.
21. Wagner P, Fuentes P, Diaz A, et al. Comparison of complications and length of hospital stay between orthopedic and orthogeriatric treatment in elderly patients with a hip fracture. Geriatr Orthop Surg Rehabil 2012;3(2):55–8.
22. Wyller TB, Watne LO, Torbergsen A, et al. The effect of a pre- and post-operative orthogeriatric service on cognitive function in patients with hip fracture. The protocol of the Oslo Orthogeriatrics Trial. BMC Geriatr 2012;12:36.
23. Biber R, Singler K, Curschmann-Horter M, et al. Implementation of a co-managed geriatric fracture center reduces hospital stay and time-to-operation in elderly femoral neck fracture patients. Arch Orthop Trauma Surg 2013;133(11):1527–31.

Lean Business Model and Implementation of a Geriatric Fracture Center

Stephen L. Kates, MD

KEYWORDS

- Geriatric fracture center • Hip fracture • Fragility fracture • Lean business methods
- Implementation • System of care • Business planning

KEY POINTS

- Lean business models are applicable to medicine.
- Lean business models allow the simultaneous improvement in quality with reduction in costs of care.
- The geriatric fracture center model of care is one example of successful implementation of a lean business model for hip fracture care.

INTRODUCTION

The population is aging rapidly, and the resulting demographic shift will create changing needs for care of older adults. One of the more common problems suffered by older adults is hip fracture.[1,2] Hip fracture is often associated with complications, disability, and death.[1] The loss of independence is also commonly associated with a hip fracture in the older adults.[3]

From an economic standpoint, hip fracture is the third most costly diagnosis in American medicine.[4] It is also common, with 330,000 hip fractures occurring annually in the United States.[5] This number is expected to increase with the increasing numbers of older adults.[6] Reported mortality in the United States is 3% inpatient mortality and 21% to 24% 1-year mortality for patients with hip fracture.[1,5,7] The average length of stay in the United States is 6.4 days, and this represents a significant use of hospital bed capacity across the country.[5] In addition, an average of 14.5% of patients discharged after hip fracture are readmitted within 30 days.[8]

Disclosures: Research grant support received from Synthes Spine, AOTrauma, NIAMS, OREF, AHRQ, paid to institution.
Consultant: Surgical excellence.

Department of Orthopaedics and Rehabilitation, University of Rochester, 601 Elmwood Avenue, Box 665, Rochester, NY 14642-0001, USA
E-mail address: stephen_kates@urmc.rochester.edu

Clin Geriatr Med 30 (2014) 191–205
http://dx.doi.org/10.1016/j.cger.2014.01.002
0749-0690/14/$ – see front matter © 2014 Elsevier Inc. All rights reserved.

From a cost and outcomes perspective, improvement of these statistics is desirable and may be achievable with improvement in the care delivery model. In this article, some methods that may be used to improve the quality, safety, and cost of care for patients with hip fracture are discussed.

WHAT IS A LEAN BUSINESS MODEL AND WHY IS IT RELEVANT TO HIP FRACTURE CARE?

Historically, there have been 3 distinct business models used in production settings around the world. These models have been used in many business settings, and an understanding of them is beginning to reach health care settings. In the following section, a brief history of these business models and why they are important considerations for care model improvement are reviewed.

Before 1911, essentially all productivity was based on craft production.[2] In craft production, individual goods and services were produced by skilled craftsmen, artisans, and service workers.[2] Each item differed from the others slightly. This model began with the site of production. Craft shops were disorganized, and often required a great deal of space. Likewise, the supply chains for such settings were best described as variable and often unreliable. Thus, the products of craft production were variable in quality and dependent on the individual craftsman. Productivity was often slow and dependent on the variable supply chain and variable workforce.

Beginning in 1911, Henry Ford introduced standardization to manufacturing by implementing standardized interchangeable parts for the cars he produced.[2] He relentlessly worked to create standardized work processes for his car assembly operations and for his supply chains. In 1914, he introduced the moving assembly line to car manufacturing.[2] During the subsequent 15 years, he was able to improve productivity, quality, and efficiency of production. During this period, he was able to reduce costs and sell his vehicles at lower prices to the public. This introduction of standardized practices to work became known as mass production.[2]

Henry Ford focused on careful use of his resources, including recycling of defective steel parts, reuse of purpose-designed shipping crates as floor boards for his Model T vehicles, and continued cycles of quality improvement during car production. Mass production plants were large, with many workers, and were also noted to require large quantities of parts and supplies on hand to dampen any variation in availability of parts for the supply chain.

Mass production was associated with problems as well. Mass production of vehicles resulted in many errors, and some vehicles at the end of the assembly line were not functional. Therefore, skilled craftsmen were required to fix the vehicles and prepare them for delivery. The assembly facilities were vast and wasted a great deal of space. Changeover times for production of different types of parts, vehicles, and services were long and expensive. There was a great deal of wasted supplies. Large quantities of supplies were required to be on hand to feed the assembly line. Quality remained variable.

Beginning in 1950, W. Edwards Deming, Taiichi Ohno, Eiji Toyoda, and Kiichiro Toyoda instituted what is now known as lean production or the Toyota Production System in Japan.[2,9] This model was first applied to motor vehicle production. Dr Deming was present in postwar Japan working for the US Department of the Army as an advisor.[2] He trained the Toyoda family and the Toyota workers to use different methods to be able to produce vehicles with limited resources, less production space, faster changeover times, and higher quality.[2] This process of vehicle production has become known as the Toyota production system. He implemented the plan, do, check, act cycle (PDCA) as a fundamental method of continuous quality improvement system. The results of the system were astonishing. Essentially, all of the vehicles started and were drivable at the end of the assembly line. There were few defects. Cars could be produced in less space and different models could be produced on a single assembly line. The supply chains became tighter, with higher-quality standardized parts. The number of wasted parts requiring recycling was reduced and waste and errors were relentlessly driven out of the production system. This model resulted in a renaissance for the Japanese automotive production industry scene in the 1960s and 1970s. Other Japanese industries adopted and successfully implemented lean business methods.[2]

Most industries, with the exception of health care, use lean business methods as the standard business model for production and for service.[9,10]

This situation raises the question: where is health care with respect to business modeling? There are mostly elements of craft production and mass production in the health care environment, with little lean production being present. By its nature, health care is the business of taking care of the health of people. People are all different, with different needs and different problems. They are certainly not standardized machines. Nonetheless, many lessons from business production can be successfully applied to health care. Some of the basic principles are useful and can result in reduction of adverse events experienced by our patients and improved efficiency of care. This result translates into reduced costs. There is an inverse relationship between improved quality and safety of care and reduced costs of care.[7] It has been estimated that there is 30% to 40% waste as a conservative estimate in health care. Some suggest that the percentage of waste could be as high as 60% in American health care.[9] This situation certainly leaves a great deal of room for improvement!

THE GERIATRIC FRACTURE CENTER (ROCHESTER MODEL) FOR CARE OF HIP FRACTURES

One example of a lean business model successfully applied to health care in some centers is the geriatric fracture center (GFC) care model.[11–13] It was initially designed as a way to improve efficiency of care of older adults with a hip fracture and uses a lean business flow model.[12] The lean flow model considers all aspects of care, from entry into the hospital until discharge from the hospital. The GFC profits from standardized work to reduce unwarranted variation.[11,12] Standardized order sets, standardized care maps, early surgical intervention, and many other standard work processes form the basis for the care model.[11,12] Another key concept is that of comanagement of the patient with orthopedic surgeons and geriatricians (or hospitalists).[11–13] Comanagement offers many advantages to the patient and their family to improve the quality and safety of care.[12,14] Comanagement permits the complementary skills of the surgeon and geriatrician or hospitalist to be combined to the benefit of the patient.[12,14] An explanation of the GFC model has been published in detail previously.[11–13] Comanagement is further discussed in the article by Drs Friedman and Mendelson elsewhere in this issue.

Basic components of a lean business model are described in **Table 1**. Any hospitalization or health care process can be broken down into a series of processes. An important lean concept is careful analysis of each process along the way to improve the process or eliminate it if it is not adding value to the overall care of the patient. Value is an interesting proposition in health care. Value can be defined as contact with care providers such as nurses and doctors, needed tests or procedures, and needed medications. Waste includes unnecessary testing or procedures, waiting, readmission, redoing procedures that could have been performed correctly the first time, and so forth. There are many different types of waste in health care. Some of

Table 1
Component tools used in a lean business model

Component	Use	Benefit	Comment
JIT (Just in Time)	Supply chain management	Inventory reduction Cost savings Reliable supply chain	Pillar of lean business
Jidoka: error proofing	Quality management Safety	Reduction of errors	Pillar of lean: used in equipment like anesthesia machine and other medical equipment
PDCA cycle	Process improvement	Repeatable, inexpensive, and essential tool for improving the quality and safety of production	Fundamental lean concept
Kaizen	Process analysis, elimination of wasteful steps and implementation of innovative ideas	Elimination of wasteful processes, cost reduction, reduction of changeover time, improved employee satisfaction	Biased for action 1- to 5-day events with involvement of employees
Process mapping: value stream mapping	Identification of steps in a given process, including those that add value and those that are waste	Allows a visual picture of the steps involved in a value stream	Essential tool of lean business
Checklists	Standard work Example: preoperative checklist, intensive care unit central line bundle	Improve quality and safety	Fundamental tool that should be used more
Kanban: signaling card or tool	Trigger reorder of supplies, movement of patients	Avoid wasted time Avoid delayed order of supplies	Fundamental tool of lean business
Standardized work	Order sets, protocols	Reduce variation and errors	Fundamental concept of lean
5S methodology: set, sort, shine (systematic cleaning), standardize, sustain	Workplace improvement for productivity and safety	Improved and safer workplace	Basic concept of workplace maintenance
Dashboard	Visual representation of system status: used as a basic management tool	Allows the employee to see the status of the system	Should be available in the workplace to see
Visual controls	See and act on the results like an oximetry machine	Safety, monitoring	Helps to improve both quality and safety

these wastes are obvious to health care providers, whereas others are more subtle and require highlighting. Different categories of waste are listed in **Table 2**.

PLANNING TO IMPLEMENT A GFC

Considerable planning is needed to properly implement a GFC to ensure that a successful program is established and maintained. Leadership is the first crucial step to success. A surgeon champion and medical champion should be identified to lead the program.[11] The surgeon and medical physician should be able to communicate well, be committed to implementing the program, and work together to resolve conflicts and overcome barriers. The leaders' relationship with the hospital administration and their colleagues should be such that the necessary steps described later can occur successfully. It is critical that the relationship with hospital administration be one of trust, honesty, community, and mutual respect.[9] Leaders should also enjoy the confidence and support of the nursing staff and medical colleagues who will support the program.

Data is the next key requirement to implement a GFC. All lean programs use data-driven performance decision making.[2,10,15] Basic data required include performance of the current system for care of patients with hip fracture. These data include length of hospital stay, time from admission to surgery, inpatient mortality, 30-day readmission and mortality, costs of care, and provision of recommendations for managing the patient's osteoporosis after discharge from the hospital. Most of these data are likely available from the hospital's administrative databases, because they are reported to the Federal Government as performance metrics already. These data are required to write an acceptable business plan and serve as control information to help gauge performance of the new program in the future.

DEVELOPMENT OF A BASIC BUSINESS PLAN

Writing a basic business plan is a skill that will be increasingly required of physicians to justify new programs, employees, and equipment in the future. A well-designed business plan increases the chances for success and serves as a blueprint for implementation for the GFC. There are many software programs available to help write a business plan, and these plans are comprehensive (and long) when all of the steps are followed. Other options are use of a standard 10-step business plan listed later or an A3 plan, which is even shorter, because it needs to fit on 1 sheet of legal size paper. These short plans are becoming increasingly popular planning systems used in industry to improve quality; they require some skill and training to write well.[16] A3 plans are also used as a PDCA quality improvement reporting system and lean thinking, known as A3 thinking. Toyota has subsequently shrunk the reports to A4 (210 × 297 mm) (8.5 × 11 in) sized paper.[16]

The following section presents a 10-step business plan. In general, the shorter plans seem to have a better chance of being read in their entirety by administrators. The business plan is a roadmap to implement the GFC and thus differs from a strategic plan, which defines the goals for the program. It is estimated that only 10% of strategic plans are successfully implemented.[17] Many organizations spend 90% of their time on the strategic plan and only 10% on the implementation of the plan, which can result in unsuccessful implementations.[17]

The 10-Step Business Plan

1. Statement of purpose: define the purpose of the program you seek to implement. Example from a previous plan I have written: "The Geriatric Fracture Program is

Table 2
Wastes in health care with examples, causes, and potential countermeasures to be used against them

The 7 Classic Wastes (Plus an Eighth)	Example	Cause	Countermeasure
Transportation	Taking a patient to radiology 3 times for 3 radiographs	Correct studies not ordered to be obtained during the first visit to radiology	Standard order sets specify the correct studies to obtain
Inventory	Too much inventory of some items but missing vital inventory in other areas	Poor inventory management	Improve supply chain with better signaling and correct par levels
Motion	Nurse gathering needed supplies for a patient because of inadequate stocking of the room/floor	Material stocking not meeting needs	Changing restocking method with appropriate signal for restocking the area
Waiting	Patients and physicians waiting for operating room availability	Scheduling system unresponsive to needs	Match the operating room availability to the demand for time
Overprocessing	Obtaining too many diagnostic studies such as laboratory tests or a computed tomography scan for a hip fracture visible on plain films	Lack of standard protocols for management of a specific diagnosis like hip fracture	Implement and follow standard orders for diagnostic testing. Highlight episodes of noncompliance
Overproduction	Repeated documentation of the same information	Misinterpretation of regulatory policies	Organization of electronic record to eliminate this waste
Defects	Readmission to the hospital or medication error: considered among worst of the wastes	Lack of emphasis on performing defect-free work	System redesign to eliminate defects Development of standard defect-free work
Wasted employee ideas: an eighth waste	The employees working in a given area usually know the problems of that area and how to fix them They are rarely asked for their ideas by their leaders	Vertical or pyramidal leadership structure: thwarts employees from sharing ideas	Use of more horizontal leadership structure, which empowers the employees to share and test their ideas to improve care

a nationally and internationally known program for care of the elderly patient with a fracture. The plan is focused on high quality, cost effective care with Total Quality Management and Lean Business principles guiding the protocol driven processes. All patients cared for in this program are co-managed with an orthopedic surgeon and a geriatrician throughout their hospital stay."

2. Five-year objectives and milestones: define where you anticipate the program implementation and progress at 1-year, 2-year, 3-year, and 5-year milestones.

Example: "At 1 year, the GFC will have been implemented with a standard set of orders, standard nursing care plan and 70% surgeon staff acceptance." This is a realistic and achievable first-year plan. Such milestones should be assessed for success in meeting them and, if necessary, for remediation of delays or roadblocks.

3. The market: description and quantification of the market you will serve including the total available market and the amount you expect to capture. Customers and segments: descriptions of the customers and the customer segments you will serve. Technology: the technology that is prevalent in the market. For example: "there are approximately 1100 hip fractures that occur annually in our catchment area. 40% of those fractures are cared for in our system and 20% in system B and 40% in system C. 80% of patients sustaining a hip fracture are admitted to the hospital from a home setting and 20% from a residential care facility or nursing home. We further estimate that with marketing and increase in capacity of our program, 15% of the volume can be shifted from the other 2 systems to our system."

4. Competition: who/where is the competition? This factor is dependent on local conditions and regional conditions. In some cases, there is no competition, and that should be stated as such. In other cases, there are 1 or more competitive health care systems vying for the business provided by these patients. In such a case, the performance and success of the competitive systems needs to be assessed and stated in the business plan. For example: "our competitive hospital system does not have an organized system for geriatric fracture care. However, their length of stay in case volume is similar to our system." In addition, there should be assessment of the level of marketing being conducted by competitive systems that could influence the success of any attempts made to increase case volume.

5. Solutions: what products and services will you provide? How will you win?: What is the plan to beat the competition or overcome the problems existent in the current system of care? How will you improve the outcome metrics at your hospital?

6. Capabilities: existing capabilities that will allow you to serve the market (research and development, clinic, doctors, staff, and so forth...). Are there enough physicians and surgeons to staff such a program? Is there bed capacity in the hospital for additional patients or is the goal of the program to better use existing bed capacity to reduce hospital overcrowding? Is there enough operating room time availability to permit timely surgery on this group of older adults? Is there a bottleneck because of lack of availability of equipment such as radiograph machines, fracture tables, or fracture fixation hardware? In some cases, all of the necessary parts of the program are present but just need to be properly organized into a smoothly functioning machine. In other cases, a deficiency needs to be remedied for successful implementation.

7. Interdependencies: what other organizations do you need to work with to be successful (internal and external). This category should include elaboration of different hospital departments that would need to cooperate for a successful program. It may also describe external partnering needed for successful implementation. This partnering could include partnerships with nursing homes, primary care physician networks, and cooperation of providers of emergency medical services. In some cases, external interdependency may refer to local or regional governmental approvals.

8. Financials: pro forma income statement (profit and loss) and maybe balance sheet and cash flow statement. These data can typically be obtained from the hospital's finance department. An explanation of why the data are required is usually

necessary. Discussions with the finance department can be helpful in forecasting future growth and estimating future expenses. The financial statements in the business plan are critical to a credible plan.

9. Issues and potential problems (discharges): what barriers there? What could go wrong? What is the mitigation plan for these issues and potential problems? Each problem and barrier should be spelled out, along with a recommended solution to overcome the problem. There have been some publications on the subject. In addition, in some cases, consultation with a business consultant who is expert in implementation science can be valuable here.

10. First-year plan and milestones: specifically, what do you plan to do in the first year? The specific plan for the first year is critical to the success of implementation. Problems should be anticipated and addressed. Specific realistic time points should be created and should be outlined. Necessary inputs, including personnel, cash, and material, should be spelled out, along with an explanation of why they are needed.

PARTNERING FOR SUCCESS

It is important to the success of a GFC to partner with the other departments involved in the care of patients with a hip fracture. These departments include the core services of geriatrics and orthopedic surgery; essential services, including anesthesiology, nursing, social work, physical therapy; and medical consulting services. Each of these groups is essential in providing necessary care to the patient with hip fracture. Once there is agreement between the medical and surgical services, it is necessary to engage each of these other services to develop agreement to work together as a team to improve the care of the patient with hip fracture. This agreement is often first addressed with a meeting between the surgical and medical champion and of each of these partners in care. Once agreement to work together has been established, it is essential to engage the remaining members of each of the services. This engagement is often achieved with an interactive presentation to the group. Description of the current state of affairs and the intended improvements to be achieved with implementation of the GFC are the primary goal of the meeting. It is important at such meetings to emphasize the benefits not only to the patient but also to the service being asked to engage in the process. The "what's in it for me?" test is important to answer for each service. Emphasis on streamlining care, standardizing care, and making efforts to simplify the process are important aspects of such a discussion.

This approach permits the providers of care to work together for the benefit of the patient and avoids development of roadblocks and barriers to successful care. Early engagement of each of these services is recommended. Before engaging the clinical services, it is important to have buy-in from hospital administration. Working with hospital administration is an essential skill and is best achieved by presenting the administrators with solutions to existing problems. It is necessary to present a business plan to the administrators to permit appropriate decisions to be made. Business plans should be based on credible and accurate predictions, using the best available data, as described earlier.

During the process of partnering with other services, it is important to establish the right tone for collaboration. This goal is achieved with an opportunity for all parties to contribute to the program in their own area. It is achieved with collegiality and respect. Respect for employees is a key lean concept.[9] A culture is thus created that is conducive to successful interdisciplinary care. It may take time to develop the right culture at some institutions to achieve this desired goal. In other institutions, such culture may already be well established.

DEVELOPMENT OF CARE MAPS AND PROTOCOLS

The development of care maps and protocols is a critical aspect of any organized health care program. By its nature, development of successful protocols requires input from all of the team members who are involved in care of the patient.[11] Such interdisciplinary development of the protocols results in success of implementation and permits a framework for modifying them in the future when that is necessary. Even if protocols are obtained from other successful programs, it is necessary to review each order in detail to be certain that they are in compliance with hospital policy and procedure as well as specific local practice styles and preferences. There is always a need to locally modify any care map or order set that is obtained externally.

When the process is started, it is important to analyze what is being done presently in the hospital for such patients. Often, a generic order set and care map are being used. This system offers an opportunity for health care providers to examine their current practices and look for opportunities to improve them. Each aspect of an order set needs to be carefully examined by multiple personnel. These personnel not only include physicians but should also include nurses, midlevel providers, therapists, dietitians, pharmacists, and (when required) specific medical consultants. Some order sets have been widely circulated, including those associated with the Rochester model of care. Even these order sets require local adaptation and examination.

Examples of necessary order sets include: emergency department orders, geriatric fracture admission order set, geriatric fracture postoperative order set and standardized discharge instructions.

When creating a standardized order set, it is important to look at opportunities to eliminate variability in patient care practices, simplify the care by removal of wasteful processes, and reduce costs (eg, generic medications). Such efforts reward both the system and the patient with better care and fewer adverse events. One side effect of standard order sets is significant cost reduction. Whenever possible, evidence-based practice should be incorporated into standard order sets. Thus, an order set reflects the current best practices when properly created. Because these best practices change with time, it is necessary to modify the order sets in keeping with new evidence.

Such order sets, of course, must take into account local, regional, and national practice guidelines, such as those established by the Joint Commission, state, and Federal Government. When necessary policies and regulations are incorporated into care maps and standard order sets, both the hospital and the program fare better during a site visit from the Joint Commission or other regulatory body. Also, health care providers are able to more easily meet such standards set by following standard order sets and care maps.

An essential component to standard protocols is a standardized process for performing a geriatric medicine consultation. This process can be a structured consultation form to be completed by the medical consultant or can be more of a checklist with free text at the end. Either way, it is essential that all necessary parts of the medical consultation be captured on the form. Such a form addresses the patient's medical fitness for the intended surgery and, ideally, should contain a description of risk stratification: low risk, medium risk, high risk, or extremely high risk for the intended surgical procedure. All of the patient's pertinent medical conditions should be described, along with whether or not the patient has been adequately optimized for the intended surgical procedure. A common problem such as dehydration should be corrected before surgery. Other conditions may be problematic but may be as good as they are going to get before surgery. Some conditions may be problematic, such as aortic stenosis, and may require active intervention during the surgery, such as maintenance of cardiac preload with fluids. Such cautions should be shared with the team before the intended procedure. In addition, a thorough medical consultation should assess the patient's preinjury functional status, which is an important predictor of outcome after surgery. Another important aspect of the presurgical assessment is referred to as the goals of care. This aspect encompasses the patient's desires for resuscitation, intubation, feeding, and other essential interventions potentially required in an emergency situation. Many states require a discussion be held with the patient or family on hospital admission to address goals of care. Locally mandated forms should be used to document the patient's goals, and the appropriate orders should be entered into the medical record for those wishes. In the event of a surgical procedure, the patient's wishes regarding resuscitation in surgery and in the postanesthesia recovery area should be made known and documented. It is important that the patient's wishes be followed and that family involvement be maintained during the course of care should their wishes change.

An important part of the presurgical medical consultation is appropriate medication reconciliation by the medical consultant. Often, patients enter the hospital on a long list of medications, often referred to as polypharmacy. It is frequently necessary to discontinue those medications that are not contributing to the welfare of the patient or are harmful to the patient's health. The medical consultant is in an ideal position to make these recommendations before surgery, and they should be reassessed after surgery as well.

It is important that the medical consultation form does not offer specific recommendations to the anesthesiologist about the type of anesthetic needed but rather permits the anesthesiologist to arrive at this plan on their own. If in doubt, it is best to review concerns as a team, which tends to lead to collegial discussions rather than confrontations.

The nursing care map should mirror the activities occurring in the order set and should take into account specific timing considerations for surgical intervention and anticipated hospital discharge. For example, if most hip fractures are operated within 24 hours of hospital admission, the nursing care map should reflect that in preparation for surgery, patient and family teaching, dietary intake, activity orders, and obtaining necessary laboratory studies. The nursing care map should be created with experienced nurses, midlevel providers, and physicians at the table to be certain that the patient's needs are being met and that there is concordance between the care map and order sets.

DEALING WITH BARRIERS TO IMPLEMENTATION

During implementation of any new care initiative, barriers and roadblocks to success are bound to occur. Some barriers are common and have occurred in many programs attempting to implement a geriatric fracture program. Others are peculiar to the local environment and less common. For successful implementation to occur, such barriers must be overcome in a way that retains engagement of participating parties in the process. Common barriers have been previously published, with suggested methods to mitigate them.[18] These barriers include physician leadership, need for a clinical case manager, lack of operating room time, anesthesia department support, lack of hospital administration support, and difficulty obtaining presurgical cardiac clearance. Each barrier needs a strategy to be developed to mitigate the problem.

For leadership, it is important to select medical and surgical leaders who are capable of building consensus and resolving differences between themselves and other services.[18] Some additional characteristics of program leaders are described earlier.

When dealing with the need for a clinical case manager, it is important to engage the hospital administration to provide necessary financing.[18] A business plan for the care manager would be helpful in such a case. An explanation of the benefits versus the costs of the care manager would be essential with such a plan. The business plan for care manager would be ideally provided in the A3 1-page format to simplify the discussion. Selection of an experienced nurse to be a care manager who is already employed by the hospital is 1 helpful strategy. Another useful strategy could be to designate a midlevel provider such as a physician's assistant or nurse practitioner to serve in such a role. The care manager is extremely important for success of a hip fracture program.

In many centers, the lack of operating room time is an issue that interferes with early surgical intervention. Some programs face competition for operating room time from cases that are considered more urgent or more interesting. In some centers, this problem can be overcome by designating a daily block of time for hip fracture fixation, whereas in other centers, the problem can be overcome with education and explanation of the importance of early surgical intervention for the elderly patient with a hip fracture.

To obtain support of the hospital administration, a different approach is beneficial. It is important to emphasize the business aspects of a geriatric fracture program, complete with a well-conceived business plan, as described earlier. It is essential to present the program as a solution to an existing problem rather than making it a problem of its own. In the current fee-for-service reimbursement model, a well-functioning and well-organized program likely results in an improvement of the net margin per case.[7,19] Early engagement of the hospital's administration is strongly recommended. In some cases, this process requires presentation of the plans to the medical center's board of directors for approval. Program leaders should be prepared to make a brief and convincing presentation to such a board if required. Such presentations are typically 10 minutes or less and should emphasize advantages of such a program in terms of cost and quality, with a brief business plan.

Another common concern that presents a barrier to hip fracture care is the need for cardiac clearance for surgery. This concern is often driven by a discomfort on the part of treating physicians with the patient's perceived high risk for surgery or poor presurgical health. The American College of Cardiology and American Heart Association have addressed this issue in a published guideline on perioperative management.[20,21] Education of the involved providers using this well-written guideline can help overcome the routine requirement for cardiology consultation or unnecessary ordering of preoperative echocardiograms.

Some barriers to implementation are local and may be challenging to manage. In some cases, employing a professional business consultant experienced in implementation of such programs can prove useful. There are many health care consulting companies. Only a few have previous experience in implementation of organized geriatric fracture programs.

DO YOU NEED A CONSULTANT?

Hospitals frequently employ consultants when the need for impartial outside guidance is required. There are many consulting firms available, and some are specialized in certain areas of hospital performance. Few are expert in implementation of geriatric fracture programs. Implementation of such a program is a mixture of implementation science and experience. Consultants can serve as organizers and managers for the implementation process. An experienced consulting service has an established process in place to implement a program. They typically are able to provide help with preparation of a business plan, organizing personnel, structuring meetings of the implementation team, assisting the team with meeting their milestones, and providing useful materials, including standard order sets and care plans, for the receiving hospital. There is a cost for such services, which, in most cases, can be readily recouped within several months of a successful implementation. Some hospitals choose to use a consultant only after failing to make progress on their own or hitting barriers that are difficult to overcome. Other hospitals choose to use a consulting service at the outset to produce a smoother and more predictable implementation process. An experienced consulting service can be useful to the hospital and the care team to overcome the problems both large and small that crop up during the process of implementation. Consultants can also help with data gathering and data management and can suggest benchmarks for the hospital to achieve. Consulting services can assist with presentations to managerial boards with the use of standardized scorecards and metrics.

Finding the right consultant is important. Often, the consultant's value is judged by their experience, which in turn dictates their costs. Some implant vendors have employed successful consulting teams as part of a value-added service to their customers to enhance their overall business. This model seems most successful if the hospital is a valued customer of the vendor to begin with. Hence, this business model could be a winning situation for both. For both parties to work together well, good open communication and a strong desire to succeed is important.

It is recommended that hospitals and physician leaders carefully examine the track record of a business consultant to be hired for implementation of such a program. Examination of services offered, the Web site, protocols, and standard products offered as well as reputation must be considered. It is also useful to ask around with other centers that have used the consultant to successfully implement a program. This strategy helps avoid disappointment and wasted resources that may otherwise occur. Typical costs for consulting services to assist with implementing a GFC are in the $30,000 to $100,000 range.

HOW MUCH DOES IT COST TO IMPLEMENT A GFC?

Costs for implementing any new program in a hospital setting are important. The business plan is most useful here. For many lean processes, the costs of implementation are revenue neutral but do consume an important resource of employee time. The geriatric fracture program would fall into this category in many cases. The process of implementation should best use existing resources, including existing medical personnel, nursing staff, therapists, operating rooms, surgical equipment, and diagnostic equipment. Some programs would require reorganization in the sense of designating an existing employee to work more closely aligned with the program, such as the care manager, as mentioned earlier. Additional costs above and beyond those costs would include fees for a consultant (if desired), costs of ongoing data collection (above and beyond standard hospital data that are already gathered), and hiring of any additional staff members to support the program.

As part of a business plan, projected cost savings realized by the lean process would typically offset any additional expenses required. In some cases, facilitators and lean business experts are already employed by the medical center and can assist in this process. In other cases, the outside consultation would be beneficial. The costs for a data manager would typically be required only for an academic research center that is focused on detailed patient level data. Few centers have a designated full-time data manager for their geriatric fracture program. Often, this function is absorbed by a quality management department, which already collects much of the needed data to complete a scorecard for performance.

HOW TO MEASURE SUCCESS OF YOUR PROGRAM

Suggested outcome parameters have been published in the literature recently.[15,22] A simple set of parameters would include: length of hospital stay, inpatient mortality, time to surgery, discharge destination, cost of care, percentage of patients meeting governmental performance measures like Surgical Care Improvement Project measures, 30-day readmission and mortality, provision of recommendations for managing the patient's osteoporosis after discharge from the hospital, and any other specific data point the hospital is particularly interested in. Many of these data points are already collected and reported to the government. Organizing them into a monthly or quarterly scorecard is an enhanced reporting process to focus attention on performance successes and problems to permit program managers to improve the outcomes.[9,17] With the study of reduced length of stay, the bed to carrying capacity of the hospital would be enhanced. In addition, measures such as cost of care may show substantial improvement in the net margin of a program. This improvement combined with reduced complications would show the substantial value of such a program to hospital leadership and help ensure its long-term success and support. It is important to use data to drive lean process improvements. Should a problem be highlighted with the collection of data, it would be important to engage in a lean process improvement process known as a Kaizen, focused on the problem, with appropriate team members needed to solve the problem.[2] Administrative support is mandatory for such process improvement efforts.

SUMMARY

Lean business processes have important usefulness in health care.[9,10] One such example is the GFC model for improvement of care of older adults with a hip fracture.[11] Such a program is collaborative and interdisciplinary in nature and uses patient centered protocol driven care.[11-13] The GFC offers standardized care to older adults with a fracture and has been reported to show improved results for quality and safety of care as well as reduced costs of care. Implementation of such a program offers many challenges specific to the individual hospital site but also offers many rewards to the patient, providers, and hospital implementing it. Such lean business processes could likely be used in many aspects of health care to reduce harmful and wasteful processes while improving quality and safety of care. Some basic business skills are beneficial to health care providers when implementing major changes in their care model. For those providers uncomfortable with these business skills, assistance from business consultants can be obtained to facilitate the process of implementation. The strong desire to implement such a program coupled with necessary resources and culture are essential for success.

REFERENCES

1. Brauer CA, Coca-Perraillon M, Cutler DM, et al. Incidence and mortality of hip fractures in the United States. JAMA 2009;302(14):1573–9.

2. Womack JP, Jones DT, Roos D, editors. The machine that changed the world. 1st edition. New York: Rawson; 1990.
3. Magaziner J, Hawkes W, Hebel JR, et al. Recovery from hip fracture in eight areas of function. J Gerontol A Biol Sci Med Sci 2000;55(9):M498–507.
4. Cutler DM, Ghosh K. The potential for cost savings through bundled episode payments. N Engl J Med 2012;366(12):1075–7.
5. Barrett M, Wilson E, Whalen D. 2007 HCUP Nationwide Inpatient Sample (NIS) comparison report. HCUP Methods Series Report # 2010-03 [Online]. 2010. p. 18–9. Available at: http://www.hcup-us.ahrq.gov/reports/methods/2010_03. pdf. Accessed June 15, 2013.
6. Cooper C, Campion G, Melton LJ 3rd. Hip fractures in the elderly: a world-wide projection. Osteoporos Int 1992;2(6):285–9.
7. Kates SL, Blake D, Bingham KW, et al. Comparison of an organized geriatric fracture program to United States government data. Geriatr Orthop Surg Rehabil 2010;1(1):15–21.
8. Goodman DC, Fisher ES, Chang CH. After hospitalization: a Dartmouth Atlas report on post-acute care for Medicare beneficiaries. Hanover (NH): Dartmouth; 2011.
9. Chalice R. 2nd edition. Improving healthcare using Toyota lean production methods, vol. 1. Milwaukee (WI): ASQ Quality Press; 2007.
10. Zidel TG. 1st edition. Lean guide to transforming healthcare, vol. 1. Milwaukee (WI): ASQ Quality Press; 2006.
11. Kates SL, Mendelson DA, Friedman SM. Co-managed care for fragility hip fractures (Rochester model). Osteoporos Int 2010;21(Suppl 4):S621–5.
12. Friedman SM, Mendelson DA, Kates SL, et al. Geriatric co-management of proximal femur fractures: total quality management and protocol-driven care result in better outcomes for a frail patient population. J Am Geriatr Soc 2008;56(7): 1349–56.
13. Friedman SM, Mendelson DA, Bingham KW, et al. Impact of a comanaged geriatric fracture center on short-term hip fracture outcomes. Arch Intern Med 2009; 169(18):1712–7.
14. Batsis JA, Phy MP, Joseph Melton L 3rd, et al. Effects of a hospitalist care model on mortality of elderly patients with hip fractures. J Hosp Med 2007;2(4):219–25.
15. Liem IS, Kammerlander C, Suhm N, et al. Literature review of outcome parameters used in studies of geriatric fracture centers. Injury 2013;44(11):1403–12. http://dx.doi.org/10.1016/j.injury.2013.06.018.
16. Sobek DK. Understanding A3 thinking. 1st edition. New York: CRC Press; 2008. Available at: http://books.google.com/books?hl=en&lr=&id=v6G1V9GdJucC& oi=fnd&pg=PP1&dq=a3+busines+plan+writing&ots=HbPVFUoZPu&sig= dta2xeqleuSNIMx3v2bNBR9_qi8#v=onepage&q=a3%20busines%20plan% 20writing&f=false. Accessed October 22, 2013.
17. Kaplan RS, Norton DP. The balanced scorecard: measures that drive performance. Boston: Harvard Business Review Press; 2010.
18. Kates SL, O'Malley N, Friedman SM, et al. Barriers to implementation of an organized geriatric fracture program. Geriatr Orthop Surg Rehabil 2012;3(1):8–16.
19. Kates SL, Mendelson DA, Friedman SM. The value of an organized fracture program for the elderly: early results. J Orthop Trauma 2011;25(4):233–7.
20. Fleischmann KE, Beckman JA, Buller CE, et al. 2009 ACCF/AHA focused update on perioperative beta blockade: a report of the American College of Cardiology Foundation/American Heart Association Task Force on Practice Guidelines. Circulation 2009;120(21):2123–51.

21. Fleisher LA, Beckman JA, Brown KA, et al. ACC/AHA 2007 guidelines on periop-
    erative cardiovascular evaluation and care for noncardiac surgery: executive
    summary: a report of the American College of Cardiology/American Heart Asso-
    ciation Task Force on Practice Guidelines (Writing Committee to Revise the 2002
    Guidelines on Perioperative Cardiovascular Evaluation for Noncardiac Surgery):
    developed in collaboration with the American Society of Echocardiography,
    American Society of Nuclear Cardiology, Heart Rhythm Society, Society of Car-
    diovascular Anesthesiologists, Society for Cardiovascular Angiography and Inter-
    ventions, Society for Vascular Medicine and Biology, and Society for Vascular
    Surgery. Circulation 2007;116(17):1971–96.
22. Liem IS, Kammerlander C, Suhm N, et al. Identifying a standard set of outcome
    parameters for the evaluation of orthogeriatric co-management for hip fractures.
    Injury 2013;44(11):1403–12.

Preoperative Optimization and Risk Assessment

Joseph A. Nicholas, MD, MPH

KEYWORDS

- Preoperative risk assessment • Preoperative care • Cardiovascular disease
- Geriatric fracture management

KEY POINTS

- Early hip fracture surgery is important for good functional outcomes.
- Most multiply comorbid geriatric patients can be safely optimized for surgery within 24 hours.
- Perioperative hypotension is common in older patients and should be anticipated and prevented.
- Advanced preoperative cardiac testing (echocardiography, stress testing) does not seem to improve outcomes and may inappropriately delay surgical repair.
- Preoperative cardiovascular medication management should be focused on preserving intravascular volume status and pain control and minimizing polypharmacy.

INTRODUCTION

There has been increasing academic and professional interest in the optimal preoperative risk assessment and perioperative care for older adults undergoing surgery. Most surgical procedures occur in older adults,[1] who as a group have higher rates of perioperative complications than the general population, even after controlling for comorbidities.[2] In addition to increased comorbidity prevalence, geriatric patients have unique physiologic risks[3] and perioperative syndromes that often complicate surgical outcomes.[4] There has been increasing emphasis on the use of standard practices and the identification of specific quality indicators to improve outcomes in older surgical patients.[5] This article summarizes the current best practices for preoperative risk assessment and preoperative optimization for older adults with osteoporotic fractures.

IMPLICATIONS OF NORMAL AGING

Normal aging of the cardiovascular,[6] pulmonary,[7] and renal[8] systems results in physiologic changes that can significantly impact cardiopulmonary stability and

Conflict of Interest: None to declare.
Division of Geriatrics, Highland Hospital, University of Rochester School of Medicine, 1000 South Avenue, Box 58, Rochester, NY 14610, USA
E-mail address: Joseph_Nicholas@urmc.rochester.edu

increase risk for perioperative complications. Normal cardiovascular aging results in a less compliant, less responsive cardiovascular system with a higher propensity for hypotension, conduction system defects, and pulmonary edema. Declines in lung compliance, vital capacity, and diffusion capacity lower the threshold for hypoxemia and hypercapnea and increase the impact of common perioperative pulmonary issues, such as atelectasis, respiratory depression, and aspiration. Renal aging processes often produce glomerulosclerosis, interstitial fibrosis, and hyalinization of the afferent arterioles and place older adults at increased risk for acute kidney injury, fluid retention, and electrolyte abnormalities. Taken together, these changes impair the older adult from maintaining physiologic homeostasis in the face of acute perioperative stressors, such as pain, anesthesia, polypharmacy, and blood loss.[9] As different patients have different degrees of physiologic aging and impairment, standardized risk assessment, medical dosing, and clinical protocols can be challenging to create.

PREOPERATIVE PRINCIPLES IN THE GERIATRIC FRACTURE PATIENT

Because there is a scarcity of prospective evidence for specific preoperative strategies, most recommendations are drawn from expert opinion guidelines, extrapolated data derived from younger patients and other surgical procedures, and the experience of high-performing geriatric fracture centers.[10,11] These centers have used preoperative strategies designed to rapidly exclude absolute contraindications to surgery and quickly optimize patients for fracture repair. Most of these centers focus on geriatric principles of empiric symptom control, anticipation of hypotension and delirium, and avoidance of polypharmacy, and do not routinely rely on subspecialty consultation or advanced diagnostic testing. Important general strategies include the following:

- Rapid optimization for early surgical fixation (<24–48 hours)
- Avoidance of perioperative hypotension
- Pain control
- Delirium prevention
- Prioritization of symptom control and functional status over extensive diagnostic evaluation

EARLY SURGERY

Early surgical repair of acute hip fractures is associated with reductions in perioperative mortality and postoperative complications, including pressure ulcers and pneumonia.[12] This reduction in mortality seems to be most prominent in frail patients with functional dependency[13] and suggests that weaker, more comorbid patients are likely to benefit most from rapid optimization for surgical fixation. However, this can be problematic for health systems and practice patterns that promote extensive preoperative diagnostic evaluation of highly comorbid patients, whereby comprehensive preoperative testing may lead to worse outcomes. This paradox may be explained by the evidence that many preoperative test abnormalities fail to correlate with postoperative complications,[14] and that for frail patients, rapid declines in functional, nutritional, and cognitive status associated with short-term immobility, pain, and delirium significantly outweigh any potential benefits of specific comorbidity evaluation and treatment. The need for efficient, focused, and goal-directed preoperative risk assessment and optimization is essential for improved outcomes.

PREOPERATIVE RISK ASSESSMENT IN OLDER PATIENTS

Although preoperative assessment in younger adults is often focused on the evaluation of cardiovascular risk, there are several other predictors of perioperative complications that should be considered in older adults. In addition to a qualitative assessment of comorbidities, additional explicit attention to cognitive, functional, and nutritional status is essential in the estimation of perioperative risk and anticipated postoperative complications.[15] In many instances, cognitive and functional status assessments are superior to cardiovascular and other comorbidity scores in predicting postoperative outcomes.[16] The American College of Surgeons and the American Geriatrics Society have collaborated to produce best practice guidelines for preoperative assessment[17] and strongly recommend several specific assessments, in addition to a complete and thorough history and physical examination (**Table 1**).

Cardiovascular Evaluation

For the geriatric fracture patient, the cardiac evaluation should be focused on ruling out serious active cardiac conditions, evaluating intravascular volume status, and anticipating perioperative hypotension. Unlike the preoperative evaluation for elective surgeries, whereby extensive testing for coronary artery disease and impaired

Table 1
Selected preoperative assessments for geriatric surgical patients

Assessment Area	Clinical Importance	Tools
Cardiac evaluation	ACC/AHA guideline supports proceeding to operating room without further risk stratification for patients without active cardiac conditions[a]	Resting electrocardiogram Revised Cardiac Risk Assessment[18] (Goldman RCRI)
Cognitive impairment	Important to establish capacity for consent Helps establish accuracy of other assessments (particularly reliability of historical details, medication compliance) Helps predict delirium, complications, and postoperative decline	Mini-Cog ADL/IADL assessment (by proxy)
Functional status	Poor functional status is associated with postoperative complications (including delirium) and after-discharge needs Functional status helps predict functional outcome	ADL/IADL assessment New mobility score (Parker mobility score)[19]
Nutritional status	Poor nutritional status is associated with increased risk for wound complications and infections	Body mass index <18.5 Albumin <3 Unintentional weight loss >10% over a 6-mo period
Polypharmacy	Identify medications that may contribute to perioperative complications (hypotension, bleeding, delirium)	Beers criteria STOPP criteria Judicious prescribing of chronic antihypertensive, diabetic, and other medications

[a] Unstable coronary syndromes, decompensated heart failure, significant arrhythmias, severe valvular disease.

ventricular function may result in changes in preoperative management and medical clearance, timely repair of acute fractures and early time to surgery are central to optimal postoperative outcomes. Other than a history and physical examination, current American College of Cardiology/American Heart Association (ACC/AHA) guidelines only explicitly recommend a resting 12-lead electrocardiogram for the typical geriatric patient undergoing orthopedic surgery. The only acute cardiac conditions recognized by the ACC/AHA that warrant more extensive evaluation and treatment before operative repair of hip fractures are unstable coronary syndromes, decompensated heart failure, significant arrhythmias, and severe valvular disease, and a general recommendation to restrict testing to patients for whom it will produce a significant change in perioperative management (**Table 2**). Because acute hip fracture patients require timely surgery to limit hemodynamic instability, pain, delirium, and immobility, it is rare for advanced cardiac testing to be of benefit. Two retrospective reviews concluded that preoperative echocardiography and stress testing did not prompt a single instance of angiography, angioplasty, or cardiac surgery, but did increase surgical delay, higher rates of invasive monitoring, and higher rates of acute medication change.[20,21]

Orthopedic surgery is considered an intermediate-risk surgery based on rates of major cardiac complications generally occurring in 1% to 5% of patients, although this may underestimate the risk for frail older adults or in patients for whom more intensive postoperative surveillance is performed. Although there are several comorbidity and risk factor indices used for patient-specific risk quantification, none of these have been validated in elderly patients in general and in hip fracture repair in particular. Studies of hip fracture patients report a wide range of adverse cardiac event rates (1%–10%),[22] a range that likely reflects differences in myocardial enzyme surveillance and case definitions.[23]

Specific issues surrounding β-blockade and other cardiovascular medication management are addressed in the Preoperative Optimization section below.

Cognitive Impairment

Cognitive impairment and dementia are highly prevalent in geriatric fracture patients[24] and are predictive of negative outcomes, including mortality, delirium, increased length of stay, and functional decline.[25] Patients without a known diagnosis of cognitive impairment can be screened in the preoperative setting. Although most comprehensive screening and diagnostic tools for cognitive impairment are too cumbersome or inappropriate for use in the acute preoperative setting, a history of

Table 2	
Active cardiac conditions that may warrant surgical delay for further evaluation and treatment	
Conditions	**Clinical Examples and Issues**
Unstable coronary syndromes	Unstable angina Acute myocardial infarction
Decompensated heart failure	New onset Class IV
Significant arrhythmias	Unstable tachycardia (rapid atrial fibrillation, supraventricular tachycardia, ventricular tachycardia) High-grade heart block (Mobitz II or third-degree AV block)
Severe valvular disease	Suspected aortic valve area <1 cm² (if it will change perioperative management)

activities of daily living/instrumental activities of daily living (ADL/IADL) deficiencies[26] or brief cognitive assessments in patients without delirium may provide an adequate assessment for clinical purposes. IADL deficiencies that may correlate with a diagnosis of dementia include impairments in telephone use, handling of finances, and medication self-administration.[27] The Mini-Cog is a brief cognitive assessment limited to a 3-item recall and a clock drawing test; this test is often not valid in the preoperative setting of the acute fracture patient in light of the high prevalence of delirium.

Functional Status

Good functional status predicts good outcomes and low rates of complications. Functional status is commonly assessed in older adults by obtaining historical features summarized as ADL/IADL, and deficits in these areas are associated with worse functional outcomes. Requiring assistance with getting out of a bed or chair, bathing and dressing, meal preparation, or shopping should prompt a full ADL/IADL assessment (**Table 3**). The New Mobility Scale has been designed and validated in geriatric hip fracture patients and can predict mortality and functional outcomes.[19] Additional historical features related to functional status include a history of falls, and the presence of vision, hearing, or swallowing deficits.

In addition to the ADL/IADL estimation of functional status, high degrees of functional capacity during moderately strenuous activities as measured by metabolic equivalents (METs) may also predict low perioperative cardiac complications. Extrapolating from ACC/AHA algorithms targeting elective surgery candidates, patients who are able to complete tasks requiring more than 4 METs (**Table 4**) are anticipated to have low rates of cardiac complications and would be unlikely to benefit from advanced cardiac testing.

Nutritional Status

Malnutrition is highly prevalent within hip fracture patients[28] and is suggested by low body mass index, low serum albumin, or significant unintentional weight loss.[17] Weight loss in older adults is disproportionately lean muscle mass and often reflects underlying sarcopenia.[29] Poor nutritional status should be identified on admission, to allow for appropriate assessment and treatment to begin as soon as possible in the postoperative period.

Polypharmacy

The risks of polypharmacy for acutely hospitalized geriatric patients are significant. Many medications that have been chronically tolerated in the stable outpatient

Table 3 Activities of daily living and instrumental activities of daily living	
ADLS	**IADLs**
Bathing	Using telephone
Toileting	Grocery shopping
Dressing	Transportation
Transferring	Cooking
Continence	Housekeeping
Feeding	Taking own medications Handling own finances

Table 4
Exercise capacity and implications

Metabolic Equivalents	Activities	Implications
1 MET	Eat, dress, use toilet	Advanced cardiac testing only if it will result in change in management
4 METs	Climb one flight of stairs Light work around the house (dusting, dishes)	No advanced cardiac testing recommended, prior orthopedic surgery
≥10 METs	Strenuous sports (swimming, skiing, singles tennis)	

setting can become dangerous in the dynamic setting of the perioperative period, and new drug interactions and other adverse reactions emerge. It is important for the geriatric fracture team to avoid conflating the long-term benefits of many chronic medications with the short-term risks of hypotension, renal failure, delirium, and sedation that can occur if medications are not adjusted and, when necessary, discontinued.

PREOPERATIVE OPTIMIZATION

Because almost all geriatric fracture patients require urgent fracture fixation for optimal outcomes, preoperative optimization is often of more practical consequence than preoperative risk assessment and should be the primary focus of the entire care team (emergency, orthopedics, medicine, and anesthesiology providers). There are 5 domains that typically require assessment, treatment, and monitoring to successfully optimize fracture patients and minimize intraoperative complications, as follows:

- Assurance of adequate intravascular volume
- Medication adjustment in anticipation of intraoperative hypotension
- Judicious continuation of β-blockers and other antiarrhythmic/chronotropic drugs for selected patients
- Pain control
- Prevention of polypharmacy and excessive testing

Preoperative Fluid Management

Almost all geriatric fracture patients will benefit from intravascular volume restoration. In addition to acute blood loss, fracture patients typically have little oral intake in the hours before fracture repair, are on chronic cardiovascular medications that promote hypotension and diuresis, and receive intravenous analgesic and anesthetic medications that result in vasodilation. This finding is true even in patients with known ventricular dysfunction, because adequate ventricular filling pressures are necessary to maintain cardiac output. The risks of intraoperative hypotension likely exceed the risks of excessive volume administration, in terms of clinical consequence and reversibility. For these reasons, liberal administration of isotonic intravenous fluids is necessary for the optimization of most patients and should be titrated with close clinical attention for pulmonary edema. Clinically significant acute congestive heart failure is not frequently reported in geriatric fracture centers, emphasizing preoperative hydration.[20]

Medication Management

Medications that promote hypotension (**Table 5**) should be withheld in the preoperative period, with an exception for chronic chronotropic medications, including β-blockers, and antihypertensives with known withdrawal consequence (eg, clonidine). In light of ongoing acute blood loss, and the reduction in blood pressure that results from most analgesics and anesthetics, most patients will not uniformly tolerate or benefit from continuation of chronic antihypertensive or afterload-reducing medications. Angiotensin-converting enzyme (ACE) inhibitors and receptor blockers have been associated with acute kidney injury in the perioperative setting,[30,31] and some advocate for routine cessation of ACE-I/angiotensin-receptor blockers in the preoperative period.[32,33] Although the long-term efficacy of ACE inhibition or blockade in managing chronic systolic cardiac dysfunction and diabetic nephropathy has been well established, use in the immediate perioperative period is likely complicated by impairment of renal compensatory mechanisms in the face of rapidly fluctuating intravascular volume status. Short-term cessation or dose attenuation in this setting is not known to cause harm and likely prevents acute kidney injury in some patients. When used for rate control for chronic stable tachyarrythmias, nondihydropyridine calcium channel blockers (eg, diltiazem or verapamil) may need to be continued in the perioperative setting, but these benefits need to be weighed against the risks of hypotension. Dihydropyridine calcium channel blockers (eg, amlodipine, felodipine) should be withheld if hypotension is anticipated or demonstrated. Loop diuretics are typically withheld in the immediate preoperative and postoperative period, until perioperative blood loss and intravascular volume have stabilized. Depending on their indications, antiplatelet and anticoagulant therapy are typically withheld and/or reversed in the preoperative period, to minimize blood loss. Condition-specific details for patients at high risk for thromboembolic disease (mechanical valve replacement, atrial thrombus) are considered elsewhere in this issue. Other noncardiac medications are also important to adjust and monitor in the

Table 5		
Common preoperative medication considerations		
Medications	**Clinical Considerations**	**Strategies**
Antihypertensives	May promote excessive hypotension in perioperative settings	Hold nonchronotropic medications until patient demonstrates a need postoperatively Continue home β-blockers, avoid hypotension
Diabetic agents	Risk for hypoglycemia with low enteral intake	Hold oral agents, reduce long-acting insulin doses, and closely monitor blood glucoses
Chronic opiate therapy	Increased tolerance may require higher opiate doses for pain control Sudden cessation may precipitate withdrawal	Monitoring for pain control, sedation, or withdrawal Consider nonpharmacologic adjunctive therapy (nerve blocks, rapid surgical fixation)
Antiplatelet and anticoagulant agents	Typically held until postoperative bleeding is controlled	

preoperative period, including chronic diabetic medications and chronic opiate and benzodiazepine therapy (see **Table 5**).

β-Blockers

Since the initial publication of data supporting the widespread use of β-blockers in the perioperative setting, several subsequent studies have suggested a more nuanced approach in patients undergoing noncardiac surgery, with many studies failing to confirm benefit.[34–36] The cardioprotective benefits of β-blockade contrast with the risks of hypotension in the acute perioperative setting, particularly in frail patients with such a physiologic tendency. There are no trials dedicated to studying the impact of β-blockers specifically, or postoperative blood pressure control in general, in patients older than 75 years. In the PeriOperative Ischemia Study Evaluation (POISE) trial,[37] the largest randomized trial of perioperative β-blockade, patients with age greater than 70 years, and those with hypotension had increased rates of stroke and death. In addition, there is a unique risk for exaggerated hypotension in the acutely bleeding hip fracture patient, and at least one retrospective analysis suggests that β-blocked patients do not tolerate surgical anemia as well as non-β-blocked patients.[38] Current ACC guidelines recommend continuing chronic β-blocker therapy in surgical patients, but also to avoid hypotension and bradycardia.[39] A recent meta-analysis[40] of secure randomized trials concluded that the risks of routine β-blockade outweighed any benefit in the general population, although this analysis was dominated by studies using relatively high doses of medications (≥100 mg metoprolol) in naive patients. Some geriatric fracture centers have reported low rates of cardiovascular complications using protocols that include low-dose β-blockade (≤25 mg metoprolol).[10]

Pain Control

Prompt and adequate pain control is an essential component of preoperative optimization and the prevention of complications.[41] Adequate preoperative pain control is associated with delirium prevention, reductions in myocardial stress and oxygen demand, and improved stability for surgical repair. The major components of expert pain control include the use of parenteral opiates and timely surgical repair and can be supplemented by local nerve blocks and other anesthetic techniques.

Laboratory Testing

Recommended preoperative laboratory testing for the typical geriatric hip fracture patient is limited to a small number of laboratory tests and essential radiographic studies (**Table 6**). Extensive testing is unlikely to benefit most patients and can

Table 6 Recommended preoperative tests for geriatric fracture patients	
Test	Indications
Complete blood count	Evaluate for anemia, provide baseline to quantify additional blood loss
Prothrombin time/International normalized ratio	For patients on warfarin therapy, or at risk for malnutrition, malabsorption, or liver disease
Electrolytes, renal function, albumin	Evaluate for acute and chronic kidney disease, malnutrition, acute electrolyte abnormalities (eg, hyponatremia, hypercalcemia)
Electrocardiogram	For patients with risk factors for atherosclerosis or cardiomyopathy or history of arrhythmia

promote complications by delaying optimization efforts, pain control, and surgical repair. Some commonly used preoperative tests (urinalysis, chest radiography) are of unclear clinical benefit and are unlikely to be beneficial for asymptomatic individuals.[42,43]

NONOPERATIVE MANAGEMENT

Compared with nonoperative management, surgical repair of hip fractures is associated with reduced mortality, improved functional status, and reduced complications.[44] Even for patients with limited life expectancy or patients with an inability to ambulate before fracture, surgical repair of hip fracture can offer improvements in pain control, edema, blood loss, and quality of life. For the small group of patients with excessive perioperative risk of mortality, nonoperative management can be considered, particularly if patients are likely to expire in the perioperative or immediate postoperative period, or if pharmacologic pain control is adequate during care needs.

Despite having higher short-term mortality rates, nonoperatively managed patients who survive 1 month seem to have 1-year mortality rates similar to those undergoing operative repair,[45,46] and a small minority can regain the ability to self-transfer and ambulate with assistive devices.[47]

Decisions for nonoperative management should reflect a confluence of the patient's goals of care, life expectancy, quality of life with pharmacologic pain control, and a realistic assessment of perioperative risk. Explicit discussions regarding end-of-life care and prognosis are typically warranted in these cases.

SUMMARY

Multiply comorbid geriatric fracture patients generally benefit from rapid optimization and surgical repair. Preoperative evaluation should be focused on exclusion of a small number of contraindications to acute surgical repair, and rapid optimization of intravascular volume status, pain control, and anticipation of hypotension. Extensive preoperative testing and consultation does not seem to be beneficial to most geriatric fracture patients and may be associated with surgical delay.

REFERENCES

1. Etzioni DA, Liu JH, Maggard MA, et al. The aging population and its impact on the surgery workforce. Ann Surg 2003;238:170–7.
2. Turrentine FE, Wand H, Simpson VB, et al. Surgical risk factors, morbidity and mortality in elderly patients. J Am Coll Surg 2006;203:865–77.
3. Cheng S, Yang T, Jeng K, et al. Perioperative care of the elderly. Int J Gerontol 2007;1(2):89–97.
4. Cicerchia M, Ceci M, Locatelli C, et al. Geriatric syndromes in peri-operative elderly cancer patients. Surg Oncol 2010;19(3):131–9.
5. McGory ML, Kao KK, Shekelle PG, et al. Developing quality indicators for elderly surgical patients. Ann Surg 2009;250:338–47.
6. Cheitlin MD. Cardiovascular physiology—changes with aging. Am J Geriatr Cardiol 2003;12(1):9–13.
7. Peterson DD, Pack AI, Silage DA, et al. Effects of aging on ventilatory and occlusion pressures responses to hypoxia and hypercapnia. Am Rev Respir Dis 1981; 124:387–91.
8. Weinstein JR, Anders S. The aging kidney: physiologic changes. Adv Chronic Kidney Dis 2010;17(4):302–7.

9. Alecu C, Cuignet-Royer E, Mertes PM, et al. Pre-existing arterial stiffness can predict hypotension during induction of anaesthesia in the elderly. Br J Anaesth 2010;105(5):585–8.

10. Friedman SM, Mendelson DA, Bingham KW, et al. Impact of a comanaged geriatric fracture center on short-term hip fracture outcomes. Arch Intern Med 2009; 169(18):1712–7.

11. Vidan M, Serra JA, Moreno C, et al. Efficacy of a comprehensive geriatric intervention in older patients hospitalized for hip fracture: a randomized, controlled trial. J Am Geriatr Soc 2005;53:1476–82.

12. Simunovic N, Devereaux PJ, Sprague S, et al. Effect of early surgery after hip fracture on mortality and complications: systematic review and meta-analysis. CMAJ 2010;182(15):1609–16.

13. Piolo G, Lauretani F, Davoli ML, et al. Older people with hip fracture and IADL disability require earlier surgery. J Gerontol A Biol Sci Med Sci 2012;67(11): 1272–7.

14. Liu LL, Dzankic S, Leung JM. Preoperative electrocardiogram abnormalities do not predict postoperative cardiac complications in geriatric surgical patients. J Am Geriatr Soc 2002;50(7):1186–91.

15. Kristjansson SR, Nesbakken A, Jordhoy MS, et al. Comprehensive geriatric assessment can predict complications in elderly patients after elective surgery for colorectal cancer: a prospective observational cohort study. Crit Rev Oncol Hematol 2010;76:208–17.

16. Penrod JD, Litke MA, Hawkes WG, et al. Heterogeneity in hip fracture patients: age, functional status, and comorbidity. J Am Geriatr Soc 2007;55(3):407–13.

17. Chow WB, Rosenthal RA, Merkow RP, et al. Optimal preoperative assessment of the geriatric patient: a best practices guideline from the American College of Surgeons National Surgical Quality Improvement Program and the American Geriatrics Society. J Am Coll Surg 2012;215(4):453–66.

18. Lee TH, Marcantonio ER, Mangione CM, et al. Derivation and prospective validation of a simple index for prediction of cardiac risk of major noncardiac surgery. Circulation 1999;100(10):1043–9.

19. Kristensen MT, Foss NB, Ekdahl C, et al. Prefracture functional level evaluated by the new mobility score predicts in-hospital outcome after hip fracture surgery. Acta Orthop 2010;81(3):296–302.

20. Ricci WM, Della Rocca GJ, Combs C, et al. The medical and economic impact of preoperative cardiac testing in elderly patients with hip fractures. Injury 2007; 38(Suppl 3):S49–52.

21. O'Heireamhoin S, Ahmed M, Mulhall KJ. The role of preoperative cardiac investigation in emergency hip surgery. J Trauma 2011;71(5):1345–7.

22. Friedman SM, Mendelson DA, Kates SL, et al. Geriatric co-management of proximal femur fractures. J Am Geriatr Soc 2008;56:1349–56.

23. Huddleston JM, Gullerud RE, Smither F, et al. Myocardial infarction after hip fracture repair: a population based study. J Am Geriatr Soc 2012;60:2020–6.

24. Seitz DP, Adunuri N, Gill SG, et al. Prevalence of dementia and cognitive impairment among older adults with hip fracture. J Am Med Dir Assoc 2011;12(8): 556–64.

25. Robinson TN, Raeburn CD, Tran ZV, et al. Postoperative delirium in the elderly: risk factors and outcomes. Ann Surg 2009;249(1):173–8.

26. Iavarone A, Milan G, Vargas G, et al. Role of functional performance in diagnosis of dementia in elderly people with low educational level living in southern Italy. Aging Clin Exp Res 2007;19(2):104–9.

27. Cromwell DA, Eagar K, Poulos RG. The performance of instrumental activity of daily living scale in screening for cognitive impairment in elderly community residents. J Clin Epidemiol 2003;56(2):131–7.
28. Lumbers M, New SA, Givson S, et al. Nutritional status in elderly female hip fracture patients: comparison with an age-match home living group attending day centers. Br J Nutr 2001;85:733–40.
29. Morley JE. Sarcopenia in the elderly. Fam Pract 2012;29(Suppl 1):i44–8.
30. Ishikawa S, Griesdale D, Lohser J. Acute kidney injury after lung resection surgery: incidence and perioperative risk factors. Anesth Analg 2012;114: 1256–62.
31. Cittanova ML, Zubicki A, Savu C, et al. The chronic inhibition of angiotensin-converting enzyme impairs post operative renal function. Anesth Analg 2001; 93:1111–5.
32. Arora P, Rajagopalam S, Ranjan R, et al. Preoperative use of angiotensin-converting enzyme inhibitors/angiotensive receptor blockers is associated with increased risk for acute kidney injury and cardiovascular surgery. Clin J Am Soc Nephrol 2008;3(5):1266–73.
33. Onuigbo MA. Reno-prevention vs. reno-protection: a critical re-appraisal of the evidence-base from the large RAAS blockade trials after ontarget—a call for more circumspection. QJM 2009;102(3):155–67.
34. Yang H, Raymer K, Butler R, et al. The effects of perioperative beta-blockade: results of the metoprolol after vascular surgery (MaVS) study, a randomized controlled trial. Am Heart J 2006;152(5):983–90.
35. Juul AB, Wetterslev J, Gluud C, et al. Effect of perioperative beta blockade in patients with diabetes undergoing major non-cardiac surgery: randomized placebo controlled, blinded multicentre trial. BMJ 2006;332(7556):1482.
36. Brady AR, Gibbs JS, Greenhalgh RM, et al. Perioperative beta-blockade (POBBLE) for patients undergoing infrarenal vascular surgery: results of a randomized double-blind controlled trial. J Vasc Surg 2005;41(4):602–9.
37. Devereaux PJ, Yang H, Yusef S, et al. Effects of extended-release metoprolol succinate in patients undergoing non-cardiac surgery (POISE trial): a randomized controlled trial. Lancet 2008;371(9627):1839–47.
38. Beattie WS, Wiieysundera DN, Karkouti K, et al. Acute surgical anemia influences the cardioprotective effects of β-blockade: a single-center, propensity-matched cohort study. Anesthesiology 2010;112(1):25–33.
39. Fleischmann KE, Beckman JA, Buller CE, et al. 2009 ACCF/AHA focused update on perioperative beta blockade: a report of the American College of Cardiology Foundation/American Heart Association Task Force on practice guidelines. Circulation 2009;120(21):2123–51.
40. Couri S, Shun-Shin MJ, Cole GD, et al. Meta-analysis of secure randomized controlled trials of β-blockade to prevent perioperative death in non-cardiac surgery. Heart 2014;100(6):456–64.
41. Morrison RS, Magaziner J, McLaughlin MA, et al. The impact of post-operative pain on outcomes following hip fracture. Pain 2003;103(3):303–11.
42. Mohammed T-LH, Kirsch J, Amorosa JK, et al. Routine admission and preoperative chest radiography. ACR Appropriateness Criteria. Reston, VA: American College of Radiology; 2011. Available at: http://www.acr.org/~/media/ACR/Documents/AppCriteria/Diagnostic/RoutineAdmissionAndPreoperativeChestRadiography.pdf. Accessed December 2, 2013.
43. Munro J, Booth A, Nicholl J. Routine preoperative testing: a systematic review of the evidence. Health Technol Assess 1997;1(12):1–62.

44. Jain R, Basinski J, Kreder H. Nonoperative treatment of hip fractures. Int Orthop 2003;27:11–7.
45. Hossain M, Neelapala V, Andrew JG. Results of non-operative treatment of hip fracture compared to surgical intervention. Injury 2009;40(4):418–21.
46. Ooi LH, Wong TH, Toh CL, et al. Hip fractures in nonagenerians—a study on operative and non-operative management. Injury 2005;36(1):142–7.
47. Gregory JJ, Kostakopoulou K, Cool WP, et al. One-year outcomes for elderly patients with displaced intracapsular fractures of the femoral neck managed non-operatively. Injury 2010;41(12):1273–6.

Preoperative Management of Anticoagulation and Antiplatelet Agents

Lauren Jan Gleason, MD[a],*, Susan M. Friedman, MD, MPH[b]

KEYWORDS

- Anticoagulation • Antiplatelet • Warfarin • Clopidogrel • Aspirin

KEY POINTS

- Given a higher frequency of comorbidities and frailty, older adults often take anticoagulants or antiplatelet agents, which present a challenge when optimizing patients for surgery.
- Actively managing reversal of anticoagulation may reduce time to surgery and complications.
- The approach to reversal of anticoagulation requires consideration of bleeding and clotting risk.

INTRODUCTION

Anticoagulants and antiplatelet agents present a unique challenge in the preoperative management of hip fractures. Assessment of bleeding risk is an important part of perioperative management. Delaying surgery to manage the effects of these medications can increase the likelihood of adverse events, such as delirium,[1] pneumonia, pressure ulceration, and mortality.[2,3] The urgency of surgery must be balanced against the increased risk of bleeding for patients on anticoagulation and antiplatelet agents.

Four variables must be considered when deciding how to manage periprocedural anticoagulation and antiplatelet agents with the goal of optimization for surgery (**Box 1**). The first is the risk of thromboembolism if the anticoagulation/antiplatelet agent is discontinued. The second is the risk of bleeding from the procedure if the anticoagulation/antiplatelet agent is continued. The third variable is the effectiveness and safety of interventions, such as receiving fresh frozen plasma or vitamin K (phytonadione). Lastly, an overriding principle is the importance of timing of surgery, because

Funding Sources: HRSA grant as support for Lauren Jan Gleason: Grant D01HP08794.
Conflict of Interest: None.
[a] Department of Internal Medicine, Beth Israel Deaconess Medical Center, LMOB 1B, 110 Francis Street, Boston, MA 02215, USA; [b] Department of Medicine, Highland Hospital, 1000 South Avenue, Box 58, Rochester, NY 14620, USA
* Corresponding author.
E-mail address: lgleason@bidmc.harvard.edu

Clin Geriatr Med 30 (2014) 219–227
http://dx.doi.org/10.1016/j.cger.2014.01.013
0749-0690/14/$ – see front matter © 2014 Elsevier Inc. All rights reserved.

Box 1
Issues to consider with reversal of anticoagulant or antiplatelet agent

1. Risk of thromboembolism if anticoagulation/antiplatelet is discontinued
2. Risk of bleeding from the procedure if anticoagulation/antiplatelet is continued
3. Effectiveness and safety of interventions to reverse anticoagulation
4. Timing of surgery

---

those on anticoagulants or antiplatelet agents often have a large number of comorbidities.

The assessment of perioperative bleeding risk in the context of anticoagulant and antiplatelet use should take into account the procedure planned for the patient. For example, percutaneous screw fixation has a much lower risk of bleeding than total hip arthroplasty.[4] The consequences of a major bleed in a patient with a total hip arthroplasty include hematoma, infection, and possibly joint removal.

ANTICOAGULANT MANAGEMENT

For patients who are admitted on anticoagulant medication, the steps in **Box 2** should be taken. The first 3 steps must be addressed preoperatively. The fourth step should be considered preoperatively, but is implemented postoperatively, and is therefore addressed in the article on Venous Thromboembolism and Postoperative Management of Anticoagulation elsewhere in this issue by Friedman and Uy.

Medications and Reason for Use

The first question to ask when a patient presents on anticoagulation is "why are is an anticoagulant being used?" Older adults are often anticoagulated for various medical conditions, including

- Atrial fibrillation (AF)
- Thromboembolic disease (venous thromboembolism, hypercoagulable states, deep vein thrombosis, pulmonary embolism)
- Prosthetic heart valves to prevent arterial or venous thrombosis

Warfarin is the most common and most studied anticoagulant used. However, 3 novel anticoagulants are being increasingly used in the older adult population: apixaban, a factor Xa inhibitor used to prevent strokes in patients with nonvalvular AF; dabigatran, a direct thrombin inhibitor approved for stroke prevention in nonvalvular AF; and rivaroxaban, a factor Xa inhibitor used for stroke prevention in patients with nonvalvular AF and for the prevention of thrombosis after total hip and knee replacement surgery.

Box 2
Anticoagulation management steps

1. Determine why the patient is taking an anticoagulation agent
2. Determine the short-term perioperative risk of thromboembolism related to the underlying condition if anticoagulation is stopped
3. Decide how to manage the patient in preparation for surgery and the timing of surgery
4. Decide whether to bridge

Risk Assessment of Stopping Anticoagulant

The second question to ask is "what is the short-term perioperative risk related to that underlying condition and to stopping the anticoagulation?" **Table 1** lists some common conditions treated with warfarin, and the embolism risk reduction conferred by the agent (both absolute and relative risk).

Nonvalvular AF is the most common reason for anticoagulant use in this population. The risk of embolism varies according to the "CHADS$_2$" score, with point scoring as follows:

- History of congestive heart failure: 1 point
- History of hypertension: 1 point
- Age 75 years or older: 1 point
- History of diabetes mellitus: 1 point
- History of stroke or transient ischemic attack: 2 points

Total scores range from 0 to 6, with a score of 0 conferring a risk of stroke of 1.9 and a score of 6 conferring risk of stroke of score of 18.2 per 100 patient-years in patients who are not anticoagulated.[5]

How to Manage Anticoagulation in Preparation for Surgery/Timing of Surgery

The next step is determining how to manage the anticoagulant in preparation for surgery. Several agents are available for reversal, and the use depends on the medication the patient is taking and the urgency of surgery. Most hip fracture surgery is considered urgent but not emergent, and therefore aiming to reverse anticoagulation within 24 to 48 hours is acceptable.

Vitamin K antagonist: warfarin

Warfarin acts as a vitamin K antagonist and prolongs the international normalized ratio (INR), which in turn makes blood coagulate more slowly and patients more prone to bleeding. To perform a surgical repair of hip fracture, the INR should be normalized to a level as safe as possible to reduce the risk of surgical bleeding. Most expert opinions recommend achieving an INR of 1.5 or less[13–15] before surgery. An elevated INR before surgery can increase the risk of bleeding and associated complications, such as neurologic dysfunction when a spinal or epidural catheter is inserted or removed,[16] hematoma, infection, and the possible need for joint removal.

Table 1
Embolism risk reduction with warfarin in several common conditions

Condition	Risk Without Warfarin	Risk with Warfarin	RRR
DVT: first 3 mo[6]	50.0%	4.0%–10.0%	80%–90%
Recurrent VTE, hypercoagulable states, cancer[7]	15.0%/y	3.0%/y	80%
CVA with cardiac source: first 2 wk[8]	12.0%	4.0%	66%
History of CVA and AF[9]	12.0%/y	4.0%/y	67%
Nonvalvular AF[10]	4.0%–5.0%/y	1.0%–2.0%/y	65%
Myocardial infarction Ejection fraction ≤28%[11]	1.5%/y 2.3%	N/A	81%
Mechanical valve[12]	4.0%/y	0.7%–1.0%	75%–82%

Abbreviations: CVA, cerebrovascular accident; DVT, deep venous thrombosis; N/A, not applicable; RRR, relative risk reduction; VTE, venous thromboembolism.

The options available to reverse warfarin include

- Administration of vitamin K
- Use of fresh frozen plasma
- Administration of recombinant factor VIIa or prothrombin complex concentrates
- Discontinuation of warfarin with a "watch and wait" approach

The watch and wait approach is a poor option. The older and more frail a person is, the longer it will take for the warfarin to be eliminated. The half-life of warfarin is approximately a day and a half but can be significantly longer. Reversal of warfarin-associated coagulopathy with a combination of vitamin K and fresh frozen plasma in patients who have sustained a hip fracture has been shown to be safe in 2 retrospective cohort studies.[17,18] **Fig. 1** shows one suggested algorithm for managing an elevated INR in patients on warfarin on admission who are safely able to be reversed.

Oral vitamin K has been shown to be more effective than subcutaneous dosing when lowering an elevated INR value.[19] Furthermore, a meta-analysis showed that oral and intravenous vitamin K have equivalent efficacies in reducing INR values over a 24-hour period in patients with an elevated INR, and there is no optimal dose of vitamin K to lower INR values.[20] The advantage of using oral vitamin K over intravenous vitamin K is that it avoids the risk of fatal anaphylaxis.[21] Subcutaneous and intramuscular vitamin K administration is associated with erratic absorption and should be avoided.

Fresh frozen plasma is an alternative and/or adjunct to vitamin K to correct coagulopathy.[9] It is human donor plasma that contains many plasma proteins, including all of

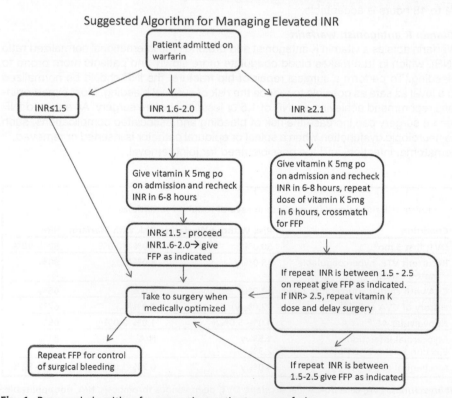

Fig. 1. Proposed algorithm for managing patients on warfarin.

the coagulation factors. One proposed formula to obtain an INR of less than 1.5 recommends

- 1 unit for an INR of 1.5 to 1.9
- 2 units for an INR of 2.0 to 3.0
- 3 units for an INR of 3.0 to 4.0
- 4 units for an INR of 4.0 to 8.0, and
- More than 4 units for an INR of greater than 8.0.[22]

Each unit of fresh frozen plasma has a volume of 190 to 240 mL. One of the challenges with fresh frozen plasma is that it only lasts approximately 6 hours, and risks include those associated with blood product transfusion (transfusion-related acute lung injury, infection) and that large volumes are often required, with the associated risk of congestive heart failure. Little evidence exists for the use of recombinant factor VIIa or prothrombin complex concentrates. Most of the studies with these products were observational in the setting of bleeding with supratherapeutic INRs. The possibility exists that they might provide an alternative to fresh frozen plasma, but more studies are necessary.[23]

There are 2 common concerns when reversing anticoagulation. The first is that a potential exists for aggressive reversal to cause increased risk of thromboembolism. The second concern is that after reversal, the patient may be warfarin-resistant and take a longer time to achieve a therapeutic level. Although it may take longer for patients to achieve a therapeutic level of warfarin after receiving reversal, this has not been shown to delay discharge.[24] Concerns about reversal should always be taken into account in the context of the clinical picture of the patient when reversing anticoagulation.

Novel Oral Anticoagulants: Dabigatran, Rivaroxaban, and Apixaban

Preoperative management of patients with AF receiving novel oral anticoagulation agents for thromboprophylaxis or stroke prevention is an important consideration for clinicians, given the increase in use of these agents.

The advantage of using these agents is their convenience, including a predictable pharmacologic profile and the lack of a need for routine monitoring, and their rapid onset of action. Nevertheless, these characteristics complicate management when surgery is needed, because the direct effect of the anticoagulant cannot be determined accurately. Therefore, determining safety for surgery can be challenging. Furthermore, no specific antidotes for reversal are currently available, limiting the ability to actively manage patients to expedite surgery, and potentially increasing the risk of preoperative blood loss.

Dabigatran

Dabigatran has an insensitive and nonlinear relationship to prothrombin time (PT) and activated partial thromboplastin time (aPTT). The aPTT may be clinically useful, because a normal aPTT is seen when the anticoagulant effect secondary to dabigatran is not present, but values often plateau at high concentrations and may underestimate supratherapeutic concentrations.[25,26] Other monitoring tests that are promising but not widely available include ecarin clotting time, hemoclot thrombin inhibitor, and thrombin clotting time. Documentation of a normal or near-normal aPTT or thrombin clotting time has been recommended to ensure that dabigatran has been adequately cleared from the circulation before surgery.

Most of dabigatran's excretion is renal (80%–85%). Given dabigatran's half-life, drug effects should decrease by approximately 50% at 12 to 18 hours after the most recent dose, and the trough levels should decrease to 25% of their previous steady state by 24 hours after stopping dabigatran in the setting of a normal creatinine clearance exceeding 50 mL/min. In moderately severe renal dysfunction (creatinine clearance of 30–50 mL/min), which is present in many older patients, the half-life is extended to approximately 18 to 28 hours. Dabigatran is potentially dialyzable. Elective procedures or surgeries with critically high bleeding are recommended to commence between 2 and 4 days after stopping the medication.[27] Currently, no guidelines or recommendations for emergent or urgent procedures exist, and the principles should be derived from elective surgeries. Additionally, because dabigatran is cleared renally, monitoring renal function and maintaining adequate hydration are important.

Rivaroxaban and apixaban

Similarly, no standard exists to monitor direct factor Xa inhibitors. Direct factor Xa inhibitors will prolong PT, INR, and aPTT in a linear, dose-dependent fashion, and these tests can be used as a qualitative assessment of exposure to direct factor Xa inhibitors.[28] However, significant interassay variability exists.

Rivaroxaban and apixaban have less renal clearance than dabigatran. These drugs have half-lives between 9 and 12 hours, which can be longer in the elderly. Rivaroxaban can affect PT values, and this can be monitored before surgery. Some evidence suggests that rivaroxaban can be reversed with prothrombin complex concentrate, but this is not widely available, and different formulations are in use. Like dabigatran, both of these medications can have a rapid onset of action, and therefore these patients should be treated with the same approach as those treated with dabigatran.

ANTITHROMBOTIC MANAGEMENT
Aspirin

Aspirin has an antiplatelet effect because it inhibits the production of thromboxane, which binds platelet molecules together to create a patch over damaged walls of blood vessels. Aspirin is often prescribed to help prevent myocardial infarction, cerebrovascular accidents, and blood clots. The 2012 guidelines from the American College of Chest Physicians (ACCP) recommend continuing aspirin around the time of surgery for patients at moderate to high risk for cardiovascular events who are undergoing noncardiac surgery.[29] As with other agents mentioned in this article, the decision to continue or withhold aspirin should reflect a balance of the consequences of perioperative hemorrhage versus the risk of perioperative vascular complications.

Antiplatelet Agents

The approach to managing patients admitted on antiplatelets is similar to that for patients taking anticoagulants, and is outlined in **Box 3**.

Determine reason for antiplatelet use

Antiplatelet agents include clopidogrel, prasugrel, ticagrelor, and ticlopidine. Indications for these medications include treatment of symptomatic atherosclerosis in

---

Box 3
Antiplatelet management steps

1. Determine why the patient is taking an antiplatelet agent
2. Determine the short-term perioperative risk associated with stopping the antiplatelet agent
3. Decide how to manage the patient in preparation for surgery and the timing of surgery

patients with acute coronary syndrome without ST segment elevation; ST elevation myocardial infarction; cerebrovascular disease; and peripheral vascular disease. The use of these agents has increased with the increase in drug-eluting coronary artery stenting procedures.

These agents work to block adenosine diphosphate receptors of subtype P2Y12 and prevent the activation of platelets and eventual cross-linking by the protein fibrin, thus preventing platelet aggregation and clot formation. Platelet inhibition can be demonstrated 2 hours after a single dose of oral clopidogrel, and the effect lasts for 5 to 9 days, which is the entire lifespan of the platelets. Less platelet aggregation may increase the risk of serious bleeding in patients undergoing surgery.

Risk assessment of stopping antiplatelet agents

The most common agent used is clopidogrel. The risk of coronary artery stent thrombosis after the premature cessation of clopidogrel is low, but stent thrombosis may be catastrophic. The ACCP recommends that for those who have undergone placement of a bare metal stent within the past 6 weeks or a drug-eluting stent in the past 6 months, both aspirin and clopidogrel should be continued perioperatively (class 2C).[29] Elective surgery should be postponed whenever possible until the minimum period of therapy with P2Y12 receptor blocker therapy is completed.

Management for surgery

Clopidogrel is different from warfarin (but similar to the newer anticoagulant agents) because no physiologic method of reversing the antithrombotic effect of this medication is known. In cases of elective surgery, clopidogrel can be discontinued well before the planned surgery, often a week before the procedure, to allow platelets to form a plug for optimal blood clotting. But in emergent or other urgent cases, such as hip fractures, the risk of increased bleeding must be carefully weighed against the benefits of the surgery.

The management of clopidogrel in patients with an acute hip fracture is often debated. One retrospective review of 21 patients showed that it was safe to operate without delay on those taking clopidogrel.[30] Another study concluded that these patients often have more comorbidities but are not at increased risk of complications such as bleeding or mortality during hip fracture repair surgery.[31] Yet another study showed that delays related to antiplatelet agents led to a higher mortality after hip fracture repair.[32]

The current challenge is to determine whether the increased risk of bleeding caused by immediate surgery is worth the risk of increased morbidity and mortality resulting from a delay of 7 to 9 days. A survey of directors of academic orthopedic programs showed a consensus for waiting 3 days or less for urgent but nonemergent surgical interventions, such as hip fractures, in patients on clopidogrel, with 23% believing that no delay was necessary. For emergent surgery, 89% believed that no delay to the operating room was indicated.[33] Recent level 2 evidence shows that patients undergoing early hip fracture surgery who are taking clopidogrel are not at a substantially increased risk for bleeding, bleeding complications, or mortality.[31] Because of the risk of bleeding, spinal anesthesia is often contraindicated in those on clopidogrel.

Additionally, no known guidelines exist for the role of platelet transfusions. Based on the reviewed physiology, one can argue that a perioperative platelet transfusion may be of some benefit, because the transfused platelets would be effective in forming a viable plug. However, the authors are unaware of any studies evaluating the effectiveness of platelet transfusion. Platelet transfusions are not standard of care and should be reserved for patients who would be expected to have bleeding problems before surgery or those who have extensive bleeding after surgery.

SUMMARY

Many patients who have sustained fragility fractures are at high risk for morbidity and mortality because of the presence of multiple comorbidities. Preoperative antithrombotic management is based on risk assessment for thromboembolic events and bleeding. Expediting time to surgery is an important goal, and therefore waiting for the INR to drift down in patients on warfarin is a poor option. Active management is less feasible in patients who are taking newer anticoagulants or antiplatelet agents. In these patients, careful monitoring and balancing of risks of thrombosis and bleeding are essential components of preoperative management.

REFERENCES

1. Juliebo V, Bjoro K, Krogseth M, et al. Risk factors for preoperative and postoperative delirium in elderly patients with hip fracture. J Am Geriatr Soc 2009;57: 1354–61.
2. Khan SK, Kalra S, Khanna A, et al. Timing of surgery for hip fractures: a systematic review of 52 published studies involving 291,413 patients. Injury 2009;40:692–7.
3. Zuckerman JD, Skovron ML, Koval KJ, et al. Postoperative complications and mortality associated with operative delay in older patients who have a fracture of the hip. J Bone Joint Surg Am 1995;77:1551–6.
4. Marsland D, Colvin PL, Mears SC, et al. How to optimize patients for geriatric fracture surgery. Osteoporos Int 2010;21:S535–46.
5. Gage BF, Waterman AD, Shannon W, et al. Validation of clinical classification schemes for predicting stroke: results from the National Registry of Atrial Fibrillation. JAMA 2001;285:2864–70.
6. Hull RD, Carter CJ, Jay RM, et al. The diagnosis of acute, recurrent, deep-vein thrombosis: a diagnostic challenge. Circulation 1983;67:901–6.
7. Levine MN, Hirsh J, Gent M, et al. Optimal duration of oral anticoagulant therapy: a randomized trial comparing four weeks with three months of warfarin in patients with proximal deep vein thrombosis. Thromb Haemost 1995;74:606–11.
8. Cardiogenic brain embolism. Cerebral Embolism Task Force. Arch Neurol 1986; 43:71–84.
9. Schulman S. Clinical practice. Care of patients receiving long-term anticoagulant therapy. N Engl J Med 2003;349:675–83.
10. Singer DE, Albers GW, Dalen JE, et al. Antithrombotic therapy in atrial fibrillation: the Seventh ACCP Conference on Antithrombotic and Thrombolytic Therapy. Chest 2004;126:429S–56S.
11. Loh E, Sutton MS, Wun CC, et al. Ventricular dysfunction and the risk of stroke after myocardial infarction. N Engl J Med 1997;336:251–7.
12. Whitlock RP, Sun JC, Fremes SE, et al. Antithrombotic and thrombolytic therapy for valvular disease: Antithrombotic Therapy and Prevention of Thrombosis, 9th ed: American College of Chest Physicians Evidence-Based Clinical Practice Guidelines. Chest 2012;141:e576S–600S.
13. Al-Rashid M, Parker MJ. Anticoagulation management in hip fracture patients on warfarin. Injury 2005;36:1311–5.
14. Kearon C, Hirsh J. Management of anticoagulation before and after elective surgery. N Engl J Med 1997;336:1506–11.
15. Jaffer AK, Brotman DJ, Chukwumerije N. When patients on warfarin need surgery. Cleve Clin J Med 2003;70:973–84.
16. Horlocker TT, Wedel DJ, Benzon H, et al. Regional anesthesia in the anticoagulated patient: defining the risks (the second ASRA Consensus Conference on

Neuraxial Anesthesia and Anticoagulation). Reg Anesth Pain Med 2003;28: 172–97.

17. Vitale MA, VanBeek C, Spivack JH, et al. Pharmacologic reversal of warfarin-associated coagulopathy in geriatric patients with hip fractures: a retrospective study of thromboembolic events, postoperative complications, and time to surgery. Geriatr Orthop Surg Rehabil 2011;2:128–34.

18. Gleason LJ, Mendelson DA, Kates SL, et al. Anticoagulation management in hip fracture patients. JAGS 2014;62(1):159–64.

19. Crowther MA, Douketis JD, Schnurr T, et al. Oral vitamin K lowers the international normalized ratio more rapidly than subcutaneous vitamin K in the treatment of warfarin-associated coagulopathy. A randomized, controlled trial. Ann Intern Med 2002;137:251–4.

20. Dezee KJ, Shimeall WT, Douglas KM, et al. Treatment of excessive anticoagulation with phytonadione (vitamin K): a meta-analysis. Arch Intern Med 2006;166: 391–7.

21. Fiore LD, Scola MA, Cantillon CE, et al. Anaphylactoid reactions to vitamin K. J Thromb Thrombolysis 2001;11:175–83.

22. Fakheri RJ. Formula for fresh frozen plasma dosing for warfarin reversal. Mayo Clin Proc 2013;88:640.

23. Leissinger CA, Blatt PM, Hoots WK, et al. Role of prothrombin complex concentrates in reversing warfarin anticoagulation: a review of the literature. Am J Hematol 2008;83:137–43.

24. Tharmarajah P, Pusey J, Keeling D, et al. Efficacy of warfarin reversal in orthopedic trauma surgery patients. J Orthop Trauma 2007;21:26–30.

25. Schulman S, Majeed A. The oral thrombin inhibitor dabigatran: strengths and weaknesses. Semin Thromb Hemost 2012;38:7–15.

26. Douxfils J, Mullier F, Robert S, et al. Impact of dabigatran on a large panel of routine or specific coagulation assays. Laboratory recommendations for monitoring of dabigatran etexilate. Thromb Haemost 2012;107:985–97.

27. Ageno W, Gallus AS, Wittkowsky A, et al. Oral anticoagulant therapy: Antithrombotic Therapy and Prevention of Thrombosis, 9th ed: American College of Chest Physicians Evidence-Based Clinical Practice Guidelines. Chest 2012;141:e44S–88S.

28. King CS, Holley AB, Moores LK. Moving toward a more ideal anticoagulant: the oral direct thrombin and factor Xa inhibitors. Chest 2013;143:1106–16.

29. Douketis JD, Spyropoulos AC, Spencer FA, et al. Perioperative management of antithrombotic therapy: Antithrombotic Therapy and Prevention of Thrombosis, 9th ed: American College of Chest Physicians Evidence-Based Clinical Practice Guidelines. Chest 2012;141:e326S–50S.

30. Sim W, Gonski PN. The management of patients with hip fractures who are taking clopidogrel. Aust J Ageing 2009;28:194–7.

31. Collinge CA, Kelly KC, Little B, et al. The effects of clopidogrel (Plavix) and other oral anticoagulants on early hip fracture surgery. J Orthop Trauma 2012;26: 568–73.

32. Harty JA, McKenna P, Moloney D, et al. Anti-platelet agents and surgical delay in elderly patients with hip fractures. J Orthop Surg (Hong Kong) 2007;15:270–2.

33. Lavelle WF, Demers Lavelle EA, Uhl R. Operative delay for orthopedic patients on clopidogrel (plavix): a complete lack of consensus. J Trauma 2008;64:996–1000.

Classification and Surgical Approaches to Hip Fractures for Nonsurgeons

Simon C. Mears, MD, PhD*

KEYWORDS

- Femoral neck fracture • Intertrochanteric hip fracture • Surgery
- Patient activity level • Fracture type

KEY POINTS

- Knowledge of hip fractures and surgical repair helps nonsurgeons develop communication with surgeons, leading to improved outcomes for elderly patients.
- Nondisplaced femoral neck fractures are treated with screw fixation, whereas displaced fractures are treated with hip replacement.
- Lower activity patients with femoral neck fractures are treated with hemiarthroplasty, whereas high activity patients have better outcomes with total hip replacement.
- Stable intertrochanteric fractures are treated with a sliding hip screw, whereas unstable fractures are treated with intramedullary hip screws.
- Subtrochanteric fractures may have typical or atypical patterns (associated with bisphosphonate use), are more difficult to reduce surgically, and are treated with an intramedullary hip screw.
- The goal of all hip fracture fixation is to allow the patient to bear weight as tolerated after surgery.

INTRODUCTION

The elderly population commonly experiences hip fractures. The care of these fractures before, during, and after the related surgery often involves many different physicians. An appreciation of the types of fractures and the surgical repair may help the nonsurgical physician build rapport with the surgeon, thus promoting better communication, which has been shown to be the crux of multidisciplinary efforts for patient care.[1,2] These team efforts have produced better results for the patient and cost savings for the health care system.[1,2]

The author has no commercial associations or sources of support that might pose a conflict of interest.
Department of Orthopaedic Surgery, The Johns Hopkins University/Johns Hopkins Bayview Medical Center, 4940 Eastern Avenue, Baltimore, MD 21224–2780, USA
* c/o Elaine P. Henze, BJ, ELS, Medical Editor and Director, Editorial Services, Department of Orthopaedic Surgery, The Johns Hopkins University/Johns Hopkins Bayview Medical Center, 4940 Eastern Avenue, #A665, Baltimore, MD 21224–2780.
E-mail address: ehenze1@jhmi.edu

Clin Geriatr Med 30 (2014) 229–241
http://dx.doi.org/10.1016/j.cger.2014.01.004
0749-0690/14/$ – see front matter © 2014 Elsevier Inc. All rights reserved.

In this review, the common types of hip fractures seen in the elderly are described, and the type of procedure used for the surgical repair of each is discussed.

ANATOMY AND FRACTURE RISK

Hip fractures typically occur as a result of a fall from standing height in a patient with osteoporosis. The elderly patient often has poor balance because of frailty and poor vision, hearing, and muscle strength. Elderly patients often have osteoporosis, resulting in less bone density. These conditions often overlap, leaving a patient with osteoporosis who is more likely to fall, with a higher risk of fracture. Individual long bones typically respond to loss in bone mass by becoming wider and thinner. The wider tube gives strength but makes the bone brittle and susceptible to fracture. For example, the proximal femur loses bone density and cortical thickness, becoming tube-shaped, with very narrow side walls.[3]

The hip joint is the articulation of the proximal femur and the acetabulum of the pelvis. The proximal femur is divided into several anatomic zones, which are used to describe fracture type, including the femoral head, the femoral neck, the intertrochanteric area, and the shaft of the femur. The proximal femur is the location of several muscle insertions that are critical to lower extremity function. The hip abductors (the gluteus medius and minimus) insert into the greater trochanter. The main hip flexor (the psoas) inserts into the lesser trochanter. The hip joint is surrounded by a thick ligamentous capsule. The capsule goes from the base of the neck to the pelvis and seals the joint. The femoral head and neck are intracapsular, whereas the trochanters are extracapsular (**Fig. 1**A).

FRACTURE TYPES

There are 3 main types of fractures in the elderly, categorized according to the anatomic position of the fracture line (**Fig. 1**B):

- Femoral neck fractures
- Intertrochanteric fractures
- Subtrochanteric fractures

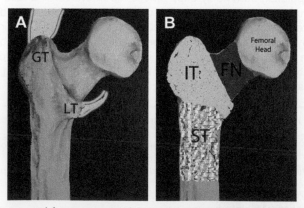

Fig. 1. Hip anatomy and fracture types. (*A*) The hip joint is pictured with the insertions of the gluteus medius and psoas muscles. GT, greater trochanter; LT, lesser trochanter. (*B*) Regions are shown identifying the areas in which femoral neck (FN), intertrochanteric (IT), and subtrochanteric (ST) fractures occur.

Each of these locations can have fracture patterns with more or less displacement or more or less fracture fragmentation. By using the fracture location and fracture pattern, and taking into account patient factors such as dementia and mobility status, the best treatment method can be determined.

- The goal of surgical treatment is to allow the patient to begin immediate full weight bearing and mobilization.

Nonoperative treatment is reserved for those at the end of life or who, secondary to severe dementia, do not have pain with their fracture (see the article elsewhere in this issue for further discussion of nonsurgical management). For most others, surgical repair offers reduced pain and return to function, with less morbidity and mortality than nonoperative treatment.

Femoral Neck Fractures

Femoral neck fractures are intracapsular and account for approximately 45% of fractures.[4,5] Decision making for these fractures is based not only on fracture type but also on the patient's activity level and frailness. In general, the decision has to be made whether to stabilize the fracture or to replace the hip. Each choice has different modality options.

Femoral neck fractures are most commonly classified using the Garden system.[6] This system takes into account the location, direction, and displacement of the fracture. Fractures that are more horizontal have more innate stability: the axial load of body weight pushes a horizontal fracture together, whereas it leads to fracture displacement for a vertical pattern. The more vertical and displaced a fracture is, the more unstable is the fracture pattern. Stage I fractures are minimally or nondisplaced, stage II fractures are very horizontal and impacted, and stage III and IV fractures are severely displaced, and the head does not line up with the remainder of the femur. In general, Garden stage I and II fractures are stable and Garden stage III and IV fractures are unstable; this definition is termed the simplified Garden system (**Fig. 2**).[7] The radiographs of Garden stage I and II fractures must be carefully examined to make sure that the femoral head is not tilted or displaced. Angulation of the femoral head, especially with weakening of the posterior cortex, makes the fracture more unstable, and screw fixation often fails.[8] An important factor in addition to stability is the

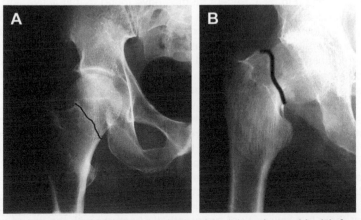

Fig. 2. Anteroposterior radiographs showing stable (*A*) and unstable (*B*) femoral neck fractures.

anatomic position of the blood supply to the femoral head. The medial femoral circumflex artery runs along the posterior side of the femoral neck.[9] Displaced fractures can interrupt the blood supply, which can lead to death of the bone in the femoral head. This condition is termed osteonecrosis, and it leads to collapse of the femoral head and arthritis, with a subsequent need for hip replacement.

The decision-making process for determining the best surgical procedure uses both the fracture type and the patient's activity level to choose between internal fixation and arthroplasty.

Internal fixation is usually performed for stable fracture patterns in the following manner under fluoroscopic guidance. The fracture is aligned by placing traction on the leg and checking biplanar fluoroscopic views. A small incision is made, and 3 guide wires are placed across the fracture. When these guide wires are correctly positioned, cannulated screws are placed across the fracture into the femoral head (**Fig. 3**A) over the top of the guide wires. Washers can increase the compressive force developed by the screws.

Arthroplasty (or joint replacement) should be the workhorse for displaced femoral neck fractures. It is reliable and leads to fewer subsequent procedures than does internal fixation, as has been shown by several long-term randomized studies.[10–14] However, within the general category of arthroplasty, there are still several decisions to be made: the arthroplasty may be partial or total and may be attached to the bone using different methods.

With a partial hip replacement (hemiarthroplasty), the femoral head is removed, and a metal replacement is inserted into the femur with or without bone cement. This replacement has a metal ball that articulates against the native acetabular cartilage (**Fig. 3**B). Current replacements have a modular head that attaches to the stem to allow for adjustment of length during surgery, which permits the surgeon to gain the correct muscle tension and leg length. Hemiarthroplasty may involve a unipolar device (1 solid head ball) or a bipolar device, in which a secondary cap is placed over a smaller head ball on the trunnion. No overall differences have been noted between these types of devices.[15] Hemiarthroplasty is a successful procedure but may lead to wear of the articular cartilage or subsequent pain.

With a total hip replacement, the acetabular cartilage is removed with a reamer and a metal acetabular component is impacted into the acetabulum. Inside the metal acetabular component, a liner is placed, which is usually made of highly cross-linked polyethylene (**Fig. 3**C). Recent studies have found that in active and younger patients, total hip arthroplasty results in less pain and better outcomes than hemiarthroplasty.[16,17] However, total hip arthroplasty has a higher risk of dislocation than partial replacement because the latter uses a larger head.[18]

Initially, replacement was performed in patients whose hip fractures had been repaired but whose uncemented devices were working poorly. A widely used historical device was called the Austin Moore replacement. These implants had no ingrowth surfaces and were wedged into the femur with little or no fixation. Overall, results were poor.[19] Current uncemented femoral implants come in many sizes, are shaped to wedge into the proximal femur, and are coated with surfaces to allow permanent bone ingrowth. For cemented implants, the device is smooth, and after it is inserted, the femur is filled with polymethylmethacrylate cement, which acts as a grout, filling in all the spaces between the bone and the implant. Results with both types of implants are excellent.[20] However, uncemented stems must be wedged into the bone and present a slightly higher risk of fractures during or after insertion.[21–24] Recent studies have shown that there is a lower risk of periprosthetic fractures with the use of cemented stems in elderly patients.[21–24]

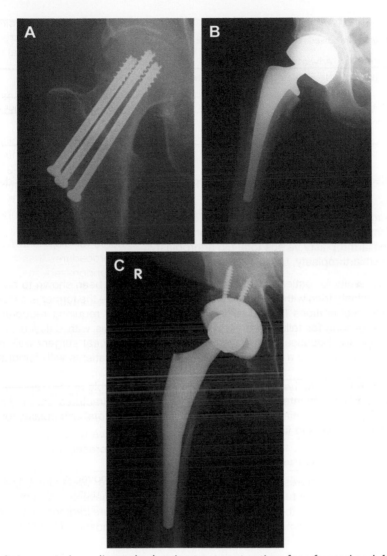

Fig. 3. Anteroposterior radiographs showing treatment options for a femoral neck fracture. (*A*) Cannulated screws. (*B*) Hemiarthroplasty. (*C*) Total hip arthroplasty.

The hip replacement may be implanted using different surgical approaches. Commonly used approaches include the posterolateral, the anterolateral, and the anterior approaches. There is no overall consensus as to the best approach for hip replacement. Each approach has a different risk and benefit profile. The posterolateral approach has a slightly higher rate of dislocation, whereas the anterolateral approach results in a slightly higher rate of limp, because of damage to the hip abductor muscles.[25–27] More recently, the anterior approaches have become more popular. The most important factor in determining approach is the experience of the surgeon. Patients with a very high dislocation risk (ie, those with contracture or neurologic disorders) may have lower dislocation rates with anterior or anterolateral approaches (**Table 1**).

Table 1
Advantages and disadvantages of the 3 surgical approaches to arthroplasty

Approach	Advantage	Disadvantage
Posterolateral	No abductor damage (low limp) Extensile	Higher dislocation risk
Anterolateral	Low dislocation risk	Possible abductor damage (higher limp)
Anterior	Low dislocation risk Low limp risk	More difficult Requires fluoroscopy

The decision-making process when selecting an arthroplasty involves consideration of:

- Surgical approach
- Cemented versus uncemented femoral component
- Hemiarthroplasty versus total hip arthroplasty
- If hemiarthroplasty, unipolar versus bipolar

Overall results for patients with displaced fractures have been shown to be better with arthroplasty than with internal fixation, primarily because the former is associated with fewer reoperations (approximately a 40% chance of requiring reoperation[13]). Common reasons for failure are nonunion or osteonecrosis with delayed need for hip arthroplasty. Because older patients do not tolerate repeat surgery well, arthroplasty is believed to be a better option for most geriatric patients with femoral neck fracture.

This finding leads to 1 common algorithm for surgery: stable or nondisplaced fractures are treated with internal fixation, whereas displaced fractures are treated with arthroplasty, that is, hemiarthroplasty for most patients and total arthroplasty for those who are very active and functional (**Fig. 4**).[28]

Intertrochanteric Fractures

Intertrochanteric fractures are extracapsular and account for approximately 45% of fractures.[4,5] These fractures have been classified using several different systems based on the position of the fracture and the amount of fracture fragmentation (comminution). The most common system used is the AO Foundation (AO)/Orthopaedic

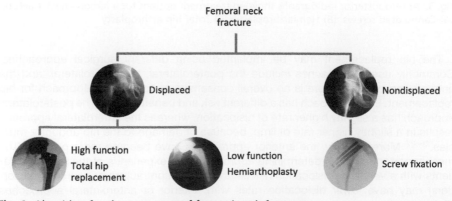

Fig. 4. Algorithm for the treatment of femoral neck fractures.

Trauma Association (OTA) system.[29] This system uses both comminution and fracture position. Overall, fractures can be divided into those that are more stable and those that are less stable. This type of classification then can drive treatment algorithms. In general, fractures with an intact lateral wall and calcar are stable (AO/OTA 31-A1.1, A1.2, A1.3, and A2.1), whereas fractures with more comminution and an unstable lateral wall are unstable (AO/OTA 31-A2.2, A2.3, A3.1, A3.2, and A3.3) (**Fig. 5**).

Fracture Stability
Stable
- Intact lateral buttress
- Few pieces (no comminution)

Unstable
- Lateral buttress is fractured
- Many pieces (comminution)
- Reverse oblique pattern
- Subtrochanteric fractures

Two main surgical procedures are used for these fractures. One is called the sliding hip screw (SHS) with side plate. With this procedure, the fracture is reduced under fluoroscopy with traction, and then a guide wire is inserted across the fracture into the center of the femoral head. The screw is placed over the guide wire, and the plate is attached to the side of the femur. The screw is thus able to slide within the barrel of the plate, which permits fracture compression, aiding in fracture fixation (**Fig. 6A**). This device has been widely adopted and is successful.[30]

The SHS is successful for fractures that have a solid buttress against which the femoral headpiece can slide. However, some fracture patterns lack this stability. One particularly unstable pattern is called the reverse oblique pattern. In this pattern, the plate does not provide a stop point for sliding, and failure rates are higher.[31] In this case, all of the pressure of walking is placed on the interface of the plate with the bone, which fails with time (**Fig. 6B**). Sometimes, fracture stability can be difficult to determine or can change intraoperatively. It is important that the lateral wall is intact for the SHS to work well.[32,33]

The other type of device used for intertrochanteric fractures is the intramedullary hip screw (IMHS). With this device, the fixation on the shaft side of the fracture is placed within the bone. First, the fracture is reduced, and then, an intramedullary nail is placed

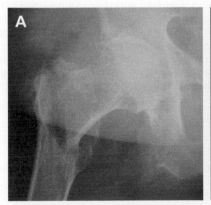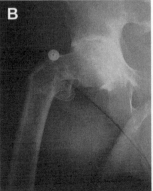

Fig. 5. Anteroposterior radiographs showing stable (*A*) and unstable (*B*) intertrochanteric fractures.

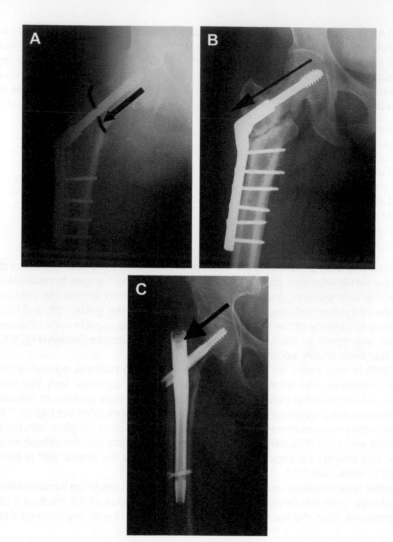

Fig. 6. Anteroposterior radiographs showing treatment options and biomechanics for intertrochanteric fractures. (*A*) SHS in a stable fracture. The arrow shows the vector of force during standing. With the lateral cortex intact, the fracture can stably impact as the screw slides within the barrel of the plate. (*B*) SHS in an unstable fracture. In this reverse oblique pattern, the plate cannot resist the sliding force in the direction of the arrow, and the device fails before fracture healing. (*C*) IMHS in an unstable fracture. The fracture impacts along the path indicated by the arrow, and the nail itself acts as a limitation to the sliding of the screw.

within the femur. It is typically inserted by making a hole in the greater trochanter. After the nail is placed in the bone, the hip screw is then placed through a hole in the nail. In general, more unstable fractures are probably best treated with an intramedullary device. The nail of the device acts as a stop point for the sliding of the screw (**Fig. 6**C).

Controversy exists as to which fracture should be treated with which device.[30] Overall, the SHS has been successful and is less expensive than the IMHS. Despite these findings, the rate of usage of the IMHS has steadily increased over the past 10 years.[34]

Some of this increase is the result of changes in design features of the IMHS. Initial designs had a propensity toward fracture at the distal end of the device.[35,36] This problem has largely been solved. Some surgeons use the IMHS for all intertrochanteric fractures, which permits less inventory in the operating room. It also protects the surgeon if the fracture pattern has been misjudged. Sometimes, it is possible to miss fracture lines that make the fracture more unstable than was initially appreciated.[37]

The rates of success for the SHS and IMHS have been shown to be related to the positioning of the hip screw within the femoral head.[38] The screw needs good purchase within the bone of the femoral head. If it does not gain purchase, the screw migrates and cuts out into the acetabulum. Then, the construct must be revised to a total hip replacement, which is a complex procedure. The screw should be centrally and deeply placed in the femoral head. A useful marker for this location is called the tip-apex distance. The distance between the end of the screw and the tip of the femoral head is measured on anteroposterior and lateral views of the hip. These measurements are added. A long measurement gives poorer fixation. For example, if the distance is greater than 24 mm, the rate of failure of the fracture to heal is significantly higher.[39] In another study, in which surgeons consciously measured this distance and made sure it was less than 24 mm, outcomes were significantly better.[40] The tip-apex distance is also believed to be important for the IMHS.[41]

Other treatments are rarely used for intertrochanteric fractures. Arthroplasty can be considered, but it is technically difficult. Although a femoral neck fracture leads to an easy hip replacement, the location of the intertrochanteric fracture is further down the femur and involves the greater and lesser trochanters, which means that there is less bone in which to insert the femoral component and may mean that a revision style implant must be used. The trochanter may also have to be repaired and anchored to the remainder of the femur. Overall, these factors make arthroplasty for intertrochanteric fractures more difficult than when it is used for a femoral neck fracture. However, there are times when arthroplasty may be the best solution for an intertrochanteric fracture. One such situation is the presence of preexisting arthritis in the hip joint. The replacement then repairs the fracture and solves the problem of the arthritic joint rather than staging a repair and subsequently replacing the hip.

Subtrochanteric Fractures

Subtrochanteric fractures are the least common type, accounting for approximately 10% of fractures,[5,42] and are located below the lesser trochanter, in the top part of the femoral shaft. These fractures can be difficult to treat, because the psoas muscle pulls on the lesser trochanter, which flexes the proximal piece of bone. Reduction can be difficult, and these fractures may need to be further surgically exposed to reduce the fracture fragments. They are treated with IMHS.

Fractures may be classified as typical or atypical. Typical fractures result from falls. Atypical fractures have now become widely recognized and are associated with bisphosphonate use.[43] They begin as a stress fracture, usually on the lateral wall of the femur in the subtrochanteric or midshaft region. The bone thickens as a result of poor turnover. A stress fracture develops and is seen as a black line in the thickened area of femur (Fig. 7). The stress fracture is susceptible to full fracture with minimal force. If a stress fracture is seen and is painful, careful consideration should be given to prophylactic treatment with an IMHS to prevent full fracture.[44] Nonoperative treatment often leads to complete fracture. In general, treatment with IMHS is successful, although healing may take longer.[45]

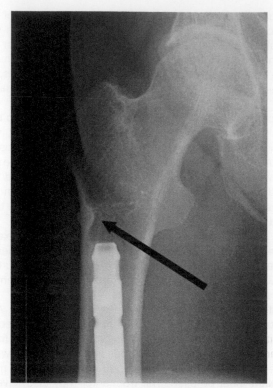

Fig. 7. Anteroposterior radiograph showing an atypical subtrochanteric fracture. The arrow points to the area of bone hypertrophy on the lateral cortex.

SUMMARY

Some appreciation for the types of hip fracture and treatment mechanisms is useful to the nonsurgeon. Surgeons treat fractures by the type of fracture and patient. Femoral neck fractures are treated with internal fixation or arthroplasty, depending on the stability of the fracture. Unstable fractures are best treated with arthroplasty; if the patient is very active, treatment should be a total hip replacement. Intertrochanteric fractures are treated with SHS or IMHS, depending on the stability of the fracture. Unstable intertrochanteric fractures and all subtrochanteric fractures should be treated with IMHS.

REFERENCES

1. Friedman SM, Mendelson DA, Kates SL, et al. Geriatric co-management of proximal femur fractures: total quality management and protocol-driven care result in better outcomes for a frail patient population. J Am Geriatr Soc 2008;56(7): 1349–56.
2. Kates SL, Mendelson DA, Friedman SM. Co-managed care for fragility hip fractures (Rochester model). Osteoporos Int 2010;21(Suppl 4):S621–5.
3. Dorr LD, Faugere MC, Mackel AM, et al. Structural and cellular assessment of bone quality of proximal femur. Bone 1993;14(3):231–42.
4. Lofman O, Berglund K, Larsson L, et al. Changes in hip fracture epidemiology: redistribution between ages, genders and fracture types. Osteoporos Int 2002; 13(1):18–25.

5. Zuckerman JD. Hip fracture. N Engl J Med 1996;334(23):1519–25.
6. Garden RS. Low-angle fixation in fractures of the femoral neck. J Bone Joint Surg Br 1961;43(4):647–63.
7. Van Embden D, Rhemrev SJ, Genelin F, et al. The reliability of a simplified Garden classification for intracapsular hip fractures. Orthop Traumatol Surg Res 2012; 98(4):405–8.
8. Clement ND, Green K, Murray N, et al. Undisplaced intracapsular hip fractures in the elderly: predicting fixation failure and mortality. A prospective study of 162 patients. J Orthop Sci 2013;18(4):578–85.
9. Gautier E, Ganz K, Krugel N, et al. Anatomy of the medial femoral circumflex artery and its surgical implications. J Bone Joint Surg Br 2000;82(5):679–83.
10. Avery PP, Baker RP, Walton MJ, et al. Total hip replacement and hemiarthroplasty in mobile, independent patients with a displaced intracapsular fracture of the femoral neck: a seven- to ten-year follow-up report of a prospective randomised controlled trial. J Bone Joint Surg Br 2011;93(8):1045–8.
11. Blomfeldt R, Tornkvist H, Ponzer S, et al. Comparison of internal fixation with total hip replacement for displaced femoral neck fractures. Randomized, controlled trial performed at four years. J Bone Joint Surg Am 2005;87(8):1680–8.
12. Chammout GK, Mukka SS, Carlsson T, et al. Total hip replacement versus open reduction and internal fixation of displaced femoral neck fractures: a randomized long-term follow-up study. J Bone Joint Surg Am 2012;94(21):1921–8.
13. Leonardsson O, Sernbo I, Carlsson A, et al. Long-term follow-up of replacement compared with internal fixation for displaced femoral neck fractures: results at ten years in a randomised study of 450 patients. J Bone Joint Surg Br 2010;92(3): 406–12.
14. Rogmark C, Johnell O. Primary arthroplasty is better than internal fixation of displaced femoral neck fractures: a meta-analysis of 14 randomized studies with 2,289 patients. Acta Orthop 2006;77(3):359–67.
15. Ong BC, Maurer SG, Aharonoff GB, et al. Unipolar versus bipolar hemiarthroplasty: functional outcome after femoral neck fracture at a minimum of thirty-six months of follow-up. J Orthop Trauma 2002;16(5):317–22.
16. Blomfeldt R, Tornkvist H, Eriksson K, et al. A randomised controlled trial comparing bipolar hemiarthroplasty with total hip replacement for displaced intracapsular fractures of the femoral neck in elderly patients. J Bone Joint Surg Br 2007;89(2):160–5.
17. Hedbeck CJ, Enocson A, Lapidus G, et al. Comparison of bipolar hemiarthroplasty with total hip arthroplasty for displaced femoral neck fractures: a concise four-year follow-up of a randomized trial. J Bone Joint Surg Am 2011;93(5): 445–50.
18. Poignard A, Bouhou M, Pidet O, et al. High dislocation cumulative risk in THA versus hemiarthroplasty for fractures. Clin Orthop Relat Res 2011;469(11): 3148–53.
19. Emery RJH, Broughton NS, Desai K, et al. Bipolar hemiarthroplasty for subcapital fracture of the femoral neck. A prospective randomised trial of cemented Thompson and uncemented Moore stems. J Bone Joint Surg Br 1991;73(2):322–4.
20. Parker MJ, Gurusamy K. Arthroplasties (with and without bone cement) for proximal femoral fractures in adults. Cochrane Database Syst Rev 2006;(3):CD001706.
21. Gjertsen JE, Lie SA, Vinje T, et al. More re-operations after uncemented than cemented hemiarthroplasty used in the treatment of displaced fractures of the femoral neck: an observational study of 11,116 hemiarthroplasties from a national register. J Bone Joint Surg Br 2012;94(8):1113–9.

22. Leonardsson O, Karrholm J, Akesson K, et al. Higher risk of reoperation for bipolar and uncemented hemiarthroplasty. 23,509 procedures after femoral neck fractures from the Swedish Hip Arthroplasty Register, 2005–2010. Acta Orthop 2012; 83(5):459–66.

23. Taylor F, Wright M, Zhu M. Hemiarthroplasty of the hip with and without cement: a randomized clinical trial. J Bone Joint Surg Am 2012;94(7):577–83.

24. Viberg B, Overgaard S, Lauritsen J, et al. Lower reoperation rate for cemented hemiarthroplasty than for uncemented hemiarthroplasty and internal fixation following femoral neck fracture: 12- to 19-year follow-up of patients aged 75 years or more. Acta Orthop 2013;84(3):254–9.

25. Hailer NP, Weiss RJ, Stark A, et al. The risk of revision due to dislocation after total hip arthroplasty depends on surgical approach, femoral head size, sex, and primary diagnosis. An analysis of 78,098 operations in the Swedish Hip Arthroplasty Register. Acta Orthop 2012;83(5):442–8.

26. Jolles BM, Bogoch ER. Posterior versus lateral surgical approach for total hip arthroplasty in adults with osteoarthritis. Cochrane Database Syst Rev 2006;(3):CD003828.

27. Mulliken BD, Rorabeck CH, Bourne RB, et al. A modified direct lateral approach in total hip arthroplasty: a comprehensive review. J Arthroplasty 1998;13(7): 737–47.

28. Callaghan JJ, Liu SS, Haidukewych GJ. Subcapital fractures: a changing paradigm. J Bone Joint Surg Br 2012;94(11 Suppl A):19–21.

29. Marsh JL, Slongo TF, Agel J, et al. Fracture and dislocation classification compendium–2007: Orthopaedic Trauma Association classification, database and outcomes committee. J Orthop Trauma 2007;21(Suppl 10):S1–133.

30. Parker MJ, Handoll HHG. Gamma and other cephalocondylic intramedullary nails versus extramedullary implants for extracapsular hip fractures in adults (review). Cochrane Database Syst Rev 2010;(9):CD000093.

31. Haidukewych GJ, Israel TA, Berry DJ. Reverse obliquity fractures of the intertrochanteric region of the femur. J Bone Joint Surg Am 2001;83(5):643–50.

32. De Bruijn K, den Hartog D, Tuinebreijer W, et al. Reliability of predictors for screw cutout in intertrochanteric hip fractures. J Bone Joint Surg Am 2012;94(14): 1266–72.

33. Hsu CE, Shih CM, Wang CC, et al. Lateral femoral wall thickness: a reliable predictor of post-operative lateral wall fracture in intertrochanteric fractures. Bone Joint J 2013;95(8):1134–8.

34. Anglen JO, Weinstein JN. Nail or plate fixation of intertrochanteric hip fractures: changing pattern of practice. A review of the American Board of Orthopaedic Surgery Database. J Bone Joint Surg Am 2008;90(4):700–7.

35. Norris R, Bhattacharjee D, Parker MJ. Occurrence of secondary fracture around intramedullary nails used for trochanteric hip fractures: a systematic review of 13,568 patients. Injury 2012;43(6):706–11.

36. Osnes EK, Lofthus CM, Falch JA, et al. More postoperative femoral fractures with the Gamma nail than the sliding screw plate in the treatment of trochanteric fractures. Acta Orthop Scand 2001;72(3):252–6.

37. Palm H, Jacobsen S, Sonne-Holm S, et al. Integrity of the lateral femoral wall in intertrochanteric hip fractures: an important predictor of a reoperation. J Bone Joint Surg Am 2007;89(3):470–5.

38. Rubio-Avila J, Madden K, Simunovic N, et al. Tip to apex distance in femoral intertrochanteric fractures: a systematic review. J Orthop Sci 2013;18(4): 592–8.

39. Baumgaertner MR, Curtin SL, Lindskog DM, et al. The value of the tip-apex distance in predicting failure of fixation of peritrochanteric fractures of the hip. J Bone Joint Surg Am 1995;77(7):1058–64.
40. Baumgaertner MR, Solberg BD. Awareness of tip-apex distance reduces failure of fixation of trochanteric fractures of the hip. J Bone Joint Surg Br 1997;79(6): 969–71.
41. Kuzyk PR, Zdero R, Shah S, et al. Femoral head lag screw position for cephalomedullary nails: a biomechanical analysis. J Orthop Trauma 2012;26(7):414–21.
42. Napoli N, Schwartz AV, Palermo L, et al. Risk factors for subtrochanteric and diaphyseal fractures: the study of osteoporotic fractures. J Clin Endocrinol Metab 2013;98(2):659–67.
43. Shane E, Burr D, Ebeling PR, et al. Atypical subtrochanteric and diaphyseal femoral fractures: report of a task force of the American Society for Bone and Mineral Research. J Bone Miner Res 2010;25(11):2267–94.
44. Banffy MB, Vrahas MS, Ready JE, et al. Nonoperative versus prophylactic treatment of bisphosphonate-associated femoral stress fractures. Clin Orthop Relat Res 2011;469(7):2028–34.
45. Egol KA, Park JH, Rosenberg ZS, et al. Healing delayed but generally reliable after bisphosphonate-associated complete femur fractures treated with IM nails. Clin Orthop Relat Res 2013. [Epub ahead of print].

Special Anesthetic Consideration for the Patient with a Fragility Fracture

Jean-Pierre P. Ouanes, DO[a],*, Vicente Garcia Tomas, MD[a], Frederick Sieber, MD[b]

KEYWORDS

- Fragility fractures • Regional anesthesia • Epidural anesthesia
- Orthopedic fractures • General anesthesia • Elderly

KEY POINTS

- Preoperative workup considerations include evaluation of associated injuries as well as comorbidities commonly found in the elderly population.
- Anesthesia options include general and regional anesthesia.
- Regional anesthesia offers the advantage of effectively anesthetizing the surgical site and avoiding some of the cardiovascular, respiratory, and cerebral physiologic alterations associated with general anesthesia.
- Regional anesthesia offers the benefit of intraoperative anesthesia, with the ability to provide analgesia into the postoperative period.

INTRODUCTION

Fragility fractures are defined by the World Health Organization as fractures caused by injury that would be insufficient to fracture a normal bone.[1] Clinically, they have been described as a low-energy fracture that occurs from minimal trauma such as a fall from a standing height or lower.[2–5] With the aging of the population, fragility fractures are becoming more common. See the article on Epidemiology of Fragility Fractures by Friedman and Mendelson elsewhere in this issue for more detailed information.

Funding Sources: Funded by NIH, Grant number RO1AG033615.

Conflicts of Interest: None.

[a] Anesthesiology and Critical Care Medicine, The Johns Hopkins Hospital, Sheik Zayed Tower 8-120, 1800 Orleans Street, Baltimore, MD 21287, USA; [b] Department of Anesthesiology and Critical Care Medicine, Johns Hopkins Bayview Medical Center, The Johns Hopkins Hospital, Johns Hopkins University School of Medicine, 4940 Eastern Avenue, Room A5W-588, Baltimore, MD 21224, USA

* Corresponding author.

E-mail address: ouanes@jhu.edu

This article focuses on special anesthesia management for fragility fractures of the extremities and hip. Vertebral fractures are common but are to be discussed with special anesthesia considerations related to spine surgery, which are beyond the scope of this article.

Initial Workup Considerations

Several principles should be kept in mind when assessing anesthetic risk in an elderly patient with a fragility fracture. A major priority is to evaluate for associated injuries to ensure that no injury takes precedence over the fracture repair.

Dementia, depression, hearing difficulties, and stroke all may interfere with the ability to make independent decisions and obtain informed consent in frail elderly patients. If a patient's ability to make decisions becomes severely impaired, then a surrogate must give consent. Advance directives, when available, can be helpful. Neurologic, pulmonary, and cardiac morbidities are the most common types of postoperative complications in the elderly, and the anesthesiologist should pay attention to these specific organ systems.

Risk Stratification

Preoperative pulmonary risk stratification

In general, what the anesthesiologist wants to know about the patient's preoperative pulmonary status is their risk for respiratory failure, pulmonary complications like pneumonia or aspiration, and difficulty in ventilator weaning or need for care in the intensive care unit. Certain physiologic parameters help predict the likelihood of postoperative pulmonary complications (**Box 1**).

Risk of hypoxia may be shown by room air saturation less than 90% or may be associated with low preoperative hemoglobin levels, although the exact level of hemoglobin at which this risk increases is controversial. Risk of postoperative CO_2 retention may be predicted by pulmonary function test, if available. Parameters such as preoperative FEV_1 (forced expiratory volume in first second of expiration) less than 50% of predicted or forced vital capacity of less than 1.7 L are associated with a higher likelihood of CO_2 retention.[6]

Preoperative cardiac risk stratification

The information of importance to the anesthesiologist when the patient has had a fall concerns whether the fall is secondary to cardiac cause. If the patient has a pacemaker, does it work? Are they in heart failure? Are they having an acute coronary syndrome? Excellent guidelines are available. The reader is referred to Figure 1 in the American College of Cardiology/American Heart Association Task Force 2007

Box 1
Physiologic parameters that help predict postoperative pulmonary complications

Predictor of pulmonary complications

Room air O_2 saturation less than 90%

Low hemoglobin levels

FEV_1 less than 50% predicted

FVC <1.7 L

Abbreviations: FEV_1, forced expiratory volume at 1 second; FVC, forced vital capacity.

guidelines on perioperative cardiovascular evaluation and care for noncardiac surgery specifically.[7]

Please refer to the article on Preoperative Optimization and Risk Assessment by Nicholas elsewhere in this issue for further details on preoperative cardiac evaluation.

Preoperative central nervous system evaluation

The anesthesiologist wishes to know that there are no active neurologic problems that may have contributed to the fall and that may, in turn, affect the patient's ability to tolerate surgery. The presence of delirium preoperatively warrants investigation to rule out serious conditions like hypoxia, hypoglycemia, electrolyte imbalances, or sepsis.[6] Neuroimaging may be necessary if history or signs point to a cerebrovascular accident (CVA). A recent CVA is associated with impaired autoregulation of the cerebral vasculature, and hemodynamic stress associated with general anesthesia could make the infarction worse.[6]

Besides the fracture itself, when evaluating the elderly, it is important to keep in mind that associated acute illness may have an atypical presentation. There may be significant differences in the presentation of disease in demented versus nondemented patients, because studies suggest that the nonspecific presentation of disease in older people is primarily linked to the presence of dementia rather than a characteristic feature of the aging process.

Elderly trauma patients should be assessed for any cervical spine fracture or injury. The result of this assessment changes how intubation is managed, or perhaps the decision may be made to avoid airway instrumentation by choosing a regional technique. However, even if a regional technique is performed, there is always the chance that it is necessary to convert to general anesthesia and secure the patient's airway secondary to inadequate anesthesia, prolonged procedure, or large fluid shifts requiring a large volume replacement.

Substance abuse, particularly alcohol, is often an underappreciated factor associated with falls. Alcohol disorders are estimated to be present in 5% to 14% of older patients in the emergency department. Alcohol abuse relates to anesthesia because the patient having delirium tremens or agitation in the recovery room can be problematic to manage.

Overall risk stratification

Preoperative assessment is performed with an eye to avoiding complications. The most important risk factors for perioperative complications in the elderly are summarized in **Box 2**.

The American Society of Anesthesiologists (ASA) has a classification system that is often used to indicate the overall physical health preoperatively (**Box 3**). This classification is often used to help predict patient risk for undergoing surgery and anesthesia.

The association between age and surgical risk is linked with increased incidence of comorbidities in the setting of decreased physiologic reserve. This situation has profound effects on the usual compensatory mechanisms. Emergency surgery is an independent predictor of adverse postoperative outcomes in older surgical patients undergoing noncardiac surgery. The consultant geriatrician would help us exclude patients from immediate surgery if they have conditions that could develop into life-threatening events with surgical stress (eg, severe blood loss and hypovolemic state, severe electrolyte derangements, oxygen supply and demand imbalances that could lead to end-organ damage). Volume status should be optimized, because the cardiovascular effects of anesthetics are exaggerated in a hypovolemic patient (see section on effects of general anesthetics).

Box 2
Factors that increase the risk of complications in the elderly

Emergency surgery

High ASA classification

Certain surgeries

  Major vascular (noncarotid)

  Thoracic (especially lung resection)

  Open colon resection or open cholecystectomy

Comorbidities

Surgical mortality in the elderly varies widely according to procedure. The current guidelines for cardiovascular evaluation of patients undergoing noncardiac surgery[7] provide a useful means of categorizing procedures into those of low, intermediate, and high risk. In general, most procedures for fragility fractures are intermediate risk.

Effects of General Anesthetics by System

The most common agents used for general anesthesia and their effects on major organ systems are reviewed (**Tables 1–3**).

Cardiovascular effects

The anesthesiologist's goal is to maintain hemodynamic stability throughout the perioperative period, ensuring adequate perfusion pressures and avoiding end-organ ischemia. Comorbidities that increase their risk for cardiovascular problems include an increase in wall thickness and stiffness of the major arteries, increase in systemic vascular resistance, decrease in myocardial compliance, and age-related decrease in activity of baroreceptors.[8] Chronic hypertension shifts the blood pressure autoregulation curve of several end organs, making it necessary to maintain the patient blood pressure within 25% to 30% of their normal baseline values to help prevent end-organ ischemia. The presence of peripheral vascular disease (PVD) or previous CVAs can decrease the patient's tolerance to hypotensive episodes.

Most intravenous anesthetics tend to cause a decrease in blood pressure by a variety of mechanisms, and the effect is exaggerated by common cardiovascular medications including angiotensin receptor blockers, angiotensin-converting enzyme

---

Box 3
ASA physical status classification

ASA physical status 1: a normal healthy patient

ASA physical status 2: a patient with mild systemic disease

ASA physical status 3: a patient with severe systemic disease

ASA physical status 4: a patient with severe systemic disease that is a constant threat to life

ASA physical status 5: a moribund patient who is not expected to survive without the operation

ASA physical status 6: a declared brain-dead patient, whose organs are being removed for donor purposes

---

Table 1 Cardiovascular physiology: effects of anesthesia					
	Propofol	Etomidate	Ketamine	Opioids	Inhalational
Blood pressure	↓↓	↓ (mild)	↑[a]	—	↓ Decrease SVR
Preload	↓	—	—	—	—
Afterload	↓	↓	↑	—	↓
Myocardial contractility	↓	—	↓ Direct effect[a]	—	—
Baroreceptor reflex	Inhibits	—	—	—	↓

Abbreviations: ↑, increase; ↓, decrease; —, unchanged; SVR, systemic vascular resistance.
[a] Net effect through centrally mediated sympathetic stimulation.
Data from Refs.[9–13]

inhibitor (ACEI), and diuretics. The cardiovascular effects of individual agents are discussed in the next section (see **Table 1**).

Propofol causes hypotension when used as an induction drug by creating arterial and venous vasodilation. It is also a direct myocardial depressant and abolishes the baroreceptor reflex, limiting the patient's ability to respond to hypotension. These effects are more pronounced with advanced age, hypovolemia, and rapid infusion. Elderly patients show increased sensitivity to the hypnotic effects of propofol, requiring smaller doses than their younger counterparts.[9] Therefore, it is important to titrate the dose to the desired effect in the elderly population.

Etomidate lacks any direct cardiodepressant effect[10] and maintains cardiovascular stability. It is an excellent induction agent for patients with known coronary artery disease (CAD), previous CVA, or pulmonary hypertension, in which cardiovascular instability may be catastrophic. Undesirable effects include adrenocortical suppression, and higher incidence of postoperative nausea and vomiting.

Ketamine is considered a direct myocardial depressant. Its net effect is an increase in blood pressure, heart rate, and cardiac output through a centrally mediated increase in sympathetic stimulation, making it a suitable agent in hypovolemic patients to avoid an exaggerated hypotensive response. The tachycardia and increase in cardiac output can be undesirable in patients with known CAD. These net effects are also blunted by the administration of β-blockers, or in critically ill patients who are unable to further stress their sympathetic system. Ketamine can have psychomimetic effects, which tend to be ameliorated by previous and concomitant benzodiazepine administration.

Opioids have a stable cardiovascular profile, unlikely to cause hypotension or myocardial depression. Morphine can stimulate histamine release, which can cause a decrease in blood pressure if administered as a rapid bolus or in high doses. Sensitivity to the analgesic effects of opioids also increases with age.[11]

Inhalational anesthetics share similar cardiovascular effects. Commonly used agents, with the exception of nitrous oxide, cause a dose-dependent decrease in mean arterial pressure. Cardiac index is not affected. Volatile agents have been shown to protect against myocardial ischemia.[12,13]

Respiratory effects

The relationship between functional residual capacity (FRC) and closing capacity (CC) plays an important role in the pulmonary mechanics of the elderly patient. FRC is defined as the lung volume at the end of normal exhalation and is reduced in the supine position as a result of decreased chest compliance from the pressure of

Table 2
Respiratory: effects of anesthesia

	Propofol	Etomidate	Ketamine	Opioids	Benzodiazepines	Inhalational
Ventilation	↓↓	↓		↓↓	↓	↓
Upper airway reflexes	↓↓	—		↓	—	↓
Response to hypercarbia	↓	—		↓	↓	↓
Other		Depression of ventilation increased in combination with inhalational/opioids	Bronchodilator Pattern ↓RR ↑V_T	Pattern ↓RR ↑V_T		Pattern ↑RR ↓V_T bronchodilator

Abbreviations: ↑, increase; ↓, decrease; —, unchanged; RR, respiratory rate; V_T, tidal volume.
Data from Refs.[9–16]

Table 3
Cerebral physiology: effects of anesthesia

	Propofol	Etomidate	Ketamine	Opioids	Benzodiazepines	Inhalational
CBF	↓↓	↓↓	↑	↓ Direct effect[a]	↓[a]	↑ Impair autoregulation at >1 MAC
CMRO$_2$	↓	↓	↑	—	↓	↓
Cerebral perfusion pressure	↓↓	↓	↑	—	↓	↑
ICP	↓	↓	↑	↓[a]	↓	↑ (>1 MAC)
Seizure foci	-/May cause	Activates/ may cause	Inhibits	—	Inhibit	—

Abbreviations: ↑, increase; ↓, decrease; —, unchanged; CBF, cerebral blood flow; ICP, intracranial pressure; MAC, minimum alveolar concentration.
[a] Hypercarbia associated with respiratory depression can cause an increase in CBF and ICP.
Data from Refs.[9–19]

abdominal contents on the diaphragm. CC refers to the volume at which small airways lacking cartilaginous support start to collapse in dependent areas of the lung, causing an intrapulmonary shunt and promoting hypoxia. CC steadily increases with age, but is not affected by posture. When CC exceeds FRC, alveoli in dependent areas of the lung collapse during normal tidal ventilation, increasing the risk of atelectasis and hypoxia. By age 66 years, CC equals or exceeds FRC in the upright position, increasing the risk of atelectasis and hypoxia.[14] General anesthesia compounds this effect by further collapsing aerated lung via a cephalad displacement of the diaphragm. Therefore, age, with its increase in CC, and general anesthesia, which further decreases the number of aerated alveoli, increase the risk of atelectasis, shunt, and hypoxia. This effect is eliminated when regional techniques are used as the main anesthetic.

Anesthesia affects the respiratory function and ventilation through a variety of mechanisms that relate to both position (as discussed earlier) and the intrinsic effects of anesthetics. Anesthesia also causes hypoventilation, increase in dead space, and increase in pulmonary shunting. Intravenous anesthetics inhibit input in multiple neurons of the respiratory system, whereas volatile agents decrease excitatory neurotransmission. Clinically, it translates into a decrease in ventilatory responses to hypoxia and hypercarbia.[15] Alveolar dead space is increased mostly during general anesthesia as a result of atelectasis and airway collapse in dependent areas of the lung. This effect can be reduced by application of positive end-expiratory pressure. Inhalational agents also inhibit hypoxic pulmonary vasoconstriction at high doses, increasing the ventilation/perfusion mismatch.

The respiratory effects of individual agents are discussed in the next section (see **Table 2**).

Propofol is a potent respiratory depressant that causes apnea at induction doses. It also reduces upper airway reflexes, making it suitable in reactive airway disease.

Etomidate has less depressant effects on respiration than propofol. For this reason, it is an acceptable agent for sedation when maintenance of spontaneous ventilation and avoiding hypoxia and hypercarbia are paramount.

Ketamine does not severely depress respiratory function. It also has bronchodilating properties, which may be beneficial in patients with reactive airways or treating bronchospasm.

Benzodiazepines are not strong respiratory depressants, although transient apnea can occur after rapid administration. This effect is exacerbated in elderly patients and in concomitant administration of opioids.[11]

Opioids decrease ventilatory responses to CO_2, which can persist for several hours. Large doses can result in apnea. Clinically, opioids result in a breathing pattern characterized by a decrease in respiratory rate, with a compensatory increase in tidal volume.[16]

Inhalational anesthetics result in an increased respiratory rate and decreased tidal volume, which leads to increased dead space ventilation. They also depress the respiratory response to hypoxia and hypercarbia, as well as hypoxic pulmonary vasoconstriction. They have bronchodilating properties.

Cerebral effects

Most intravenous anesthetics decrease both cerebral blood flow (CBF) and cerebral metabolic rate (CMRO$_2$), with the exception of ketamine.

The cerebral effects of individual agents are discussed in the next section (see **Table 3**).

Propofol decreases CBF and CMRO$_2$, resulting in a decrease in intracranial pressure (ICP). However, the systemic hypotension associated with its administration can compromise cerebral perfusion pressure. Propofol may be neuroprotective against focal ischemia (not global ischemia). Excitatory responses such as muscle twitching can be observed after administration of propofol. Most studies support an anticonvulsant effect of propofol.[17]

Etomidate shares a similar profile with propofol. However, it can activate seizure foci and can also cause myoclonus during administration.

In contrast to most intravenous anesthetics, ketamine is a cerebral vasodilator causing an increase in CBF, CMRO$_2$, and ICP and is therefore not recommended in patients with intracranial hypertension.

Opioids are considered cerebral vasoconstrictors. However, the respiratory depression associated with them can lead to significant hypercarbia, which in turn causes an increase in CBF and ICP. When administered in high doses, opioids can cause severe skeletal muscle rigidity (stiff chest syndrome), which may interfere with adequate mechanical ventilation. The dose for volatile anesthetics is decreased in the presence of opioids.[18]

Benzodiazepines also cause a reduction of CBF and CMRO$_2$, but to a lesser extent. Similar to the case with opioids, caution must be taken when administering benzodiazepines to patients with decreased intracranial compliance because of the transient respiratory depression caused after their administration. Benzodiazepines are also strong anticonvulsants.

Inhalational anesthetics do not abolish cerebral vascular responses to CO_2, but do impair cerebral autoregulation of blood flow. Nitrous oxide causes cerebral vasodilation and increases CMRO$_2$, whereas the potent inhalational agents decrease CMRO$_2$. Increases in CBF and ICP occur at concentrations greater than average dosing.[19]

Effects of Regional Anesthetics

Regional anesthesia is an anesthetic technique that renders a portion of the patient's body insensate to pain, allowing for the surgical procedure to take place and maintaining normal cognitive function. Regional anesthesia is accomplished by depositing local anesthetics perineurally. Local anesthetics provide anesthesia and analgesia by blocking voltage gated sodium channels, leading to an interruption of the transmission of pain sensation along the nerve. The degree of nerve blockage depends on local anesthetic drug choice as well as drug concentration and volume. These local anesthetics vary from short-acting anesthesia (30 minutes) to long-acting anesthesia (8 hours) and have variable analgesia from 30 minutes to 12 to 24 hours, depending how quickly the patient clears the drug. Additives may be beneficial to increase the duration of block by decreasing systemic absorption of the drug as well as providing an indicator of intravascular injection with placement of the block. In the absence of continuous perineural catheters, prolongation of the local anesthetic may be achieved with additives.

Examples of regional anesthesia include spinals, epidurals, and peripheral nerve blocks. Each is discussed in detail in the following sections.

There are many advantages of regional anesthesia.

The use of regional anesthesia instead of general anesthesia with volatile agents has been shown to reduce postoperative nausea and vomiting and lead to a reduced need for postoperative analgesics.[20–23] It has also been associated with decreased blood loss during surgery.[24]

Peripheral nerve blocks provide the additional benefit of affecting only the extremity that they are performed on and they are not associated with major hemodynamic shifts, which can be seen with general anesthesia.

As with any anesthetic, there are risks associated with regional anesthesia; however, serious complications are rare.[25]

The advantages of regional anesthesia in preventing cognitive dysfunction have been reviewed many times. This is a controversial topic, and a recent meta-analysis[26] was unable to show that the use of intraoperative neuraxial anesthesia reduces the incidence of postoperative cognitive dysfunction when compared with general anesthesia.

Neuraxial: spinal and epidural

Neuraxial anesthesia is divided into spinal anesthesia, epidural anesthesia, or a combination of the 2.

Onset of spinal anesthesia begins shortly after the injection of drug in the intrathecal space, regardless of the local anesthetic used. However, the time of onset of spinal anesthesia varies depending on the drug used, with shorter-acting local anesthetics taking 10 to 15 minutes and longer-acting local anesthetics taking greater than 20 minutes.

Epidural anesthesia requires the same block height as the spinal anesthesia but requires more time for onset, and there can be greater variability with the spread. There is greater spread in older patients, which is believed to be related to a less compliant epidural compartment.[27]

Differential nerve block is the phenomenon describing nerve fibers with varying sensitivity to local anesthetic blockade. The order of nerves blocked is sympathetic nerve fibers followed by pain, touch, proprioception, and motor. This phenomenon happens in peripheral nerves blocks, spinals, and epidurals. It is more of a temporal phenomenon in the peripheral nerve blocks and a spatial phenomenon in neuraxial blocks. Chamberlain and Chamberlain[28] described a sympathetic block extending 2 to 6 dermatomes higher than pinprick sensation. The significance of this finding is that there may be cardiovascular side effects during spinal and epidural anesthesia. The blockade of the sympathetic fibers is the principal mechanism for hypotension and bradycardia in neuraxial anesthesia. Hypotension is the result of both arterial and venodilation. Venodilation generally leads to a decrease in preload, which can be compensated with intravenous fluid bolus and vasopressors.

The renin-angiotensin system helps offset the hypotensive event from neuraxial anesthesia, and therefore, special consideration should be given when administering neuraxial anesthesia to patients taking ACEIs or angiotensin II receptor blockers. The effect of neuraxial anesthesia on respiratory physiology is minimal. Lung volumes, resting minute ventilation, dead space, and arterial blood gas tensions show little or no change with neuraxial anesthesia. However, high blocks can affect active exhalation.[29]

Complications of Neuraxial Anesthesia

Postdural puncture headache (PDPH) is a common complication of spinal anesthesia, with variable reported incidence depending on needle size. The headache is classically described as virtually nonexistent in the supine position and severe fronto-occipital headache with associated symptoms, which disappear when the patient is supine again. The incidence of PDPH decreases with age.[30] Inadvertent spinal anesthesia higher than the dermatome level of C4 leads to profound hypotension, bradycardia, and respiratory arrest. If cardiovascular and respiratory functions are adequately supported, then the spinal anesthetic resolves without sequelae.

Epidural and spinal hematoma are rare but devastating complications. The incidence is reported as less than 1 in 150,000.[29] The leading risk factor for neuraxial hematoma is anticoagulation use. For guidelines concerning administration in patients who are anticoagulated, the reader is referred to the American Society for Regional Anesthesia and Pain Medicine consensus statement on neuraxial anesthesia and anticoagulation.[31]

Spinal and epidural anesthesia has been shown to decrease intraoperative blood loss[24] and mortality in surgical patients by one-third.[32] The mechanism of the decreased blood loss is likely secondary to arterial and venous hypotension lower than the level of the neuraxial blockade. Investigators from a 2000 review article were not certain about the mechanism for the decreased mortality.[32]

Like peripheral nerve blocks, epidural anesthesia can extend into the postoperative period to provide analgesia with superior analgesia to parenteral opioids.[33]

Peripheral nerve blocks

This section is dedicated to specific techniques. An overview of the indications and brief description of the blocks are provided (**Table 4**).

Complications that apply to all peripheral nerve blocks are hemorrhagic, infectious, and neurologic. The focus here is on specific complications based on region of the body where the block took place. The overall risk of a serious adverse event after peripheral nerve block has been reported as 0.04%.[34]

Upper extremity

There are many techniques describing blocks of the brachial plexus. These blocks are reviewed in the categories of above the clavicle and below the clavicle (**Fig. 1**).

Above the clavicle: interscalene and supraclavicular nerve blocks are techniques named for their approach to the brachial plexus. The interscalene nerve block blocks the brachial plexus between the anterior and medial scalene muscles at the trunk level. This block reliably covers the upper and middle trunks and often misses ulnar distribution.[25]

Side effects and complications

Side effects and complications may be a result of spread of the local anesthetic to surrounding structures or by accidental placement of the needle to an incorrect location or damage from placement.

The overall incidence of short-term and long-term complications is 0.4%.[35,36]

Complications or side effects with upper extremity blocks arise from effects of local anesthetic on surrounding structures or as the result of inappropriate needling **Box 4**.

Table 4
Regional anesthesia by fragility fracture type

Fracture	Technique	Anesthesia Agent	Considerations and Comments
Upper Extremity Humerus Radius/ulnar	Single-shot or catheter brachial plexus block above or below clavicle depending on fracture location and patient comorbidities	Choice of agent based on anesthetic goal (ie, goal of intraoperative ± postoperative anesthesia and analgesia vs intraoperative anesthesia alone vs postoperative analgesia alone)	May leave a perineural catheter for postoperative pain control Blocks the brachial plexus above the clavicle associated with: a. Ipsilateral phrenic nerve block 50%–100% of the time b. Horner syndrome c. Hoarseness d. Potential for pneumo-thorax (1%–6%)
Hip/femur	Spinal CSE Epidural	Choice of anesthesia based on estimated duration of surgery and need for postoperative analgesia	Contraindicated in patients receiving antithrombotic or thrombolytic therapy See ASRA guidelines[31] Hip fractures pain generally controlled with acetaminophen after repair Cautious management of epidural for postoperative pain with concomitant anticoagulation See ASRA guidelines[31]
Lower Extremity Foot/ankle	Spinal CSE Epidural Single-shot or catheter femoral or sciatic nerve blocks	Choice of anesthesia based on estimated duration of surgery and need for postoperative analgesia	Neuraxial contraindication same as above for hip/femur Peripheral nerve blocks are acceptable in patients on antithrombotic or thrombolytic therapy; must consider risk benefit of regional and visualization of the vessels with ultrasonography and compressibility of the vasculature of the purposed site

Abbreviations: ASRA, American Society of Regional Anesthesia; CSE, combined spinal epidural anesthesia.

These complications are likely dependent on the skill of the person performing the regional technique. Serious infections associated with single-shot or continuous blocks are rare.[25]

A supraclavicular approach targets the brachial plexus at the trunk or division level, depending on the insertion site. This approach has similar risks as the interscalene, with the incidence of phrenic nerve paresis ranging from 50% to 100%,[25] likely depending on insertion site and volume of drug given. The incidence of pneumothorax is approximately 6%, based on all published literature, but likely more rare in experts trained in regional anesthesia using ultrasound guidance.[25]

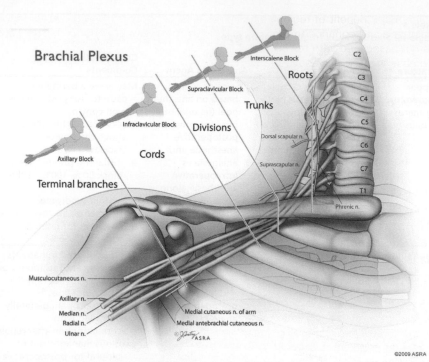

Fig. 1. Peripheral nerve block approaches at the brachial plexus and corresponding sensory distributions. Copyright © 2009 American Society of Regional Anesthesia and Pain Medicine. Used with permission. All rights reserved.

Box 4
Complications or side effects with upper extremity blocks from effects of local anesthetic on surrounding structures or inappropriate needling

Local anesthetic spread[37–40]

  Transient blockade of the phrenic nerve with subsequent hemidiaphragmatic paresis with an incidence of 100%,[37] leading to reduction in spirometric measurements by 25% to 32%

  Blockade of the cervical sympathetic chain with an incidence of 20% to 90%,[38] leading to Horner syndrome

  Hoarseness secondary to recurrent laryngeal nerve blockade[39,40]

Inappropriate needling[25]

  Intravascular injection 0% to 11%

  Subarachnoid or epidural injection

  Pneumothorax 6%

  Infection

Data from Neal JM, Gerancher JC, Hebl JR, et al. Upper extremity regional anesthesia: essentials of our current understanding, 2008. Reg Anesth Pain Med 2009;34(2):134–70.

One major benefit of regional anesthesia is that it may provide the initial surgical anesthesia and continue to provide postoperative analgesia. Peripheral nerve blocks are not associated with major respiratory changes, except for a pulmonary function decrease with blocks above the clavicle transiently affecting the phrenic nerve and in turn leading to a transient hemidiaphragm paresis.

Brachial plexus blocks below the clavicle
Infraclavicular, axillary, and distal terminal branch blocks are shown in **Fig. 1**.

The infraclavicular approach targets the brachial plexus at the cord level in the lateral aspect of the chest. It has a small risk of pneumothorax (0.6%)[25] and no chance of phrenic nerve blockade, allowing the patient to maintain normal respiratory function. The anesthesia associated with this block is mid humerus and distal.

Axillary nerve block targets the brachial plexus at the terminal branches. The risks associated with this block are bleeding, infection, damage to underlying tissue, and intravascular injection of drug.

Lower extremity
The lumbar plexus gives rise to the femoral nerve, which turns into the saphenous nerve and provides innervation of the skin over the medial leg and ankle.

The remainder of the leg receives innervations from branches from the sciatic nerve. The sciatic nerve can be anesthetized anywhere along its course from proximally to distally but is often blocked proximally under the gluteus maximus muscle or distally before the split into common peroneal and tibial nerves in the popliteal fossa. If a thigh tourniquet is going to be used, this requires a neuraxial or a proximal sciatic and femoral nerve block to provide anesthesia for the tourniquet discomfort in addition to the surgical site.

Risks of the femoral and sciatic nerve blocks are bleeding, intravascular injection, infection, and damage to the nerve.

Choice of Anesthetic by Fracture

The anesthetic options are based on location of fracture as well as the patient comorbidities and preferences.

The choice of anesthetic is less of a concern in ASA I-II patients. ASA III and IV patients with significant cardiovascular or respiratory comorbidities may benefit from avoidance of general anesthesia and the hemodynamic derangements associated with it.

Extremity fracture
Extremity fractures are amenable to regional anesthesia for the intraoperative anesthetic and a peripheral nerve catheter for postoperative pain control. Upper extremity anesthesia can be accomplished with a single brachial plexus injection or placement of a peripheral nerve catheter (see **Table 4**).

Regional anesthesia choice for lower extremity fractures depends on the location of the fracture, patient comorbidities, duration of surgery, location of the tourniquet, and patient preference. Branches of the sacral plexus as well as branches of the lumbar plexus need to be anesthetized for the primary anesthesia. This goal can be accomplished with a neuraxial technique or peripheral nerve techniques (see **Table 4**).

Hip fracture
Our anesthetic of choice is neuraxial anesthesia assuming no contraindications (see **Table 4**). In our center, 42% of procedures are performed under spinal, often because of relative and absolute contraindications for regional anesthesia and anesthesiologist

preference. These patients are in pain and often deteriorate the longer it takes to fix the fracture. Early fracture repair helps with cognitive function and earlier mobilization.

Researchers from Cornell University reviewed data from 400 US hospitals to determine whether neuraxial anesthesia or general anesthesia had better outcomes after primary hip or knee replacements.[40] These investigators reviewed 382,236 cases from 2006 to 2010 comparing neuraxial with general anesthesia. It was found that the neuraxial group had an 80% lower 30-day mortality and 30% to 50% lower risk of major complications, including stroke, renal failure, pneumonia, or need for mechanical ventilation.

Strategies for postoperative pain management

Undertreatment of postoperative pain can lead to adverse physiologic and psychological consequences, which can lead to increased morbidity and mortality and prolong patient recovery time.[41] Suboptimal pain management leads to inadequate ambulation and increased complications, including greater lengths of hospital stay and costs associated with those.[42]

Multimodal analgesia The pain management objective is to maximize patient recovery and function and minimize the associated side effects. A multimodal approach can best accomplish this.[43] First-line agents are nonopioid agents like acetaminophen, and targeted local anesthetics. Acetaminophen is likely the agent of choice for mild to moderate pain in the elderly patient with normal hepatic function, because of its effective analgesic properties and minimal side effects. Peripheral nerve blocks, either single-shot or catheter techniques, offer the unique ability to provide superior pain control to opioid alone and the ability to do so over an extended period.

Peripheral nerve catheters, a technique gaining popularity in the United States, can be placed preoperatively or postoperatively and provide extended pain relief while the infusion is running. Patients may be discharged home with peripheral nerve catheters in place and remove them at home or return to the hospital for removal. This practice is hospital specific.

SUMMARY

Older adults presenting with fragility fractures often require special preoperative management. Medical optimization before surgery is often a team approach. Anesthetic considerations for intraoperative management are based on patient comorbidities and preferences. Regional anesthesia may be preferable to general because of reduced negative cardiovascular, pulmonary, and possible cognitive effects.

REFERENCES

1. Guidelines for preclinical evaluation and clinical trials in osteoporosis. Geneva (Switzerland): World Health Organization; 1998.
2. Brown JP, Josse RG. 2002 clinical practice guidelines for the diagnosis and management of osteoporosis in Canada Scientific Advisory Council of the Osteoporosis Society of Canada. CMAJ 2002;167(Suppl 10):S1–34.
3. Vanasse A, Dagenais P, Niyonsenga T, et al. Bone mineral density measurement and osteoporosis treatment after a fragility fracture in older adults: regional variation and determinants of use in Quebec. BMC Musculoskelet Disord 2005;6:33.
4. American Academy of Orthopaedic Surgeons. Position Statement (1159) 2009. Available at: http://www.aaos.org/about/papers/position/1159.asp. Accessed September 14, 2013.

5. Holroyd C, Cooper C, Dennison E. Epidemiology of osteoporosis. Best Pract Res Clin Endocrinol Metab 2008;22(5):671–85.
6. Wong GT, Sun NC. Providing perioperative care for patients with hip fractures. Osteoporos Int 2010;21:S547–53.
7. Fleisher LA, Beckman JA, Brown KA, et al, American College of Cardiology/ American Heart Association Task Force on Practice Guidelines (Writing Committee to Revise the 2002 Guidelines on Perioperative Cardiovascular Evaluation for Noncardiac Surgery), American Society of Echocardiography, American Society of Nuclear Cardiology; Heart Rhythm Society, Society of Cardiovascular Anesthesiologists, Society for Cardiovascular Angiography and Interventions, Society for Vascular Medicine and Biology, Society for Vascular Surgery. ACC/AHA 2007 guidelines on perioperative cardiovascular evaluation and care for noncardiac surgery: a report of the American College of Cardiology/American Heart Association Task Force on Practice Guidelines (Writing Committee to Revise the 2002 Guidelines on Perioperative Cardiovascular Evaluation for Noncardiac Surgery): developed in collaboration with the American Society of Echocardiography, American Society of Nuclear Cardiology, Heart Rhythm Society, Society of Cardiovascular Anesthesiologists, Society for Cardiovascular Angiography and Interventions, Society for Vascular Medicine and Biology, and Society for Vascular Surgery. Circulation 2007;116(17):e418–99 [Erratum appears in Circulation 2008;117(5):e154; Erratum appears in Circulation 2008;118(9): e143–4].
8. Leung JM. Elderly patients. In: Stoelting RK, Miller RD, editors. Basics of anesthesia. 5th edition. Philadelphia: Churchill Livingstone; 2007. p. 518–9.
9. Dundee JW, Robinson FP, McCollum JS, et al. Sensitivity to propofol in the elderly. Anaesthesia 1986;41:482–5.
10. Eilers H. Intravenous anesthetics. In: Stoelting RK, Miller RD, editors. Basics of anesthesia. 5th edition. Philadelphia: Churchill Livingstone; 2007. p. 109.
11. Lortat-Jacob B, Servin F. Pharmacology of intravenous drugs in the elderly. In: Sieber F, editor. Geriatric Anesthesia. 1st edition. McGraw-Hill; 2007. p. 95–8.
12. DeHert SG, Cromheeke S, ten Broecke PW, et al. Effects of propofol, desflurane, and sevoflurane on recovery of myocardial function after coronary surgery in the elderly high-risk patients. Anesthesiology 2003;99:314–23.
13. DeHert SG, Van Der Linden PJ, Cromheeke S, et al. Cardioprotective properties of sevoflurane in patients undergoing coronary surgery and cardiopulmonary bypass are related to the modalities of its administration. Anesthesiology 2004; 101:299–310.
14. Morgan ME, Mikhail MS, Murray MJ. Respiratory physiology: the effects of anesthesia. In: Murry M, Morgan G, Mikhail M, editors. Clinical anesthesiology. 4th edition. McGraw-Hill; 2006. p. 546.
15. Feiner J. Clinical cardiac and pulmonary physiology. In: Stoelting RK, Miller RD, editors. Basics of anesthesia. 5th edition. Philadelphia: Churchill Livingstone; 2007. p. 62.
16. Stoelting R. Opioids. In: Stoelting RK, Miller RD, editors. Basics of anesthesia. 5th edition. Philadelphia: Churchill Livingstone; 2007. p. 116.
17. Stoelting RK, Hillier SC. Nonbarbiturate intravenous anesthetic drugs. In: Pharmacology and physiology in anesthetic practice. 4th edition. Philadelphia: Lippincott Williams & Wilkins; 2006. p. 155–78.
18. Lang E, Kapila A, Schlugman D, et al. Reduction of isoflurane minimal alveolar concentration by remifentanyl. Anesthesiology 1996;85:721–8.

19. McKay RE, Sonner J, McCay WR. Inhaled anesthetics. In: Stoelting RK, Miller RD, editors. Basics of anesthesia. 5th edition. Philadelphia: Churchill Livingstone; 2007. p. 93–4.

20. Pavlin DJ, Rapp SE, Polissar NL, et al. Factors affecting discharge time in adult outpatients. Anesth Analg 1998;87(4):816–26.

21. Hadzic A, Kerimoglu B, Loreio D, et al. Paravertebral blocks provide superior same-day recovery over general anesthesia for patients undergoing inguinal hernia repair. Anesth Analg 2006;102(4):1076–81.

22. Williams BA, Kentor ML, Vogt MT, et al. Femoral-sciatic nerve blocks for complex outpatient knee surgery are associated with less postoperative pain before same-day discharge: a review of 1,200 consecutive cases from the period 1996-1999. Anesthesiology 2003;98(5):1206–13.

23. Williams BA, Kentor ML, Vogt MT, et al. Economics of nerve block pain management after anterior cruciate ligament reconstruction: potential hospital cost savings via associated postanesthesia care unit bypass and same-day discharge. Anesthesiology 2004;100(3):697–706.

24. Richman JM, Rowlingson AJ, Maine DN, et al. Does neuraxial anesthesia reduce intraoperative blood loss? A meta-analysis. J Clin Anesth 2006;18(6): 427–35.

25. Neal JM, Gerancher JC, Hebl JR, et al. Upper extremity regional anesthesia: essentials of our current understanding, 2008. Reg Anesth Pain Med 2009;34(2): 134–70.

26. Wu CL, Hsu W, Richman JM, et al. Postoperative cognitive function as an outcome of regional anesthesia and analgesia. Reg Anesth Pain Med 2004; 29(3):257–68.

27. Burn JM, Guyer PB, Langdon L. The spread of solutions injected into the epidural space. Breast J 1973;45:338.

28. Chamberlain D, Chamberlain B. Changes in skin temperature of the trunk and their relationship to sympathetic block during spinal anesthesia. Anesthesiology 1986;65:139.

29. Bernards CM. Epidural and spinal anesthesia. In: Barash PG, Cullen BF, Stoelting RK, editors. Clinical anesthesia. 6th edition. Philadelphia: Lippincott Williams & Wilkins; 2009. p. 946.

30. Lybecker H, Møller JT, May O, et al. Incidence and prediction of postdural puncture headache. A prospective study of 1021 spinal anesthesias. Anesth Analg 1990;70(4):389–94.

31. Horlocker TT, Wedel DJ, Rowlingson JC, et al. Regional anesthesia in the patient receiving antithrombotic or thrombolytic therapy: American Society of Regional Anesthesia and Pain Medicine Evidence-Based Guidelines (third edition). Reg Anesth Pain Med 2010;35(1):64–101.

32. Rodgers A, Walker N, Schug S, et al. Reduction of postoperative mortality and morbidity with epidural or spinal anaesthesia: results from overview of randomised trials. BMJ 2000;321:1493.

33. Block BM, Liu SS, Rowlingson AJ, et al. Efficacy of postoperative epidural analgesia: a meta-analysis. J Am Med Assoc 2003;290:2455.

34. Auroy Y, Benhamou D, Bargues L, et al. Major complications of regional anesthesia in France. The SOS regional anesthesia hotline service. Anesthesiology 2002;97:1274–80.

35. Borgeat A, Ekatodramis G, Kalberer F, et al. Acute and nonacute complications associated with interscalene block and shoulder surgery. A prospective study. Anesth Analg 2001;95:875–80.

36. Urmey W, McDonald M. 100% incidence of hemidiaphragmatic paresis associated with interscalene brachial plexus anesthesia as diagnosed by ultrasonography. Anesth Analg 1991;72:498–503.
37. Borgeat A, Blumenthal S. Unintended destinations of local anesthetics. In: Neal JM, Rathmell JP, editors. Complications in regional anesthesia and pain medicine. Philadelphia: Saunders Elsevier; 2007. p. 157–63.
38. Seltzer JL. Hoarseness and Horner's syndrome after interscalene brachial plexus block. Anesth Analg 1977;56:585–6.
39. Capdevila X, Pirat P, Bringuier S, et al. Continuous peripheral nerve blocks in hospital wards after orthopedic surgery. Anesthesiology 2005;103:1035–45.
40. Memtsoudis SG, Sun X, Chiu YL, et al. Perioperative comparative effectiveness of anesthetic technique in orthopedic patients. Anesthesiology 2013;118(5):1046–58.
41. Wu CL, Cohen SR, Richman JM, et al. Efficacy of postoperative patient-controlled and continuous infusion epidural analgesia versus intravenous patient-controlled analgesia with opioids: a meta-analysis. Anesthesiology 2005;103:1079–88.
42. Karani R, Meier DE. Systemic pharmacologic postoperative pain management in the geriatric orthopaedic patient. Clin Orthop Relat Res 2004;(425):26–34.
43. Hanna MN, Ouanes JP, Tomas VG. Postoperative pain and other acute pain syndromes. In: Benzon HT, Rathmell JP, Wu CL, et al, editors. Practical management of pain. 5th edition. Philadelphia: Elsevier; 2014. p. 271.

Management of Postoperative Complications: General Approach

V. Ana Sanguineti, MD[a],*, Jason R. Wild, MD[b], Mindy J. Fain, MD[c]

KEYWORDS

- Physiological changes of aging • Postoperative complications • Early mobility
- Urinary catheters • Malnutrition and pressure ulcers • Pain management
- Postoperative cognitive dysfunction • Pneumonia and urinary track infections

KEY POINTS

- An aging-sensitive environment of care can reduce postoperative complications.
- Understanding and anticipating the physiologic changes of aging can help to avoid postoperative complications.
- General approach involves early mobility; freedom from tethers (indwelling urinary catheters and other devices); effective pain control; treating malnutrition; preventing pressure ulcers; reducing risk for pulmonary, urinary, and wound infections; and managing cognition.

INTRODUCTION

Effective management of the postoperative period following hip repair requires attention to four key components: an aging-friendly environment that addresses physical and social needs; team care that includes patient and family preferences, goals and values; the collaboration of physicians and other providers who are skilled in geriatric principles of care; and processes and procedures that are engineered into daily practice to assure full adherence to the best of care.

The goal of postoperative management is to promote early mobility and avoid postoperative complications, recognizing the potentially devastating impact of complications on the recovery of elderly hip fracture patients. The recommended approach involves aggressive early mobilization; freedom from tethers (indwelling urinary catheters and other devices); effective pain control; treating malnutrition; preventing pressure ulcers; reducing risk for pulmonary, urinary, and wound infections; and managing

Conflict of Interest: none to declare.
[a] Division of Geriatrics, General Internal Medicine and Palliative Medicine, Department of Medicine, University of Arizona College of Medicine, 1501 N. Campbell Avenue, P.O. Box 245036, Tucson, AZ 85724-5036, USA; [b] Department of Orthopaedic Surgery, University of Arizona College of Medicine, 1609 N Warren Street, Suite 108, P.O. Box 245064, Tucson, AZ 85724-5064, USA; [c] Division of Geriatrics, General Internal Medicine and Palliative Medicine, Department of Medicine, University of Arizona College of Medicine, 1821 E Elm Street, Tucson, AZ 85719, USA
* Corresponding author.
E-mail address: asanguineti@deptofmed.arizona.edu

Clin Geriatr Med 30 (2014) 261–270
http://dx.doi.org/10.1016/j.cger.2014.01.005
0749-0690/14/$ – see front matter © 2014 Elsevier Inc. All rights reserved.

cognition. This carefully structured and patient-centered management provides older, vulnerable patients their best chance of returning to their previous level of functioning as quickly and safety as possible.

Keys to effective management
- Aging-friendly environment
- Patient-and-family–centered care
- Collaborative interdisciplinary team
- Processes and procedures engineered into care.

Goals of postoperative management
- Promote mobility and avoid postoperative complications
- Return patient to their highest level of functioning.

OVERVIEW OF THE POSTOPERATIVE PERIOD

The postoperative period is characterized by several challenges for the elderly patient. The normal decline in physiologic reserve seen in the cardiovascular, pulmonary, renal, and neurocognitive systems of the elderly is further affected by the physiologic stress of surgery, anesthesia, and immobility.[1,2] Furthermore, this decreased functional reserve, coupled with accumulated comorbidities and impairments in functional status often found in the elderly, predisposes the patient to an increased risk for postoperative complications. These complications delay recovery and result in an increased length of stay, loss of function, and risk of subsequent decline that threatens the patient's ability to transition to the highest level of independent living in the home and community.

Morbidity and mortality surge in the week following surgery.[3] Criteria from the American Heart Association and the American Society of Anesthesiologists have been developed to predict perioperative risk; however, these criteria are imperfect in assessing the surgical risk for elderly patients. Other markers for postoperative risk are now recognized as equally valuable. These include the presence of frailty, malnutrition, and functional status. A clearly outlined approach to assess and manage risk is required to achieve the best outcomes.[4–6] In addressing the approach to the management of patients in the postoperative period, it is worthwhile to specifically examine the organ systems affected by this stress to best understand the recommendations.

IMPLICATIONS OF PHYSIOLOGIC CHANGES OF AGING ON POSTOPERATIVE COMPLICATIONS

An understanding of the physiology of the elderly patient allows the team managing hip fractures to direct care with the aim of mitigating adverse events that develop.

Respiratory System

- Pulmonary morbidity is the most common complication following noncardiac surgery.
- Physiologic aging leads to lowered Pao_2, increased work of breathing, and decline in central hypoxic drive.
- Postoperative narcotics and immobility lead to atelectasis, hypoxia, and hypercarbia.

Pulmonary morbidity, along with cardiac events, is the most common complication following non-cardiac surgery in elderly patients.[7] Several well-known aging-related physiologic changes in the respiratory system result in a patient who is vulnerable to postoperative pulmonary complications. With aging, there is stiffening of the ribcage, decreased elasticity of the lungs, and reduced number and function of the cilia along the respiratory tract. In the lung parenchyma, alveolar surfaces are reduced. These changes lead to impaired cough, increased work of breathing, decreased lung volumes, and an overall greater dependence on the diaphragm. The aging lung has a lowered Pao_2 and increased dead space, leading to a mismatch of ventilation and perfusion. Compounding these changes is the decline in the central hypoxic drive for respiration.[8]

Perioperative immobility causes suppression of ribcage expansion and reduced effectiveness of diaphragmatic excursions. This leads to atelectasis and ventilation-perfusion (V/Q) mismatch. Narcotics administered in the postoperative period contribute to hypercarbia from irregular and weakened respirations, and is another common pathway to atelectasis. There is further lowering of the Pao_2, which causes hypoxia, which may be profound and yet clinically subtle. Atelectasis and impaired cough are commonly seen in the postoperative patient. These increase the patient's chances of aspirating or developing pneumonia.[9]

Cardiovascular System

- Physiologic changes of cardiovascular aging results in a patient more prone to dehydration, orthostasis, dyspnea, and falls.
- Diminished baroreceptor sensitivity and increased vascular stiffness compromise the older patient's ability to respond to volume changes.
- General anesthesia may further compromise cardiac output.
- Hypotension may develop quickly in the vulnerable older patient.

Age-related changes of the heart have been well studied and, because of these changes, the patient is more prone to dehydration, orthostasis, dyspnea, and falls. Changes to the anatomy include an increase in fibrosis within the myocardium and stiffening of the walls leading to conduction disturbances, diastolic dysfunction, and left ventricular hypertrophy. Valves tend toward calcification and resulting stenosis may lead to ischemia or congestive heart failure.

The heart also declines physiologically with decreases in baroreceptor sensitivity and reduced elasticity of the arterial walls. Peripheral vascular resistance increases and systolic hypertension can result from these changes.

There is a decrease in plasma volume that, along with aging-related renal changes, makes the body vulnerable to volume changes. The expected compensatory change in heart rate to accommodate volume changes is muted. Hypotension develops quickly due to the heart's reduced ability to respond to volume loss. Although the heart rate loses its responsiveness to catecholamines, the cardiac output is not affected by normal aging. However, in response to stressors such as immobility, as well as several medications used for general anesthesia, cardiac output will be lowered.[10]

Recently, a previously unrecognized incidence of postoperative myocardial infarctions among elderly subjects with hip fracture repair was documented. In this study, approximately 14% of subjects experienced an myocardial infarction after hip fracture repair, 75% of which were asymptomatic.[11] This study underscores the need to define the cumulative stressors to the cardiovascular system following surgery to reduce this serious and silent complication.

Renal System

- Renal changes with aging have important implications in the management of postoperative fluids and medications.

- Overestimation of glomerular filtration rate (GFR) results in adverse medication effects, so the Cockcroft-Gault equation should be used to dose medications.

Known physiologic changes of the renal system with aging have important implications for the management of postoperative fluids and medications. With aging, the kidneys experience a decline in the number of functioning glomeruli and nephrons. There is decreased blood flow across the capillary bed and decreased filtration such that the GFR is reduced. Unfortunately, this decline in GFR is often unrecognized by the clinician because the age-related loss of skeletal muscle mass affects serum creatinine, a key component of the calculated or estimated GFR (eGFR). Relying on a low or normal serum creatinine in an elderly patient as a measure of renal function can result in an overestimation of the GFR. A more accurate estimate of the GFR is obtained with the Cockcroft-Gault method, which identifies potential adverse effects of renally excreted medications. Be aware, however, that most laboratory systems use a method other than Cockcroft-Gault to calculate the eGFR, one that often overestimates renal function in the elderly.

These predictable changes in renal function have important implications for the management of postoperative older patients. It is common for the elderly patient to experience volume overload in the postoperative period if close attention is not paid to renal status and the cardiac output.[12] Electrolyte imbalances, especially hyponatremia, are seen frequently, as are the body's accumulation of drugs due to unrecognized renal impairment. Medications that are excreted via the kidneys should be monitored closely. The Cockcroft-Gault equation is recommended when measuring GFR in the elderly.[13]

Skin

- Aging skin has less subcutaneous tissue, decreased cell turnover, and less moisture.
- Aging skin is more susceptible to pressure, shear, friction, and moisture.
- Pressure ulcers are a serious and avoidable postoperative complication.

The skin is not immune from the aging process. With age comes the loss of epidermal and dermal thickness, as well as a decrease in the underlying support of subcutaneous tissue. The skin also loses moisture and has decreased cellular turnover, making it more susceptible to the effects of shear, friction, and pressure forces. Moisture that accumulates contributes to the resultant breakdown in skin. Skin health is negatively affected by malnutrition.[14,15] Pressure ulcers are often seen in the patient who is recovering from a hip fracture. However, there is a concerted effort by hospitals to lower the incidence in recent years because of government mandates affecting Medicare reimbursement when acute ulcers develop while hospitalized. These ulcers can cause pain and infection that can be localized or systemic, increase the length of hospital stay, influence the postdischarge level of care, and affect overall morbidity and mortality.

GENERAL APPROACH

The following approaches are described separately for ease of discussion; however, they are highly interconnected and should be considered in association with each other. For example, early mobility, a goal of postoperative management, is difficult to achieve without effective pain control or a reduction in the number of tethering devices, such as indwelling urinary catheters or cardiac telemetry.

Early Mobility

- Immobility is associated with serious pulmonary complications and skin breakdown.
- Surgical repair within 48 hours of injury results in reduced mortality at 30 days and 1 year.
- Rapid mobilization postoperatively is associated with decreased complications, shorter hospital stays, and decreased costs of care.
- The treatment plan, including weight-bearing status, should be tailored to allow for early mobility.

Immobility as an injurious factor cannot be overstated. Immobility is frequently associated with postoperative complications and is a significant factor in the development of many, particularly pulmonary events and skin breakdown. Immobility is implicated in thromboembolism, pneumonia, and respiratory failure. It contributes to the development of pressure ulcers following hip repair, loss of bone mineral density, fatigue, and orthostatic hypotension, while increasing the risk of delirium.[1] Furthermore, in patients with hip fractures, immobility negatively impacts functional status at 2 months post repair.[16]

A shortened time to mobilization is thought to affect several important factors in geriatric hip fracture patients; notably, decreased risks of infection, venous thromboembolism, pressure ulcers, shorter hospital stays, and decreased cost of care.[17] Timing of surgical management of older adults with hip fractures is an important determinant of morbidity and mortality. Patients who experience a delay in surgery greater than 48 hours from admission demonstrate a statistically higher mortality at 30 days and 1 year.[17,18] The addition of comprehensive geriatric care with a particular focus on mobilization has shown to increase the amount of time that patients spend in upright positions and has improved lower limb function scores, when compared with standard orthopedic care.[19–22]

It is best to emphasize early mobility and initiation of physical therapy beginning day one following surgery. Effective pain management is critical to achieving early optimal mobility. In general, the treatment plan for a geriatric patient is usually tailored to allow for early weight bearing and mobilization, albeit occasionally with activity precautions depending on the type of surgery.

Freedom from Tethers

- The average patient will be confined by four different restraints, limiting mobility and increasing the risk for delirium.
- Reevaluate the need for all lines and devices daily.

On average, the patient recovering from a hip fracture repair will be confined by four restraints: oxygen tubing, sequential compression devices, an intravenous line, and an indwelling urinary catheter. In several institutions, cardiac monitors are also used during the first 48 hours following surgery. Additionally, the patient may frequently have a pulse oximeter, a wound drain, and a second intravenous line for the first 24 to 48 hours after surgery. The net result is to effectively immobilize the patient. For an elderly patient with limited vision, hearing, and cognition, this situation can be frightening, lead to agitation, and is a modifiable risk factor for the development of delirium. All lines and devices constraining the patient should be reevaluated daily, with a mind toward eliminating these tethers.

Pain Management

- Effective pain control is essential for mobilization, and for reducing the risk of delirium.

- There is a delicate balance between pain control and oversedation, and daily assessment is required.
- Be sure to monitor for side effects of narcotics, including urinary retention and constipation.

Pain accompanies a hip fracture and its repair. Pain can be a cause of immobility and precipitate delirium. When patients receive no opioid or a very low dose of opioid, their risk of developing delirium increases ninefold.[23,24] There is a delicate balance of pain control versus oversedation. It is critical to reassess pain daily and, in general, recommendations are to use scheduled doses if the patient is unable to ask or self-manage.

There are several choices when selecting a pain-management strategy. Early in the postoperative period, intravenous analgesics may be required. Morphine is well accepted and effective, although hydromorphone is a preferable choice when the GFR is around 30 mL/min or less, due to the active metabolites of morphine that linger and cause prolonged sedation in patients with chronic kidney disease.

Epidural anesthesia can also be considered when there is difficulty in controlling the immediate postoperative pain.[25] There is some evidence for the beneficial effects of pain control using epidural analgesia with bupivacaine and morphine.[26] Other combinations studied in noncardiac surgeries include ropivacaine and hydromorphone or fentanyl delivered via an epidural route. The combination of an epidural analgesic and local anesthetic allows for lower doses and possibly earlier recovery of the patient's mental status when compared with the effects of intravenous opioids.[25–27]

When the patient is tolerating oral intake, oxycodone or its equivalent can be effective in controlling pain and allowing for early ambulation. Acetaminophen should also be part of the regimen as pain diminishes in intensity, limiting the daily dose to 3 g or less per day. When implementing a narcotic pain regimen, it is necessary to monitor and manage the common and predictable side effects, such as constipation and urinary retention.

Malnutrition and Pressure Ulcers

- The highest rates of pressure ulcers occur in hospitalized orthopedic patients.
- Malnutrition is a risk factor for pressure ulcers.
- A structured assessment and management of the patient's nutrition and skin can mitigate some of the most common complications of hip fracture repair.

The development of pressure ulcers in the postoperative period is a well-known complication of hip fracture repair. Pressure on the skin from prolonged immobility leads to ischemic tissue and subsequent skin breakdown. The highest rates of pressure ulcers occur in hospitalized orthopedic populations, ranging from 9% to 40%.[28]

The prevalence of protein-caloric malnutrition in the elderly is significant in those with multiple illnesses, as well as in hospitalized patients, and the preexisting nutritional status of the patient contributes to the development of pressure ulcers. Malnutrition also affects wound healing, and can lead to infection and prolonged hospitalization.[29,30] Serum albumin levels less than 3.5 g/dL, a body mass index (BMI) less than 19, and total lymphocyte counts less than 1500 cells/μL are used to identify patients with malnutrition and those at risk for wound healing complications.

Several studies have looked at malnutrition as a risk factor for poor outcomes after hip fracture surgery and have noted a relationship between malnutrition and pressure ulcer development. A few studies show a direct link between the levels of a patient's BMI and serum albumin with pressure ulcer presence. The incidence of pressure ulcers can be minimized with the addition of nutritional supplementation containing a calorie-rich and protein-rich preparation.[28,29] Therefore, although the urgent nature of a hip fracture does not allow a patient's nutritional status to be optimized before surgery, intervention with nutritional supplementation in the postoperative period may help to lower the rates of infection and shorten the hospitalization. Malnourished patients benefit from a nutritional consult and patients with poor oral intake can benefit from calorie-dense supplements such as Ensure or Boost.[31,32]

A multipronged approach to help prevent pressure ulcers includes formally assessing and managing the patient's nutritional status and skin condition, and promoting early mobility. These structured interventions may prevent some of the most common complications associated with hip fractures.[33,34]

Prevention of Infections

- Pneumonia and urinary tract infections are the most common postoperative infections, related to immobility and use of indwelling urinary catheters.
- Good pulmonary hygiene and avoidance of oversedation can reduce pneumonia.
- Management of perioperative stress-induced hyperglycemia through structured insulin protocols can shorten hospital stays.

Pneumonia and urinary tract infections continue to be the most common postoperative infections in hip fracture patients. Their prevalence relates to the physiologic changes that occur with immobility and the use of indwelling urinary catheters. These infections predict a higher morbidity and mortality in the 30 days following hospitalization and are associated with further decline in the elderly patient's functional status.[1]

Several studies have demonstrated the increased risk of bacteriuria and urinary tract infections with indwelling catheters in place more than 2 days following surgery.[1] Therefore, the removal of indwelling urinary catheters within 2 days should decrease nosocomial urinary tract infections. This is a common recommendation to prevent perioperative urinary tract infections.[35] Avoiding certain medications, such as anticholinergic medications, managing constipation, and promoting early mobility can help to reduce urinary retention in elders, and allow for early removal of catheters.

More complicated is the management of the respiratory system. Attention to good pulmonary practices with the use of effective positioning, a bedside incentive spirometer to prevent atelectasis, and avoidance of oversedation are beneficial measures to prevent pneumonia.[36] Oxygen supplementation can minimize the effects of hypoxia.

Orthopedic wound infections are also an important cause of morbidity and mortality in the older patient. Perioperative stress-induced hyperglycemia, even in patients who are not diabetic, has been implicated as an independent risk factor for 30-day surgical infection.[37] Perioperative glucose levels greater than 220 mg/dL have been associated with a sevenfold increased infection risk.[38] Additionally, diabetic patients admitted to the hospital often have poor glycemic control, not only secondary to stress but also because they have been taken off their home regimen and placed on sliding-scale protocols, which provides suboptimal glycemic control. Early postoperative initiation of a basal bolus insulin regimen with long-acting insulin is advised. After an initial set dose, insulin doses are changed daily based on the previous day's results of blood glucose measurements. This protocol has been shown to decrease hyperglycemia events and has shortened hospital stays by an average of 2 days when compared with sliding scale insulin regimen alone.[39,40]

Management of Cognition

- Older adults are at higher risk for postoperative cognitive dysfunction (POCD).
- POCD manifests as difficulty with memory, concentration, attention, learning, and speed of response, but more research is needed to clarify this syndrome.

- It is unclear which anesthetic agents may minimize risk of POCD.

Aside from acute postoperative delirium, general anesthesia can be associated with persistent disturbances in cognitive function known as POCD. Neurophysiologic testing has shown postoperative difficulty with memory, concentration, attention, learning, and the speed of mental and motor response.[41]

Whereas most research has focused on POCD after cardiac surgery, many newer studies are examining POCD after noncardiac surgery. Unfortunately, most have been underpowered and the vague definition of POCD makes it difficult to study via meta-analysis. Further research is required in this area but some conclusions can be made. Elderly patients are at higher risk for development of POCD. Those patients with POCD persisting at 3 months had a higher mortality rate at 2 years.[42]

Recommendations as to which anesthetic agents may minimize risk of POCD are lacking. Some studies have indicated that regional and general anesthesia carry the same risk for POCD at 3 months, making the cause unclear. Although our understanding of the effects of anesthesia is evolving, it is clear that postoperative cognitive dysfunction may necessitate changes to after-hospital disposition and care requirements.

Other Considerations

As with other factors that affect a patient's recovery, constipation, sleep deprivation, and depression are underrecognized and undertreated in the hospitalized geriatric patient. These conditions are especially common in the hip fracture patient due to narcotic medications, pain, loss of function, and premorbid comorbidities. Through early recognition of these additional disorders, it is also possible to improve outcomes and lower the risk of delirium.

SUMMARY

The management of the aging patient in the postoperative setting requires consideration of several problems unique to, or of greater consequence, in the elderly. The aging-related physiologic changes discussed previously describe the vulnerable older adult and predict the increased risk of several postoperative complications. Added stresses include the hip fracture and the surgical repair process, as well as the physical and cognitive demands of recovery, and are the source of subsequent and predictable risks for anemia, delirium, and venous thromboembolism. Optimal management of the elderly hip fracture patient requires full attention to these problems to promote the best outcomes, and reduce morbidity and mortality.

REFERENCES

1. Beliveau MM, Multach M. Perioperative care for the elderly patient. Med Clin North Am 2003;87:273–89.
2. Potter JF. The older orthopaedic patient: general considerations. Clin Orthop Relat Res 2004;(425):44–9.
3. Pedersen SJ, Borgbjerg FM, Schousboe B, et al, Hip Fracture Group of Bispebjerg Hospital. A comprehensive hip fracture program reduces complication rates and mortality. J Am Geriatr Soc 2008;56(10):1831–8.
4. Makary MA, Segev DL, Pronovost PJ, et al. Frailty as a predictor of surgical outcomes in older patients. J Am Coll Surg 2010;210(6):901–8.
5. Potter J, Klipstein K, Reilly JJ, et al. The nutritional status and clinical course of acute admissions to a geriatric unit. Age Ageing 1995;24:131–6.

6. Penrod JD. Heterogeneity in hip fracture patients: age, functional status, and comorbidity. J Am Geriatr Soc 2007;55(3):407–13.
7. Lawrence VA, Hilsenbeck SG, Mulrow CD. Incidence and Hospital Stay for cardiac and pulmonary complications after abdominal surgery. J Gen Intern Med 1995;10:671–8.
8. Enright PL. Chapter 82. Aging of the respiratory system. In: Halter JB, Ouslander JG, Tinetti ME, et al, editors. Hazzard's Geriatric Medicine and gerontology. 6th edition. New York: Mcgraw-Hill; 2009. p. 984.
9. Janssens JP, Pache JC, Nicod LP, et al. Physiological changes in respiratory function associated with ageing. Eur Respir J 1999;13(1):197–205.
10. Kitzman DW, Taffet G. Chapter 74. Effect of aging on cardiovascular structure and function. In: Halter JB, Ouslander JC, Tinetti ME, et al, editors. Hazzard's geriatric medicine and gerontology. 6th edition. New York: McGraw-Hill; 2009. p. 885–8, 890–1.
11. Gupta BP, Huddleston JM, Kirkland LL, et al. Clinical presentation and outcome of perioperative myocardial infarction in the very elderly following hip fracture surgery. J Hosp Med 2012;7:713–6.
12. Wiggins J, Patel SR. Chapter 85, page 1009–10, Chapter 88, page 1048–54, 1057. Changes in kidney function. In: Halter JB, Ouslander JC, Tinetti ME, et al, editors. Hazzard's geriatric medicine and gerontology. 6th edition. New York: McGraw-Hill; 2009.
13. Loran DB, Hyde BR, Zwischenberger JB. Perioperative management of special populations: the geriatric patient. Surg Clin North Am 2005;85:1259.
14. Siebers MJ. Chapter 20. Pressure ulcers. Duthie: practice of geriatrics. 4th edition. USA: Saunders; 2007.
15. Bates-Jensen BM, MacLean CH. Quality indicators for the care of pressure ulcers in vulnerable elders. J Am Geriatr Soc 2007;55:S409–16.
16. Siu AL. Early ambulation after hip fracture: effects on function and mortality. Arch Intern Med 2006;166(7):766.
17. Shiga T, Wajima Z, Ohe Y. Is operative delay associated with increased mortality of hip fracture patients? Systematic review, meta-analysis, and meta-regression. Can J Anaesth 2008;55:146–54.
18. Bottle A, Aylin P. Mortality associated with delay in operation after hip fracture: observational study. BMJ 2006;332:947–51.
19. Taraldsen K, Sletvold O, Thingstad P, et al. Physical behavior and function early after hip fracture surgery in patients receiving comprehensive geriatric care or orthopedic care–a randomized controlled trial. J Gerontol A Biol Sci Med Sci 2013. [Epub ahead of print]. http://dx.doi.org/10.1093/gerona/glt097.
20. Kamel HK, Iqbal MA, Mogallapu R, et al. Time to ambulation after hip fracture surgery: relation to hospitalization outcomes. J Gerontol A Biol Sci Med Sci 2003;58: 1042–5.
21. Pashikanti L, Von Ah D. Impact of early mobilization protocol on the medical-surgical inpatient population: an integrated review of literature. Clin Nurse Spec 2012;26:87–94.
22. Kostuj T, Smektala R, Schulze-Raestrup U. The influence of timing of surgery on mortality and early complications in femoral neck fractures, by surgical procedure: an analysis of 22,566 cases from the German External Quality Assurance Program. Unfallchirurg 2013;116(2):131–7.
23. Inouye SK, Borgardus ST Jr, Charpentier PA, et al. A multicomponent intervention to prevent delirium in hospitalized older patients. N Engl J Med 1999; 340(9):669.

24. Morrison RS, Magaziner J, Gilbert M, et al. Relationship between pain and opioid analgesics on the development of delirium following hip fracture. J Gerontol 2003; 58:76–81.

25. White JJ, Khan WS, Smitham PJ. Perioperative implications of surgery in elderly patients with hip fractures: an evidence-based review. J Perioper Pract 2011; 21(6):1467.

26. Foss NB, Kristensen MT, Kristensen BB, et al. Effect of postoperative analgesia on rehabilitation and pain after hip fracture surgery: a randomized double-blind, placebo-controlled trial. Anesthesiology 2005;102(6):1197.

27. Mann C, Pouzeratte Y, Boccara G, et al. Comparison of intravenous or epidural patient controlled analgesia in the elderly after major abdominal surgery. Anesthesiology 2000;92(2):433.

28. Bates-Jensen BM. Chapter 58. Pressure ulcers. In: Halter JB, Ouslander JG, Tinetti ME, et al, editors. Hazzard's geriatric medicine and gerontology. 6th edition. New York: McGraw-Hill; 2009. p. 703–4.

29. Koval KJ, Maurer SG, Su ET, et al. The effects of nutritional status on outcome after hip fracture. J Orthop Trauma 1999;13(3):164–9.

30. Montero PB. Malnutrition as a prognostic factor in elderly patients with hip fractures. Med Clin (Barc) 2007;128(19):721–5.

31. Avenell A, Handoll HH. Nutritional supplementation for hip fracture aftercare in older people. Cochrane Database Syst Rev 2006;(4):CD001880.

32. Gunnarsson AK. Does nutritional intervention for patients with hip fractures reduce postoperative complications and improve rehabilitation? J Clin Nurs 2009;18(9):1325–33.

33. Koren-Hakim T. The relationship between nutritional status of hip fracture operated elderly patients and their functioning, comorbidity and outcome. Clin Nutr 2012;31(6):917–21.

34. Pioli G, Barone A, Giusti A, et al. Predictors of mortality after hip fracture: results from 1-year follow-up. Aging Clin Exp Res 2006;18(5):381–7.

35. Ksycki MF, Namias N. Nosocomial urinary tract infection. Surg Clin North Am 2009;89:475–81.

36. Lo IL. Pre-operative pulmonary assessment for patients with hip fracture. Osteoporos Int 2010;21(Suppl 4):S579–86.

37. Richards JE, Kauffmann RM, Obremskey WT, et al. Stress-induced hyperglycemia as a risk factor for surgical-site infection in nondiabetic orthopedic trauma patients admitted to the intensive care unit. J Orthop Trauma 2013;27(1):16–21. http://dx.doi.org/10.1097/BOT.0b013e31825d60e5.

38. Karunakar MA, Staples KS. Does stress-induced hyperglycemia increase the risk of perioperative infectious complications in orthopaedic trauma patients? J Orthop Trauma 2010;24(12):752–6. http://dx.doi.org/10.1097/BOT.0b013e3181d7aba5.

39. Richards JE. Relationship of hyperglycemia and surgical site infection in orthopedic surgery. J Bone Joint Surg Am 2012;94(13):1181–6.

40. Rizvi AA. Undergoing orthopedic surgery. J Am Acad Orthop Surg 2010;18: 426–35.

41. van Dijk D, Keizer AM, Diephuis JC, et al. Neurocognitive dysfunction after coronary artery bypass surgery: a systematic review. J Thorac Cardiovasc Surg 2000; 120:632–9.

42. Steinmetz J, Christensen KB, Lund T, et al, ISPOCD Group. Long-term consequences of postoperative cognitive dysfunction. Anesthesiology 2009;110(3): 548–55. PMID: 19225398.

Management of Common Postoperative Complications

Delirium

Houman Javedan, MD*, Samir Tulebaev, MD

KEYWORDS

- Delirium • Management • Prevention • Complications • Antipsychotics

KEY POINTS

- Delirium is a common postoperative surgical complication.
- The cause of delirium is frequently multifactorial.
- Prevention is better than treatment.
- Look for the highest-yield interventions at each stage.
- Differentiate treating symptoms from treating the cause(s).

INTRODUCTION

Delirium is a common postoperative complication that increases both mortality and morbidity in elderly patients.[1,2] Delirium on its own has been associated with higher in-hospital mortality (4%–17%)[1,3,4] and postdischarge mortality (22.7-month mortality hazard ratio, 1.95).[2] In orthopedic patients the prevalence and incidence are 17% and 12% to 51% respectively.[5] Addressing delirium involves prevention, surveillance, and early treatment in order to mitigate the detrimental effects on vulnerable elderly patients with hip fractures.

DIAGNOSIS

Delirium is a diagnostic concept that evolved over many years from astute clinical observations that somatic illnesses cause distinct abnormalities in brain function. After years of uncertain terminology, it was eventually codified in the Diagnostic and Statistical Manual of Mental Disorders (DSM).[6] In the first edition the syndrome was under the heading acute brain syndrome associated with various insults, then organic brain syndrome, and eventually becoming delirium with specific diagnostic criteria in the revised third edition of the DSM (DSM-III-R).[7–9] Delirium remains a clinical diagnosis, therefore the reference standard for delirium is a psychiatric evaluation in accordance

Division of Aging, Brigham and Women's Hospital, 1620 Tremont Street, Boston, MA 02120, USA
* Corresponding author.
E-mail address: hjavedan@partners.org

Clin Geriatr Med 30 (2014) 271–278
http://dx.doi.org/10.1016/j.cger.2014.01.015
0749-0690/14/$ – see front matter © 2014 Elsevier Inc. All rights reserved.

with evolving DSM criteria. The current gold standard is DSM-V, which provides the following diagnostic criteria[10]:

1. A disturbance in attention (ie, reduced ability to direct, focus, sustain, and shift attention) and awareness (reduced orientation to the environment).
2. The disturbance develops over a short period of time (usually hours to a few days), represents a change from baseline attention and awareness, and tends to fluctuate in severity during the course of a day.
3. An additional disturbance in cognition (eg, memory deficit, disorientation, language, visuospatial ability, or perception).
4. The disturbances in criteria 1 and 3 are not better explained by another preexisting, established, or evolving neurocognitive disorder and do not occur in the context of a severely reduced level of arousal, such as coma.
5. There is evidence from the history, physical examination, or laboratory findings that the disturbance is a direct physiologic consequence of another medical condition, substance intoxication or withdrawal (ie, caused by a drug of abuse or a medication), or exposure to a toxin, or has multiple causes.

However, a complete psychiatric evaluation is labor intensive. In one study, the psychiatric evaluation took a mean of 90 minutes.[11] Moreover, psychiatric resources are scarce in comparison with the number of patients with delirium. As the medical community increasingly recognized the impact of delirium on morbidity, mortality, functional status, and length of hospital stay, there was a need for more efficient instruments to diagnose delirium. This need led to a proliferation of screening instruments, with more than 24 of them described in published studies.[6] One of the most widely used clinical algorithms is the confusion assessment method (CAM), which was developed from criteria based on DSM-III-R.[11] It has been used in 4000 published studies, extensively validated, and has sensitivity of 94%, specificity of 89%, and high reliability compared with expert psychiatric evaluation.[6]

CAM has been validated in surgical patients.[1] It consists of the following criteria:

1. Acute onset and fluctuating course
2. Inattention
3. Disorganized thinking
4. Altered level of consciousness

For the diagnosis of delirium, the presence of the first 2 criteria is required in addition to either criterion 3 or 4.[11] Once there are at least 3 criteria, the diagnosis of delirium is established.

Acute onset and fluctuating course are historical data that are obtained from caregivers or health care professionals. Therefore, knowledge of baseline cognitive status is important. Sometimes detailed history is not available during initial evaluation, and diagnosis of delirium is presumed. However, it underscores that the clinician should make every effort to contact the primary caregiver or the patient's known health professionals. Fluctuating course is also assessed during daily clinical evaluations in the postoperative period.

Complex attention is one of the neurocognitive domains and describes ability to focus, sustain, and divide and shift attention.[10] It also describes processing speed. Careful clinical observation during the interview is important to assess an individual's attention. Is the patient easily distractible, do questions need to be repeated because the patient's attention wanders, or does the patient perseverate with an answer to a previous question rather than appropriately shift attention?[11] However, simple observation is not enough. Formal evaluation of attention must be done to decrease interobserver variability. A task, such as naming days of the week backwards or months of the year backwards, can serve as tests of attention.[6] Other commonly used methods are forward digit span (4 or more random digits) or serial sevens.[6] Attention can be preserved in dementia and the test should be congruent to the person's cognitive ability.

Disorganized thinking is characterized by illogical flows of ideas, irrelevant or rambling conversation, and frequent switches from one topic to another.[10] Disorganized thinking is likely driven in part by disturbances of complex attention and also perceptual abnormalities that might include misinterpretations, illusions, and hallucinations in one or more sensory modalities.[10] There is no formal scale to quantify disorganized thinking and it is mostly based on the experience of the clinician.

In addition, altered level of consciousness is an observer's impression of whether a patient looked alert (normal), vigilant (hyperalert), lethargic (drowsy, easily aroused), stuporous (difficult to arouse), or comatose.[11] Altered level of consciousness may be formally assessed using the Richmond Agitation and Sedation Scale, which is a validated measure.[12] In addition, there are 3 variants of delirium based on psychomotor activity and level of consciousness.[10] Hyperactive delirium is easily diagnosed and is what most clinician mean when they mention delirium. It is characterized by psychomotor agitation and disturbed emotional state with patients calling out, screaming, cursing, muttering, moaning, or making other sounds. Psychomotor agitation may significantly interfere with patient care and safety, as well as the safety of health care personnel, and is a frequent reason for indiscriminate administration of antipsychotic medications or sedatives. The less recognized form of delirium is the hypoactive variant with decreased level of consciousness and apathy; however, the hypoactive form has been shown to carry poorer prognosis.[13] In addition, delirium may fluctuate between hyperactive and hypoactive forms, which is referred to a mixed delirium.

MANAGEMENT GOALS

- Prevent delirium
- Minimize length of delirium
- Minimize severity of delirium

NONPHARMACOLOGIC STRATEGIES

Nonpharmacologic measures have always been a foundation of delirium management. Pharmacologic management consisting of antipsychotic medications is mostly directed toward agitation, which is a symptom of hyperactive delirium or mixed delirium. Antipsychotic medications and benzodiazepines do not treat underlying causes of delirium and, in the case of benzodiazepines, may trigger delirium. In contrast, nonpharmacologic management attempts to address the multifactorial nature of delirium by early identification and elimination of risk factors.

One of the earliest landmark multicomponent intervention studies conducted on general medical wards, by Inouye and colleagues,[14] focused on 6 components that were chosen because of known association with the risk of delirium and amenability to treatment. The interventions were directed toward management of:

- Cognitive impairment
- Sleep deprivation
- Immobility
- Visual impairment
- Hearing impairment
- Dehydration

This strategy was able to decrease incidence of delirium by 40% and duration by 35%, but not the severity or recurrence rates.[14] It became known as the Hospital Elder Life Program (HELP) and was disseminated in the United States and abroad with some variations tailored to individual institutions. HELP required an interdisciplinary team and staff dedicated to implementation of the program.

Another landmark study, by Marcantonio and colleagues,[18] used proactive geriatric consultation on patients with hip fracture that also targeted multiple components. Interventions included:

- Adequate oxygen delivery
- Correcting fluid and electrolyte balance
- Providing adequate nutritional intake
- Identification and elimination of medications that could potentially trigger delirium
- Early mobility
- Appropriate environmental stimuli

This study showed reduction of the incidence of delirium by one-third and reduction of the severity of delirium by one-half.[6]

Reorganization of medical care, appropriate resource allocation, and education of staff with the focus on delirium prevention has also been shown to reduce duration of delirium and mortality in delirious patients.[15] The nonpharmacologic measures are usually done by trained medical staff, but even intervention by family members who have been briefly educated about some aspects of delirium has been shown to be effective.[16] Most studies in nonpharmacologic management used different variations and combinations of the following strategies:

- Removal of deliriogenic medications, such as:
  ○ Antihistamines (eg, diphenhydramine)
  ○ Antiemetics that affect dopamine (eg, metoclopramide, prochlorperazine)
  ○ Benzodiazepines (eg, lorazepam, clonazepam)
  ○ Antimuscarinics (eg, oxybutynin)
  ○ Muscle relaxants (eg, baclofen)
- Cognitive stimulation
  ○ Frequent reorientation
  ○ Provision of clocks, calendars; name of providers prominently displayed
  ○ Family present at bedside
- Improving sensory impairment
  ○ Provide glasses
  ○ Provide hearing aids
  ○ Provide dentures
- Mobility
  ○ Out of bed for meals
  ○ Reducing tethers (eg, telemetry, catheters, feeding tubes)
  ○ Early physical therapy
- Correction of metabolic abnormalities
  ○ Maintain adequate hydration (encourage oral intake)
- Education of staff, with focus on recognition of delirium and implementation of preventive measures
- Evaluating for other acute issues (eg, infection, hypoxia, urinary retention)

In the context of delirium, it is hard to separate preventive measures from nonpharmacologic treatment. Once delirium occurs, preventive measures become treatment modalities because of the multifactorial nature of delirium and the incomplete understanding of the pathophysiology of delirium.[17] A nonpharmacologic approach requires a multidisciplinary team that simultaneously attempts to address and manage multiple risk factors for delirium. It can only be implemented through education, reallocation of resources, and reorganization of care for elderly adults by all those involved.

Controversies

- Blood transfusion to a hemoglobin of 10 g/dl in a multicomponent intervention was helpful[18] but, in isolation, did not show any improvement.[19] Furthermore, increased delirium was observed with intraoperative blood transfusions greater than 1000 mL red blood cells.[20]

PHARMACOLOGIC STRATEGIES

The multifactorial nature of delirium makes medications another tool to help with addressing many of the driving and exacerbating factors. Pharmaceutical interventions are traditionally thought of as antipsychotics. Antipsychotics in delirium do not treat the underlying cause but address the symptoms. For example, agitation is a symptom that can escalate to a level that is detrimental to the patient and dangerous to caregivers. Treating pain and sleep deprivation with an appropriate medication addresses one of the underlying causes and can be more effective than antipsychotics.

As a result, the medication, timing, and dosing of the medication need to be tailored to the specific patient with constant monitoring and adjustment because all of these medications carry risks and side effects. At present, data for long-term risks of antipsychotics are well established, but smaller retrospective studies have shown that use in short-term acute circumstances is likely to be safe.[21,22]

- Treating causes
  - Pain
    - Standing acetaminophen addresses pain and reduces opiate requirement[23,24]
    - Dosing of opiates is important because too much can cause delirium, but poor pain control can also cause delirium[25-27]
    - A retrospective study in hip fractures highlights the importance of 24-hour opiate dosing (0.15 mg/kg intravenous [IV] morphine in 24 hours was not associated with delirium)[28]
  - Sleep deprivation
    - Consider trazodone 25 mg at bedtime, as needed[29]
    - Consider quetiapine 12.5 to 25 mg at bedtime if agitation of delirium also needs to be treated
    - Avoid use of diphenhydramine or benzodiazepines
- Treating symptoms (**Table 1**)[30]
  - Agitation/hallucinations
    - Haloperidol
      - Pros: oldest and most accumulated historical evidence, IV/intramuscular (IM) and oral availability
      - Cons: QT prolongation, documented torsades de pointes with IV administration, extrapyramidal symptoms greater than 4.5 mg daily
    - Quetiapine
      - Pros: most sedating; helpful for sleep, some evidence of safety in Lewy body dementia and Parkinson dementia
      - Cons: no IV/IM/sublingual (SL) form, QT prolongation

Table 1 Dosing regimens	
Drug	**Dosage**
Haloperidol	0.25–1.0 mg PO/IM to be repeated every 30–60 min if needed. Maximum dose of 3.0 mg in 24 h to minimize side effects[34]
Risperidone	0.25–0.5 mg PO; repeat every 30–60 min if needed
Quetiapine	12.5–50 mg PO; repeat every 30–60 min if needed. Consider maximum dose of 175 mg/d[35]
Olanzapine	2.5–5.0 mg PO/SL/IM; repeat every 30–60 min if needed
Lorazepam[a]	0.25 mg-1.0 mg PO/IM repeat every 30–60 min if needed

Abbreviation: PO, by mouth.

[a] The authors recommend this as a choice of last resort because no good evidence supports use in elderly. If a benzodiazepine must be used, recommend shorter acting formulations with no active metabolites.

- Olanzapine
  - Pros: SL/IM form
  - Cons: most anticholinergic, QT prolongation
- Lorazepam
  - Pros: not QT prolonging, benzodiazepine without active metabolites
  - Cons: can induce delirium, causes cognitive impairment, increases risk of falls, no good evidence to support its use in non–alcohol-associated delirium

Maximal Effective Dose

Haloperidol has been in use the longest and studies have shown that doses of more than 3.0 mg increase medication side effects without significant added benefit to duration or severity of delirium.

There is not enough evidence to definitively identify the maximal effective dose in other antipsychotic medications. However, from geriatric pharmacokinetic principles it is best to use the least effective dose.

Timing

The authors recommend evaluating the pattern of agitation throughout the day and giving a low dose of medication at the beginning of the agitation before it escalates. This method prevents escalation to a point at which even maximum dosing is ineffective and allows the overall 24-hour dosing to stay at a minimum.

Cholinesterase Inhibitors

- Anticholinesterases have not been effective in treating delirium.[31]

Controversies

- There have been no adequate controlled trials in non–alcohol-withdrawal delirium to support use of benzodiazepines.[32]
- One meta-analysis supports possible perioperative prophylactic use of antipsychotics.[33]

SUMMARY/DISCUSSION

Delirium can be addressed with nonpharmacologic and pharmacologic interventions that prevent and treat delirium with its associated detrimental effects on vulnerable elderly patients with hip fractures. However, the multifactorial nature of delirium demands that each patient be assessed and a tailored series of interventions be implemented. Furthermore, continued monitoring and adjustment by the health care team throughout the perioperative stay addresses the continued complexity of the syndrome.

REFERENCES

1. Marcantonio ER, Goldman L, Mangione CM, et al. A clinical prediction rule for delirium after elective noncardiac surgery. JAMA 1994;271(2):134–9.
2. Witlox J, Eurelings LS, de Jonghe JF, et al. Delirium in elderly patients and the risk of postdischarge mortality, institutionalization, and dementia: a meta-analysis. JAMA 2010;304(4):443–51.
3. Rudolph JL, Jones RN, Rasmussen LS, et al. Independent vascular and cognitive risk factors for postoperative delirium. Am J Med 2007;120:807–13.
4. Norkiene I, Ringaitiene D, Misiuriene I, et al. Incidence and precipitating factors of delirium after coronary artery bypass grafting. Scand Cardiovasc J 2007;41:180–5.
5. Inouye SK, Westendorp RG, Saczynski JS. Delirium in elderly people. Lancet 2013. http://dx.doi.org/10.1016/S0140-6736(13)60688-1.
6. Lipowski ZJ. Delirium, clouding of consciousness and confusion. J Nerv Ment Dis 1967;145(3):227–55.
7. American Psychiatric Association Committee on Nomenclature and Statistics. Mental disorders; diagnostic and statistical manual. Washington, DC: American Psychiatric Association; 1952.
8. American Psychiatric Association Committee on Nomenclature and Statistics. Diagnostic and statistical manual of mental disorders. 2d edition. Washington, DC: American Psychiatric Association; 1968.
9. American Psychiatric Association, American Psychiatric Association Work Group to Revise DSM-III. Diagnostic and statistical manual of mental disorders: DSM-III-R. 3rd edition. Washington, DC: American Psychiatric Association; 1987.
10. American Psychiatric Association, DSM-5 Task Force. Diagnostic and statistical manual of mental disorders: DSM-5. 5th edition. Washington, DC: American Psychiatric Association; 2013.
11. Inouye SK, van Dyck CH, Alessi CA, et al. Clarifying confusion: the confusion assessment method. A new method for detection of delirium. Ann Intern Med 1990;113(12):941–8.
12. Ely EW, Truman B, Shintani A, et al. Monitoring sedation status over time in ICU patients: reliability and validity of the Richmond Agitation-Sedation Scale (RASS). JAMA 2003;289(22):2983–91.
13. Meagher DJ, Leonard M, Donnelly S, et al. A longitudinal study of motor subtypes in delirium: relationship with other phenomenology, etiology, medication exposure and prognosis. J Psychosom Res 2011;71(6):395–403.
14. Inouye SK, Bogardus ST Jr, Charpentier PA, et al. A multicomponent intervention to prevent delirium in hospitalized older patients. N Engl J Med 1999;340(9): 669–76.
15. Lundstrom M, Edlund A, Karlsson S, et al. A multifactorial intervention program reduces the duration of delirium, length of hospitalization, and mortality in delirious patients. J Am Geriatr Soc 2005;53(4):622–8.
16. Martinez FT, Tobar C, Beddings CI, et al. Preventing delirium in an acute hospital using a non-pharmacological intervention. Age Ageing 2012;41(5):629–34.
17. Inouye SK. Delirium in older persons. N Engl J Med 2006;354(11):1157–65.

18. Marcantonio ER, Flacker JM, Wright RJ, et al. Reducing delirium after hip fracture: a randomized trial. J Am Geriatr Soc 2001;49(5):516–22.
19. Gruber-Baldini AL, Marcantonio E, Orwig D, et al. Delirium outcomes in a randomized trial of blood transfusion thresholds in hospitalized older adults with hip fracture. J Am Geriatr Soc 2013;61(8):1286–95.
20. Behrends M, DePalma G, Sands L, et al. Association between intraoperative blood transfusions and early postoperative delirium in older adults. J Am Geriatr Soc 2013;61(3):365–70.
21. Mittal V, Kurup L, Williamson D, et al. Risk of cerebrovascular adverse events and death in elderly patients with dementia when treated with antipsychotic medications: a literature review of evidence. Am J Alzheimers Dis Other Demen 2011; 26(1):10–28.
22. Hatta K, Kishi Y, Wada K, et al. Antipsychotics for delirium in the general hospital setting in consecutive 2453 inpatients: a prospective observational study. Int J Geriatr Psychiatry 2013. http://dx.doi.org/10.1002/gps.3999.
23. Available at: http://www.who.int/cancer/palliative/painladder/en/. Accessed October 15, 2013.
24. Tsang KS, Page J, Mackenney P. Can intravenous paracetamol reduce opioid use in preoperative hip fracture patients? Orthopedics 2013;36(Suppl 2):20–4. http://dx.doi.org/10.3928/01477447-20130122-53.
25. Morrison RS, Magaziner J, Gilbert M, et al. Relationship between pain and opioid analgesics on the development of delirium following hip fracture. J Gerontol A Biol Sci Med Sci 2003;58A:76–81.
26. Marcantonio ER, Juarez G, Goldman L, et al. The relationship of postoperative delirium with psychoactive medications. JAMA 1994;272:1518–22.
27. Marino J, Russo J, Kenny M, et al. Continuous lumbar plexus block for postoperative pain control after total hip arthroplasty. A randomized controlled trial. J Bone Joint Surg Am 2009;91:29–37.
28. Sieber FE, Mears S, Lee H, et al. Postoperative opioid consumption and its relationship to cognitive function in older adults with hip fracture. J Am Geriatr Soc 2011;59(12):2256–62.
29. Miura LN, DiPiero AR, Homer LD. Effects of a geriatrician-led hip fracture program: improvements in clinical and economic outcomes. J Am Geriatr Soc 2009;57(1):159–67.
30. Mittal V, Muralee S, Williamson D, et al. Review: delirium in the elderly: a comprehensive review. Am J Alzheimers Dis Other Demen 2011;26(2):97–109.
31. Overshott R, Karim S, Burns A. Cholinesterase inhibitors for delirium. Cochrane Database Syst Rev 2008;(1):CD005317.
32. Lonergan E, Luxenberg J, Areosa Sastre A. Benzodiazepines for delirium. Cochrane Database Syst Rev 2009;(4):CD006379.
33. Teslyar P, Stock VM, Wilk CM, et al. Prophylaxis with antipsychotic medication reduces the risk of post-operative delirium in elderly patients: a meta-analysis. Psychosomatics 2013;54(2):124–31.
34. Lonergan E, Britton AM, Luxenberg J, et al. Antipsychotics for delirium. Cochrane Database Syst Rev 2007;(2):CD005594.
35. Tahir TA, Eeles E, Karapareddy V, et al. A randomized controlled trial of quetiapine versus placebo in the treatment of delirium. J Psychosom Res 2010;69(5): 485–90.

Management of Postoperative Complications: Anemia

Laura Rees Willett, MD[a],*, Jeffrey L. Carson, MD[b],*

KEYWORDS

- Anemia • Hip fracture • Blood transfusion

KEY POINTS

- Anemia is extremely common following hip fracture surgery.
- Evaluation should include important comorbidities, symptoms, and vital signs in addition to hemoglobin level.
- Consistent evidence from randomized trials favors a restrictive transfusion strategy, leading to utilization of less blood with at least equivalent clinical outcomes.
- The optimal restrictive transfusion threshold is unknown, but there is a preponderance of published experience using a hemoglobin threshold of 8 g/dL in the elderly hip fracture population.
- The most common serious risk of transfusion in this population is circulatory overload.
- Further work is needed to define the optimal transfusion threshold for general postoperative elderly patients, as well as those with comorbid acute coronary syndrome or chronic kidney disease.

INTRODUCTION

Anemia is extremely common following hip fracture. More than 80% of patients have a hemoglobin concentration less than 11 g/dL.[1] Most hip fracture patients are elderly and suffer from multiple comorbidities. In decades past, standard postoperative practice was to maintain hemoglobin levels of greater than 10 g/dL, especially in elderly patients or those with coexisting cardiovascular disease. Over the past several years, new data from randomized trials evaluating thresholds for transfusion have become available, resulting in new guidelines,[2] which recommend lower, or more restrictive, hemoglobin thresholds than those used in the past. Randomized trials of transfusion therapy were necessary because the results of observational studies are confounded by severity of underlying illness.[3]

[a] Division of Education, Rutgers Robert Wood Johnson Medical School, 1 RWJ Place, MEB-486, New Brunswick, NJ 08903, USA; [b] Division of General Internal Medicine, Rutgers Robert Wood Johnson Medical School, 125 Paterson Street, New Brunswick, NJ 08901, USA
* Corresponding authors.
E-mail addresses: willetlr@rwjms.rutgers.edu; jeffrey.carson@rutgers.edu

Clin Geriatr Med 30 (2014) 279–284
http://dx.doi.org/10.1016/j.cger.2014.01.006
0749-0690/14/$ – see front matter © 2014 Elsevier Inc. All rights reserved.

PATIENT EVALUATION

In addition to the current hemoglobin level, the following should be assessed:

- Preinjury hemoglobin level
- Cardiac and renal comorbid conditions
- Signs of continuing active bleeding
- Cardiovascular symptoms
- Vital signs
- Coagulation abnormalities

Although unproven, these factors could play a role in choosing a transfusion threshold, deciding to transfuse despite a hemoglobin level over the threshold, or considering alternative or adjunctive therapies for anemia.

MANAGEMENT GOALS

The randomized controlled trials of transfusion compare the outcomes of patients randomized to more restrictive (ie, lower) transfusion thresholds to those assigned more liberal or traditional thresholds. **Table 1** summarizes the data from selected large trials of transfusion thresholds in adults. The largest trial (FOCUS) is of greatest applicability, because it included adult hip fracture patients with a hemoglobin level less than 10 g/dL.[4] All patients had either cardiovascular disease or multiple cardiac risk factors. Patients (n = 2016) with an average age of 82 years were randomized to a restrictive hemoglobin threshold of 8 g/dL or a liberal threshold of 10 g/dL. The protocol allowed for patients to be transfused at a hemoglobin level higher than their assigned threshold in the event of serious symptoms attributed to anemia, including chest pain due to cardiac ischemia, congestive heart failure, or hypotension or tachycardia unresponsive to fluid challenge. Patients randomized to the restrictive threshold (vs the liberal threshold)

- Received a median of 0 units (vs 2 units) of blood
- Had a hemoglobin before transfusion of 7.9 g/dL (vs 9.2 g/dL)
- Experienced a 30-day mortality of 4.3% (vs 5.2%)
- Experienced a 60-day rate of inability to walk unassisted of 28.1% (vs 27.6%)

No important clinical outcomes were significantly different between the 2 groups. Importantly, about one-fifth of patients in the restrictive group received transfusion despite having a hemoglobin level greater than 8 g/dL, due to symptoms, signs, or protocol violations. The most common indication for such a transfusion was hypotension or tachycardia unresponsive to fluid replacement.

The other large trials summarized in **Table 1**[5–8] are less applicable to the typical after-hip fracture population. Each of these had a patient population with an average age between 58 and 70 years and varying clinical scenarios. However, all of these trials as well as a recent Cochrane review[9] and guidelines[2] reached the same overall conclusion: a restrictive threshold is preferable to the more traditional liberal threshold. Although exposing patients to the lower risk and lower cost of fewer transfusions, the restrictive strategy achieves similar or even improved[8] clinical outcomes.

Several caveats come along with this conclusion. Important subgroups of patients are not well represented in these trials:

- Acute coronary syndrome (generally excluded)
- Chronic kidney disease (11% or fewer)

Further data will be needed to assess the transfusion needs of these populations.[10,11] The rates of transfusion at hemoglobin levels higher than the assigned

Table 1
Selected large randomized trials of restrictive versus liberal transfusion thresholds in adults

Trial Setting	Number of Patients	Average Age (y)	Cardiac Disease (%)	Restrictive vs Liberal Threshold Hemoglobin (g/dL)	Restrictive Group Transfused When Over Threshold Hemoglobin (%)	Mortality
Postcardiac surgery (TRACS)[6]	502	59	100	8.0 vs 10.0	1.6 with symptoms	At 30 d R = 6% L = 5% (NS)
Postelective joint replacement (So-Osman)[7]	603	70	Not available (69 high risk)	Risk-tailored threshold vs local standard	Not available	At 14 d R = 0% L = 1% (NS)
Intensive care (TRICC)[5]	836	58	26	7.0 vs 10.0	1.4	At 30 d R = 19% L = 23% (NS)
Acute upper gastrointestinal bleed (Villanueva)[8]	921	65	Not available	7.0 vs 9.0	9 without symptoms 8 with symptoms	At 45 d R = 5% L = 9% (P = .02)
After-hip fracture (FOCUS)[4]	2016	82	40	8.0 vs 10.0	6 without symptoms >12 with symptoms	At 30 d R = 4% L = 5% (NS)

Abbreviations: L, liberal group; NS, not statistically significant; R, restrictive group.

threshold, for symptoms or protocol violation, are quite different in different trials. It is unclear whether transfusion in these circumstances acted as an important safety mechanism or simply led to unnecessary blood use. Most importantly, the optimal transfusion threshold remains unknown. The trials with the largest numbers of elderly hip fracture and cardiac patients chose a restrictive threshold of 8 g/dL, whereas the trials with patients in the intensive care unit or with acute gastrointestinal bleeding chose a restrictive threshold of 7 g/dL. It is possible that the optimal threshold might be lower still.

Nontransfusion management of anemia will be mentioned only briefly here. Clearly, patients with substantial premorbid anemia, coagulopathies, or severe ongoing bleeding will need additional evaluation and therapy. Anticoagulant therapy is common in the elderly. Ongoing bleeding related to warfarin may require vitamin K and fresh-frozen plasma or 4-factor prothrombin complex administration.[12] Prothrombin complex may be preferred to plasma therapy, but current recommendations are based on small studies, which were underpowered to assess important clinical outcomes. Also, prothrombin complex may be unavailable in many hospital pharmacies. Other coagulopathies will likely require hematologic consultation. If hip fracture occurs in a severe multiple trauma setting, other therapies such as autologous blood salvage, tranexamic acid,[13] and massive transfusion protocols may be needed and are beyond the scope of this article.[14]

RISKS OF TRANSFUSION

The risks of transfusion are summarized in **Table 2**. The risk of transfusion causing an infection with known agents, which was quite high in decades past, is currently miniscule. Noninfectious risks of transfusion occur at much higher rates. Transfusion-associated circulatory overload (TACO) is particularly common, occurring in 1% to 4% of transfusions.[15–17] Risk factors include chronic kidney disease and congestive heart failure,[15,18] both of which are common in elderly patients with hip fracture.[1] The other major causes of red blood cell transfusion–associated mortality are acute hemolysis, usually due to the infusion of incompatible blood, and transfusion-related acute lung injury (TRALI).[19] TRALI is most commonly associated with infusion of plasma from parous female donors; its incidence may be decreased with changes in blood-banking practice.[16,20] For the typical hip fracture patient, transfusion-associated circulatory overload is by far the most common serious adverse outcome related to transfusion. It is usually easily treated with diuresis, but may cause further morbidity or occasional mortality.

Table 2 Approximate risks of transfusion	
Transfusion-Associated Outcome	**Approximate Risk**
HIV infection	<1 in 1 million
Hepatitis C infection	<1 in 1 million
Hepatitis B infection	<1 in 200,000
Severe hemolytic reaction	<1 in 100,000
TRALI	<1 in 10,000 (estimates quite variable)
Transfusion-associated circulatory overload	1%–4%
Minor febrile reactions	1%–2%

Data from Refs.[2,15,17,20–22]

EVALUATION AND ADJUSTMENT

Patients will require frequent reassessment, not just of their hemoglobin level but also of their clinical status. It may be particularly challenging to assess whether shortness of breath, chest pain, hypotension, and tachycardia are due to blood loss or its treatments. For example, dyspnea occurring within a few hours after transfusion could be due to circulatory overload or TRALI. Alternatively, it could be a manifestation of severe anemia causing ischemia, an unrelated complication such as pulmonary embolism, or an underlying comorbid condition. Many patients in the randomized trials received transfusion for such signs and symptoms, despite hemoglobin levels higher than their assigned restrictive threshold. It is unclear if this practice is a useful addition to their care.

SUMMARY

Anemia is an exceptionally common complication of hip fracture and repair. Current guidelines recommend utilization of a more restrictive transfusion strategy in postoperative patients.[2] In the typical hip fracture patient, elderly and often with cardiovascular comorbidities, there is much more published experience establishing the safety of a hemoglobin threshold of 8 g/dL than any alternative restrictive threshold. In the absence of active ongoing bleeding, hypotension or tachycardia unresponsive to fluids, or cardiac decompensation thought to be secondary to anemia, clinicians should avoid transfusing patients with hemoglobin levels greater than 8 g/dL. Use of a lower threshold diminishes serious transfusion risks, the most common of which is circulatory overload. Future work may allow the adoption of even lower transfusion thresholds and elucidate whether important subgroups of patients, such as those with acute coronary syndrome or chronic kidney disease, would be better served by thresholds different from those of the general after-hip fracture population.

REFERENCES

1. Carson JL, Duff A, Berlin JA, et al. Perioperative blood transfusion and postoperative mortality. J Am Med Assoc 1998;279(3):199–205.
2. Carson JL, Grossman BJ, Kleinman S, et al. Red blood cell transfusion: a clinical practice guideline from the AABB*. Ann Intern Med 2012;157(1):49–58.
3. Carson JL, Hebert PC. Here we go again-blood transfusion kills patients?: comment on "Association of blood transfusion with increased mortality in myocardial infarction: a meta-analysis and diversity-adjusted study sequential analysis". JAMA Intern Med 2013;173(2):139–41.
4. Carson JL, Terrin ML, Noveck H, et al. Liberal or restrictive transfusion in high-risk patients after hip surgery. N Engl J Med 2011;365(26):2453–62.
5. Hebert PC, Wells G, Blajchman MA, et al. A multicenter, randomized, controlled clinical trial of transfusion requirements in critical care. Transfusion Requirements in Critical Care Investigators, Canadian Critical Care Trials group. N Engl J Med 1999;340(6):409–17.
6. Hajjar LA, Vincent JL, Galas FR, et al. Transfusion requirements after cardiac surgery: the TRACS randomized controlled trial. JAMA 2010;304(14):1559–67.
7. So-Osman C, Nelissen R, Brand R, et al. The impact of a restrictive transfusion trigger on post-operative complication rate and well-being following elective orthopaedic surgery: a post-hoc analysis of a randomised study. Blood Transfus 2013;11(2):289–95.

8. Villanueva C, Colomo A, Bosch A, et al. Transfusion strategies for acute upper gastrointestinal bleeding. N Engl J Med 2013;368(1):11–21.
9. Carson JL, Carless PA, Hebert PC. Transfusion thresholds and other strategies for guiding allogeneic red blood cell transfusion. Cochrane Database Syst Rev 2012;(4):CD002042.
10. Cooper HA, Rao SV, Greenberg MD, et al. Conservative versus liberal red cell transfusion in acute myocardial infarction (the CRIT Randomized Pilot Study). Am J Cardiol 2011;108(8):1108–11.
11. Carson JL, Brooks MM, Abbott JD, et al. Liberal versus restrictive transfusion thresholds for patients with symptomatic coronary artery disease. Am Heart J 2013;165(6):964–71.e1.
12. Holbrook A, Schulman S, Witt DM, et al. Evidence-based management of antico-agulant therapy: antithrombotic therapy and Prevention of Thrombosis, 9th ed: American College of Chest Physicians evidence-based clinical practice guide-lines. Chest 2012;141(Suppl 2):e152S–84S.
13. Roberts I, Shakur H, Afolabi A, et al. The importance of early treatment with tra-nexamic acid in bleeding trauma patients: an exploratory analysis of the CRASH-2 randomised controlled trial. Lancet 2011;377(9771):1096–101, 1101.e1–2.
14. Holcomb JB. PROPPR—Pragmatic, randomized optimal platelet and plasma ra-tios. 2012. Available at: http://cetir-tmc.org/research/proppr. Accessed November 30, 2012.
15. Li G, Rachmale S, Kojicic M, et al. Incidence and transfusion risk factors for transfusion-associated circulatory overload among medical intensive care unit patients. Transfusion 2011;51(2):338–43.
16. Gajic O, Rana R, Winters JL, et al. Transfusion-related acute lung injury in the crit-ically ill: prospective nested case-control study. Am J Respir Crit Care Med 2007; 176(9):886–91.
17. Bierbaum BE, Callaghan JJ, Galante JO, et al. An analysis of blood management in patients having a total hip or knee arthroplasty. J Bone Joint Surg Am 1999; 81(1):2–10.
18. Murphy EL, Kwaan N, Looney MR, et al. Risk factors and outcomes in transfusion-associated circulatory overload. Am J Med 2013;126(4):357.e29–38.
19. Fatalities reported to FDA following blood collection and transfusion: Annual Summary for fiscal year 2010. 2011. Available at: http://www.fda.gov/biologicsbloodvaccines/safetyavailability/reportaproblem/transfusiondonation fatalities/ucm254802.htm. Accessed December 13, 2011.
20. Toy P, Gajic O, Bacchetti P, et al. Transfusion related acute lung injury: incidence and risk factors. Blood 2011;119(7):1757–67.
21. Zou S, Dorsey KA, Notari EP, et al. Prevalence, incidence, and residual risk of hu-man immunodeficiency virus and hepatitis C virus infections among United States blood donors since the introduction of nucleic acid testing. Transfusion 2010;50(7):1495–504.
22. Popovsky MA. Transfusion-associated circulatory overload: the plot thickens. Transfusion 2009;49(1):2–4.

Venous Thromboembolism and Postoperative Management of Anticoagulation

Susan M. Friedman, MD, MPH*, Joshua D. Uy, MD

KEYWORDS

- Deep venous thrombosis • Pulmonary embolism • Prevention

KEY POINTS

- The incidence of venous thromboembolism (VTE) after fracture repair has decreased over time, as a result of improved surgical technique and earlier mobilization.
- Hip fracture patients are considered to be in the highest risk category for VTE.
- All hip fracture patients should receive VTE prophylaxis, which may include pharmacologic and nonpharmacologic approaches.
- There are many pharmacologic options for VTE prophylaxis, and the choice should be based on each patient's characteristics and circumstances.
- Optimizing VTE prophylaxis requires consideration of both the risk of thromboembolism and bleeding risk.

INTRODUCTION/EPIDEMIOLOGY

The reported risk of venous thromboembolism (VTE) following hip fracture repair is substantial, but varies depending on how it was measured and when the study was completed. Earlier studies, which were placebo-controlled, showed that the incidence of VTE without prophylaxis ranged from 46% to 75%[1–4]; however, many of these cases were determined through screening and were asymptomatic. The incidence of proximal deep venous thrombosis (DVT) is 27% without prophylaxis,[5] and the rate of fatal pulmonary embolism (PE) has been estimated previously at 1.9%.[6] VTE is the second most common complication following hip fracture surgery.[7] Because of this, the American College of Chest Physicians (ACCP) puts hip fracture patients in the highest risk group.[8]

The incidence of VTE has decreased over time, as a result of improved surgical techniques, reductions in time to surgery, and earlier mobilization. Still, without

Department of Medicine, Division of Geriatrics, University of Rochester School of Medicine and Dentistry, 1000 South Avenue, Box 58, Rochester, NY 14620, USA
* Corresponding author.
E-mail address: susan_friedman@URMC.rochester.edu

Clin Geriatr Med 30 (2014) 285–291
http://dx.doi.org/10.1016/j.cger.2014.01.007
0749-0690/14/$ – see front matter © 2014 Elsevier Inc. All rights reserved.

prophylaxis, current estimates for symptomatic VTE are 4.3% within 35 days of surgery, with symptomatic DVT and PE incidence of 1.8% and 1%, respectively, in the first 10 to 14 days following surgery.[9] With low molecular weight heparin (LMWH) treatment for 35 days, the incidence of symptomatic VTE is reduced to 1.8% (ie, a number needed to treat [NNT] of 40).

The rationale for thromboprophylaxis is multifold.[8] As described previously, VTE following hip fracture surgery is common, and usually silent. Screening patients who are at risk is neither effective nor cost-effective. Morbidity (including symptomatic DVT and PE and postphlebitic syndrome) and mortality are high. Finally, thromboprophylaxis is effective at preventing symptomatic VTE and fatal PE, and has repeatedly been shown to be cost-effective.

The process of developing VTE starts early. In 1 study, 62% of those who waited 48 hours or more for surgery had venographic evidence of DVT.[10] However, the presentation of symptoms is often delayed until after the initial hospitalization.[11] In 1 study, patients presented with DVT or PE a median of 24 days and 17 days after surgery, respectively.[12]

Hip fracture patients have many reasons for being at risk for VTE. Virchow triad requires the development of at least one of the following: venous stasis, vascular intimal injury, and hypercoagulable state.[13] Following a hip fracture, patients can develop venous stasis due to immobility, as well as from supine positioning for surgery. Vascular intimal injury may occur at the time of the fracture or during surgery. A transient hypercoagulable state may occur from the release of tissue factors.

PATIENT EVALUATION OVERVIEW

The first step in evaluating patients for postoperative anticoagulation is to determine both their risk of VTE as well as their risk of bleeding. In addition to the risks common to all hip fracture patients, other factors increase risk further (**Box 1**). A history of malignancy increases risk of VTE, and metastatic disease confers higher risk than localized disease.[14] Certain malignancies, such as pancreatic and stomach malignancies,

---

Box 1
Risk factors for VTE

Patient characteristics

- Age ≥85
- Malignancy
- Previous VTE
- Obesity
- Congestive heart failure
- Charlson comorbidity score ≥3
- Paralysis
- Presence of an inhibitor deficiency state

Surgical characteristics

- Surgical delay
- Prolonged surgery
- Extracapsular fracture

are associated with particularly high risk of VTE.[15] A history of VTE, especially recent and/or unprovoked, increases risk. Presence of an inhibitor deficiency state, such as protein C, protein S, or antithrombin deficiency, increases the relative risk of VTE recurrence by up to threefold.[16] The type of fracture may be important; in 1 large series, patients with extracapsular fractures (intertrochanteric or subtrochanteric) were twice as likely to develop symptomatic VTE as those with intracapsular fractures.[17]

The risk of bleeding is also important to consider. Different classification schemes have been developed to evaluate bleeding risk.[18–21] The HAS-BLED scale[20] evaluates 1-year risk of major bleeding (defined as intracranial bleeding, bleeding requiring hospitalization, hemoglobin decrease >2 g/L, and/or transfusion) in patients with atrial fibrillation (**Table 1**). Most patients in the study cohort were taking oral anticoagulation medications, but the predictive capability was similar for those who were taking them and those who were not.

Table 1
HAS-BLED score for determining risk of major bleed

	Condition	Points	Total	Bleeds Per 100 Patient-years
H	Hypertension	1	0	1.13
A	Abnormal liver or kidney function	1 or 2	1	1.02
S	Stroke	1	2	1.88
B	Bleeding tendency	1	3	3.74
L	Labile international normalized ratio	1	4	8.70
E	Elderly (≥65)	1	5–9	Insufficient data
D	Drugs or alcohol	1 or 2		

Hypertension is defined as systolic blood pressure >160 mm Hg. Abnormal kidney function is defined as the presence of chronic dialysis or renal transplantation or serum creatinine ≥200 μmol/L. Abnormal liver function is defined as chronic hepatic disease (eg, cirrhosis) or biochemical evidence of significant hepatic derangement (eg, bilirubin >2× the upper limit of normal, in association with aspartate transaminase/alanine transaminase/alkaline phosphatase >3× the upper limit of normal). Bleeding refers to previous bleeding history or predisposition to bleeding (eg, bleeding diathesis, anemia). Labile international normalized ratio refers to unstable/high international normalized ratios or poor time in therapeutic range (eg, <60%). Drugs/alcohol use refers to concomitant use of medications, such as antiplatelet agents and nonsteroidal anti-inflammatory drugs.

PHARMACOLOGIC TREATMENT OPTIONS

The ACCP recommends routine VTE prophylaxis in hip fracture patients.[9] Several options are available, based on the patient's individual characteristics (**Table 2**). LMWH is recommended as the preferred agent (grade of evidence 2B), and should be started at least 12 hours before surgery, or 12 or more hours postoperatively (grade 1B). Aspirin was added to the list of options since 2008,[5] and there was not consensus within the panel. Aspirin has been shown to be effective in reducing VTE risk in hip fracture, but less effective than LMWH.[22]

Because many patients with hip fractures are already taking aspirin and/or clopidogrel for other comorbidities, the benefits of adding another anticoagulant medication need to be weighed against the additional risk of bleeding. A patient taking aspirin in addition to warfarin has almost twice the risk of bleeding, and a patient on both aspirin and clopidogrel in addition to warfarin has 4 times the risk.[23]

The optimal duration of prophylaxis is unclear. One study comparing 1 week versus 4 weeks of anticoagulation following a hip fracture using fondaparinux showed

Table 2	
ACCP 2012 recommendations for VTE pharmacologic prophylaxis	
Agent	**Grade of Evidence**
Low molecular weight heparin	1B
Fondaparinux	1B
Low-dose unfractionated heparin	1B
Warfarin	1B
Aspirin	1B

a reduction of VTE from 35.0% to 1.4%.[24] However, most of these cases were asymptomatic. The reduction in symptomatic VTE was more modest, at 2.7% versus 0.3%, for an NNT of 42. The rate of significant bleeding was 0.6% versus 2.4%, for a number needed to harm (NNH) of 56, although the rate of bleeding requiring reoperation was equivalent in the 2 groups. Because of the ongoing risk for symptomatic VTE after hospital discharge, the ACCP recommends extending thromboprophylaxis for up to 35 days after surgery.[9]

NONPHARMACOLOGIC TREATMENT OPTIONS

The most recent ACCP guidelines include intermittent pneumatic compression devices (IPCDs) as an alternative to pharmacologic prophylaxis (grade 1C).[9] In patients with increased bleeding risk, either IPCDs or no prophylaxis is recommended. Patients who use IPCDs should wear the devices for 18 hours per day. Dual prophylaxis with pharmacologic treatment and an IPCD during hospitalization (grade 2C) is recommended for those who do not place a high value on the undesirable consequences of dual prophylaxis, such as discomfort and the potential for delirium. The NNT for symptomatic VTE is 63.[9] Patients who receive LMWH will sustain 10 fewer symptomatic VTEs per 1000 patients (NNT 100) than those who are treated with IPCDs, at the expense of 10 additional major bleeds per 1000 patients (NNH 100).[9]

In patients who have contraindications to both pharmacologic and mechanical thromboprophylaxis, inferior vena cava (IVC) filter placement is sometimes considered. In a trauma population, the efficacy of PE prevention is high, with an NNT of 24.[25] However, this is balanced by the potential harms, including DVT at the insertion site, IVC occlusion, and filter migration. In a study of orthopedic patients with IVC filters placed for prophylaxis, 5% developed DVT.[26]

Comprehensive VTE prophylaxis includes more than merely deciding what agent to use and how long to use it (**Box 2**). Other interventions, such as minimizing time to surgery, eliminating restraints, and early physical therapy, all help to reduce the time of immobility, thereby reducing venous stasis and limiting VTE risk. A systemic approach

Box 2
Comprehensive VTE prophylaxis includes
• Prompt surgery
• Early weight bearing
• Elimination of restraints
• Delirium prevention
• Pain management

that incorporates these elements, including pharmacologic and nonpharmacologic components, has been associated with low rates of VTE.[27]

TO BRIDGE OR NOT TO BRIDGE

For patients who are admitted on warfarin and will be resuming warfarin after surgery, the question of whether to bridge with a short-acting anticoagulant arises. The goal of bridging is to minimize the time that a patient is not anticoagulated, but this must be balanced by early postsurgical bleeding risks.

The ACCP recommends resuming warfarin 12 to 24 hours after surgery, when hemostasis is achieved (grade 2C).[28] Patients can be divided into high (>10% annual risk of thromboembolism), intermediate (5%–10% annual risk) and low (<5%) risk patients. High-risk patients should receive bridging (grade 2C).[28] These patients include mechanical valve patients with mitral valve, caged-ball, tilting disc prosthesis or stroke or transient ischemic attack (TIA) within 6 months; atrial fibrillation patients with CHADS2 (Congestive heart failure, hypertension, age >75, diabetes, stroke/TIA)[18] score of 5 or 6, stroke or TIA within the past 3 months, or rheumatic heart disease; or VTE patients with VTE within the past 3 months or severe thrombophilia.

Data to support the approach to such patients are few; therefore, an individualized approach is required, based on a patient's specific comorbidities and risks, as well as the surgical procedure. For example, the ACCP lists joint arthroplasty as a procedure at high risk of bleeding during perioperative antithrombotic medication administration, so these risks must also be considered.

The use of bridging must also be considered within the context of the overall plan of care. If bridging would cause a significant delay to rehabilitation placement, the harms of a prolonged hospitalization could outweigh the incremental benefit of bridging a few more days.

SUMMARY

Fragility fracture patients are at high risk of postoperative VTE, both because of their injury and surgery, as well as their underlying frailty. Hip fracture patients are considered to be the highest risk group for VTE. Because of the high incidence and significant consequences of VTE, all patients should receive prophylaxis, which may include both pharmacologic and nonpharmacologic approaches. A comprehensive approach is multifaceted, and includes getting patients to surgery expeditiously and early mobilization. The decision of how to optimize prophylaxis is determined by evaluating the patient's risk of VTE and of bleeding, as well as his or her goals of care.

REFERENCES

1. Powers PJ, Gent M, Jay RM, et al. A randomized trial of less intense postoperative warfarin or aspirin therapy in the prevention of venous thromboembolism after surgery for fractured hip. Arch Intern Med 1989;149(4):771–4.
2. Agnelli G, Cosmi B, Di Filippo P, et al. A randomised, double-blind, placebo-controlled trial of dermatan sulphate for prevention of deep vein thrombosis in hip fracture. Thromb Haemost 1992;67(2):203–8.
3. Hamilton HW, Crawford JS, Gardiner JH, et al. Venous thrombosis in patients with fracture of the upper end of the femur. A phlebographic study of the effect of prophylactic anticoagulation. J Bone Joint Surg Br 1970;52(2):268–89.

4. Rogers PH, Walsh PN, Marder VJ, et al. Controlled trial of low-dose heparin and sulfinpyrazone to prevent venous thromboembolism after operation on the hip. J Bone Joint Surg Am 1978;60(6):758–62.

5. Geerts WH, Bergqvist D, Pineo GF, et al. Prevention of venous thromboembolism: American College of Chest Physicians Evidence-Based Clinical Practice Guidelines (8th edition). Chest 2008;133(Suppl 6):381S–453S.

6. Dahl OE, Caprini JA, Colwell CW Jr, et al. Fatal vascular outcomes following major orthopedic surgery. Thromb Haemost 2005;93(5):860–6.

7. McLaughlin MA, Orosz GM, Magaziner J, et al. Preoperative status and risk of complications in patients with hip fracture. J Gen Intern Med 2006;21(3):219–25.

8. Geerts WH, Pineo GF, Heit JA, et al. Prevention of venous thromboembolism: the seventh ACCP Conference on Antithrombotic and Thrombolytic Therapy. Chest 2004;126(Suppl 3):338S–400S.

9. Falck-Ytter Y, Francis CW, Johanson NA, et al. Prevention of VTE in orthopedic surgery patients: antithrombotic therapy and prevention of thrombosis, 9th edition: American College of Chest Physicians Evidence-Based Clinical Practice Guidelines. Chest 2012;141(Suppl 2):e278S–325S.

10. Zahn HR, Skinner JA, Porteous MJ. The preoperative prevalence of deep vein thrombosis in patients with femoral neck fractures and delayed operation. Injury 1999;30(9):605–7.

11. Hitos K, Fletcher JP. Venous thromboembolism and fractured neck of femur. Thromb Haemost 2005;94(5):991–6.

12. Bjornara BT, Gudmundsen TE, Dahl OE. Frequency and timing of clinical venous thromboembolism after major joint surgery. J Bone Joint Surg Br 2006;88(3): 386–91.

13. Bagot CN, Arya R. Virchow and his triad: a question of attribution. Br J Haematol 2008;143(2):180–90.

14. Maraveyas A, Johnson M. Does clinical method mask significant VTE-related mortality and morbidity in malignant disease? Br J Cancer 2009;100(12):1837–41.

15. Chew HK, Wun T, Harvey D, et al. Incidence of venous thromboembolism and its effect on survival among patients with common cancers. Arch Intern Med 2006; 166(4):458–64.

16. Kearon C. Long-term management of patients after venous thromboembolism. Circulation 2004;110(9 Suppl 1):I10–8.

17. McNamara I, Sharma A, Prevost T, et al. Symptomatic venous thromboembolism following a hip fracture. Acta Orthop 2009;80(6):687–92.

18. Gage BF, Waterman AD, Shannon W, et al. Validation of clinical classification schemes for predicting stroke: results from the National Registry of Atrial Fibrillation. JAMA 2001;285(22):2864–70.

19. Gage BF, Yan Y, Milligan PE, et al. Clinical classification schemes for predicting hemorrhage: results from the National Registry of Atrial Fibrillation (NRAF). Am Heart J 2006;151(3):713–9.

20. Pisters R, Lane DA, Nieuwlaat R, et al. A novel user-friendly score (HAS-BLED) to assess 1-year risk of major bleeding in patients with atrial fibrillation: the Euro Heart Survey. Chest 2010;138(5):1093–100.

21. Friberg L, Rosenqvist M, Lip GY. Evaluation of risk stratification schemes for ischaemic stroke and bleeding in 182 678 patients with atrial fibrillation: the Swedish Atrial Fibrillation cohort study. Eur Heart J 2012;33(12):1500–10.

22. Gent M, Hirsh J, Ginsberg JS, et al. Low-molecular-weight heparinoid orgaran is more effective than aspirin in the prevention of venous thromboembolism after surgery for hip fracture. Circulation 1996;93(1):80–4.

23. Hansen ML, Sorensen R, Clausen MT, et al. Risk of bleeding with single, dual, or triple therapy with warfarin, aspirin, and clopidogrel in patients with atrial fibrillation. Arch Intern Med 2010;170(16):1433–41.
24. Eriksson BI, Lassen MR. Duration of prophylaxis against venous thromboembolism with fondaparinux after hip fracture surgery: a multicenter, randomized, placebo-controlled, double-blind study. Arch Intern Med 2003;163(11):1337–42.
25. Rajasekhar A, Lottenberg R, Lottenberg L, et al. Pulmonary embolism prophylaxis with inferior vena cava filters in trauma patients: a systematic review using the meta-analysis of observational studies in epidemiology (MOOSE) guidelines. J Thromb Thrombolysis 2011;32(1):40–6.
26. Bass AR, Mattern CJ, Voos JE, et al. Inferior vena cava filter placement in orthopedic surgery. Am J Orthop (Belle Mead NJ) 2010;39(9):435–9.
27. Friedman SM, Mendelson DA, Kates SL, et al. Geriatric co-management of proximal femur fractures: total quality management and protocol-driven care result in better outcomes for a frail patient population. J Am Geriatr Soc 2008;56(7): 1349–56.
28. Douketis JD, Spyropoulos AC, Spencer FA, et al. Perioperative management of antithrombotic therapy: antithrombotic therapy and prevention of thrombosis, 9th ed: American College of Chest Physicians Evidence-Based Clinical Practice Guidelines. Chest 2012;141(Suppl 2):e326S–50S.

Management of Postoperative Complications

Cardiovascular Disease and Volume Management

Joseph A. Nicholas, MD, MPH

KEYWORDS

- Postoperative complications • Cardiovascular disease
- Geriatric fracture management

KEY POINTS

- Cardiovascular comorbidity is common with fragility fracture.
- Perioperative hypotension is common and should be anticipated and prevented.
- Perioperative cardiovascular medication management should be focused on preserving or improving intravascular volume status, avoiding tachyarrhythmias, and minimizing polypharmacy.
- The potential benefits of antiplatelet and anticoagulant therapy must be balanced with the risk for postsurgical bleeding and transfusion.

INTRODUCTION

Many patients who experience fragility fractures have high degrees of comorbidity that place them at risk for a variety of postoperative cardiovascular complications. In addition to any personal medical history of coronary artery disease, congestive heart failure, and atrial fibrillation, typical age-related changes to the cardiovascular system place older adults at risk for perioperative hypotension, coronary ischemia, and acutely depressed cardiac output. Although significant academic attention has been directed to quantifying preoperative risk of cardiovascular complications in the perioperative setting, less rigorous study has been done on how to best manage common postoperative cardiovascular complications. Nonetheless, substantial observational data from existing geriatric fracture centers can provide guidance on the prevention and management of cardiovascular complications in the postoperative setting.

Conflict of Interest: None to declare.
Division of Geriatrics, Highland Hospital, University of Rochester School of Medicine, 1000 South Avenue Box 58, Rochester, NY 14610, USA
E-mail address: Joseph_Nicholas@urmc.rochester.edu

Clin Geriatr Med 30 (2014) 293–301
http://dx.doi.org/10.1016/j.cger.2014.01.008
0749-0690/14/$ – see front matter © 2014 Elsevier Inc. All rights reserved.

IMPLICATIONS OF NORMAL CARDIOVASCULAR AGING

Normal aging of the cardiovascular system results in physiologic changes[1] that can significantly impact hemodynamic stability in the postoperative setting. In general, normal cardiovascular aging results in a less compliant and less responsive cardiovascular system with a higher propensity for hypotension, conduction system defects, and pulmonary edema (**Table 1**). These changes make extrapolating clinical data derived from studies of younger subjects problematic. Taken together, these changes impair the older adult from maintaining physiologic homeostasis in the face of acute stressors, including those commonly found in the perioperative setting, such as pain, anesthesia, and blood loss. This aging of the cardiovascular system also makes some chronically administered cardiovascular medications less well tolerated over time, and less well tolerated in specific settings. Because different patients have different degrees of physiologic aging and impairment, standardization of medication doses and administration protocols for cardiovascular medications is challenging. In addition to using protocols that respect these physiologic changes, frequent patient-specific clinical evaluation and reassessment is likely necessary to achieve optimal outcomes.

CORE PRINCIPLES FOR POSTOPERATIVE MANAGEMENT IN OLDER PATIENTS

In light of the significant physiologic differences between older adults with fragility fractures and the younger, more functional, and less comorbid study subjects on whom most existing perioperative clinical recommendations are based, extrapolating from most existing postoperative guidelines to this population is difficult and dangerous. Additionally, conflating the long-term benefits of some chronic cardiovascular therapies with the short-term risks and benefits of these therapies is not appropriate in the physiologically dynamic postoperative setting. Finally, older adults who are frail and have multiple comorbidities are at high risk for excessive diagnostic testing, numerous subspecialty consultations, polypharmacy, and iatrogenic harm when traditional single-disease guidelines are integrated into postoperative treatment plans. For these reasons, the most valid existing data to guide standard postoperative recommendations can be drawn from the observational experience of high-performing fragility fracture centers, most of which use geriatric comanagement as a cornerstone of their programs. In general, these programs have placed a high priority

Table 1
Selected age-related cardiovascular changes

Physiologic Change	Clinical Consequence
Decreased elasticity/increased stiffness of arterial system	LVH, isolated systolic hypertension, widened pulse pressure
Myocardial cell hypertrophy, dropout, interstitial fibrosis	Delayed ventricular relaxation, diastolic dysfunction, and heart failure Aortic valve calcification, sclerosis, and stenosis
Decreased responsiveness to β-adrenergic stimulation	Increased circulating catecholamines
Decreased sensitivity to baroreceptors, chemoreceptors	Increased circulating catecholamines
Loss of atrial pacemaker cells	Reduced resting heart rate Reduced maximal heart rate

Abbreviation: LVH, left ventricular hypertrophy.

on certain general strategies: avoidance of hypotension, pain control, avoidance of polypharmacy, and the prevention and treatment of delirium. Although most have not used or studied uniform strategies for specific cardiovascular comorbidities or complications, they do report lower rates of adverse outcomes. The major strategies that seem to be relevant for avoiding cardiovascular complications in frail older adults are as follows:

- Anticipation of postoperative hypotension
- Assurance of adequate intravascular volume
- Judicious use of β-blockers and other antiarrhythmic/chronotropic drugs for selected patients
- Cessation or dose attenuation for most chronic antihypertensive medications until patients show a need
- Recognition of diuretic dependence when evaluating oliguria and volume status
- Prevention of polypharmacy and excessive testing

COMMON CARDIOVASCULAR RESPONSES TO UNCOMPLICATED ORTHOPEDIC SURGERY

It is important for all care team members to understand the most common cardiovascular responses that occur in the perioperative setting. In general, significant drops in blood pressure can occur on induction of either general or regional anesthesia, and may require intraoperative fluids and vasopressor medications to attenuate.[2] Postoperatively, exaggerated drops in blood pressure can be expected when patients are upright or participating in therapy. Lastly, multiple neurohumoral stress responses lead to water and salt conservation, oliguria, and expansion of the intravascular and extravascular volume, much of which may be necessary to maintain postoperative blood pressure and cardiac output.[3] This can also result in transient hyponatremia related to antidiuretic hormone secretion.[4] In short, geriatric patients should be expected to require hydration and a positive fluid balance in the immediate postoperative period, and to be able to tolerate a natural or pharmacologically induced diuresis once the effects of anesthesia and acute blood loss have subsided.

COMMON CARDIOVASCULAR COMPLICATIONS AND STRATEGIES

In the absence of large and rigorous trials evaluating specific postoperative strategies for older patients with fragility fractures in the postoperative setting, current practice is best informed through applying the strategies used in current geriatric fracture centers that report good overall outcomes. In general, care has focused on hemodynamic stability, early mobility, and symptom control, rather than strict adoption of disease-specific treatment guidelines for these conditions (Table 2).[5]

Hypotension

Hypotension is a common consequence of physiologic stress on the older adult, and should be anticipated in the postoperative setting.[6,7] In addition to the physiologic aging of the cardiovascular system described previously, many other predictable factors contribute to postoperative hypotension, including prolonged anesthetic effects (seen in general and regional anesthesia techniques), opiate effects (parenteral and enteral administration), acute blood loss, and poor oral intake of fluids. Many cardiovascular medications can contribute to hypotension and impair appropriate neurocardiovascular compensation in this setting. Many noncardiovascular medications (sedatives, antiemetics) also produce hypotension as a side effect. For these reasons, even

Table 2
Chronic cardiovascular diseases and common postoperative strategies

	Chronic Stable Disease Therapies	Common Postoperative Strategies
Poor systolic heart function	β-blockade	Continue β-blockade
	Afterload reduction with ACE inhibitor or ARB	Holding or attenuating afterload reducing agents until stable blood pressure
	Aldosterone antagonism	Holding aldosterone antagonists until metabolically stable
	Loop diuretics	Holding loop diuretics until stable anemia and renal function, and resumption of oral intake
	Fluid restriction	Volume administration with close attention to pulmonary status
Hypertension	Multiple agents for goal SBP	Holding nonchronotropic blood pressure medications
		Allowing modest hypertension during admission
		Evaluating for orthostasis, treating to standing blood pressure goal
Secondary prevention of CAD	Antiplatelet agents (ASA, clopidogrel)	Resumption of ASA during postoperative period

Abbreviations: ACE, angiotensin-converting enzyme; ARB, angiotensin receptor blockers; ASA, acetylsalicylic acid; CAD, coronary artery disease; SBP, systolic blood pressure.

long-standing cardiovascular medications and goals can be problematic in a typical postoperative course. Although a small number of these antiadrenergic medications (eg, β-blockers, clonidine) can have rebound phenomena when abruptly discontinued, many others, including calcium channel blockers, angiotensin-converting enzyme (ACE) inhibitors, and diuretics, can often be held or dose-attenuated without known adverse effects.[8,9] In addition, preadmission antihypertensives that have not been continued in the postoperative period should not be resumed on discharge until the patient demonstrates an indication. Many patients will not be able to tolerate their pre-surgical medication regimen until they have resolved their postoperative anemia, stopped opiate therapy, and recovered from surgery.

Atrial Fibrillation

New, recurrent, or uncontrolled atrial fibrillation can complicate the postoperative period. Contributors to the development of unstable atrial fibrillation include inadequate intravascular volume resuscitation, acute blood loss, poor pain control, or the abrupt discontinuation of chronic antiadrenergic agents or chronic opiate or benzodiazepine therapy.[10] Alcohol withdrawal, myocardial ischemia, pulmonary embolism, and fat emboli syndrome should also be considered. Routine low-dose perioperative β-blockade may limit this complication but must be balanced against the risk of drug-induced hypotension.

Heart Failure and Volume Assessment

Intravenous fluid administration, cessation of diuretics, blood loss and transfusion, and myocardial stress can all contribute to the development of acute pulmonary edema in the postoperative period. Many classic physical examination findings (ie, rales, edema, elevated jugular venous pressure) and laboratory results (elevated

B-type natriuretic peptide [BNP]) have decreased specificity for detecting acute heart failure in the older adult, and must be taken into context when arriving at a diagnosis (**Table 3**).[11,12] Serial BNP testing should be cautiously interpreted in light of normal biologic variation in results seen in stable patients.[13,14] A trial of diuresis may be necessary to fully assess for a response to therapy. A new diagnosis of heart failure may warrant evaluations for ischemia, arrhythmia, or valvular disease, and echocardiography and cardiology consultation may be helpful in select patients.

Urine output is often a centerpiece of postoperative volume assessment, but the significance of oliguria in the older adult can be confusing to medical and surgical providers. In the early postoperative period, oliguria is more likely to represent intravascular volume depletion, bleeding, or vasodilation, and can be managed with fluid or blood administration as indicated. Persistent oliguria despite an adequate trial of fluid replacement and evaluation for anemia may be caused by acute urinary retention as a result of prostatic hypertrophy, opiate therapy, or acute renal failure, or may reflect loop diuretic dependence in patients who have not yet resumed their home medications (**Table 4**). The presence of oliguria and subsequent administration of volume or diuretics require patient-specific decision making, and close reevaluation of hemodynamics, renal function, and pulmonary edema.

Myocardial Ischemia

Clinically detected myocardial infarction in the postoperative period occurs in fewer than 1% of patients who have experienced a hip fracture,[15,16] although a higher incidence can be seen with more routine trending of biomarkers.[17] Whether many of these reported events either represent a conventional myocardial event or reflect physiologic stress in the frail patient is unknown. Cardiac biomarkers, including creatinine kinase (total and MB fraction) and cardiac-specific troponin levels, can be elevated without ongoing myocardial ischemia,[18] because of traumatic muscle damage and renal insufficiency, respectively. Other than minimizing physiologic stress and instability, routine low-dose β-blocker administration in patients with adequate blood pressure may offer some additional protection, although relevant interventional studies are limited.[19] Perioperative elevation in myocardial enzymes is a marker for increased mortality at 6 months.[20]

Patients with recently placed cardiac stents on dual antiplatelet therapy should be managed in consultation with cardiology; in general, dual antiplatelet therapy is continued[21] even in the perioperative setting until 6 weeks (for bare metal stents) to 6 months (for drug eluting stents) after stent placement, as long as bleeding is not severe.

Table 3
Selected heart failure symptoms and findings in older adults

Symptoms and Findings	Common Geriatric Conditions Other Than Left Heart Failure
Edema	Venous insufficiency Postoperative edema Venous thrombosis Cor pulmonale
Elevated jugular venous pressure	Pulmonary hypertension Cor pulmonale
Pulmonary rales, hypoxia, dyspnea	Atelectasis Pulmonary fibrosis Bacterial pneumonia

Table 4 Common causes of oliguria in the postoperative setting	
	Common Causes of Oliguria
Early postoperative period (<48 h)	Inadequate volume restoration Acute blood loss
Late postoperative period (>48 h)	Urinary retention Diuretic dependence Renal failure Heart failure

PERIOPERATIVE CONSIDERATIONS WITH COMMON CHRONIC CARDIOVASCULAR MEDICATIONS
β-Blockers

Since the initial publication of data supporting the widespread use of β-blockers in the perioperative setting, several subsequent studies have suggested a more nuanced approach in patients undergoing noncardiac surgery, with many studies failing to confirm benefit.[22–24] The cardioprotective benefits of β-blockade contrast with the risks of hypotension in the acute perioperative setting, particularly in frail patients with this physiologic tendency. No trials have been dedicated to studying the impact of β-blockers specifically, or postoperative blood pressure control in general, in patients older than 75 years. In the PeriOperative Ischemic Evaluation (POISE) trial,[25] the largest randomized trial of perioperative β-blockade, patients older than 70 years and those with hypotension had increased rates of stroke and death. Additionally, acutely bleeding patients with hip fractures have a unique risk for exaggerated hypotension, and at least one retrospective analysis suggests that patients taking β-blockers do not tolerate surgical anemia as well as those who are not.[26] Current American College of Cardiology guidelines recommend continuing chronic β-blocker therapy in surgical patients, and avoiding hypotension and bradycardia.[27] A recent meta-analysis[28] of secure randomized trials concluded that the risks of routine β-blockade outweighed any benefit in the general population, although this analysis was dominated by studies using relatively high doses of medications (metoprolol ≥100 mg) in β-blocker naïve patients. Some geriatric fracture centers have reported low rates of cardiovascular complications using protocols that include low-dose β-blockade (metoprolol ≤25 mg).[29]

ACE Inhibitors

ACE inhibitors and angiotensin receptor blockers (ARBs) have been associated with acute kidney injury in the postoperative setting in some studies,[30,31] and some investigators advocate for routine cessation of ACE inhibitors/ARBs in the preoperative period.[32,33] Although the long-term efficacy of ACE inhibition or blockade in managing chronic systolic cardiac dysfunction and diabetic nephropathy have been well established, use in the immediate postoperative period is likely complicated by impairment of renal compensatory mechanisms in the face of rapidly fluctuating intravascular volume status.[34,35] Short-term cessation or dose attenuation in this setting is not known to cause harm, and likely prevents acute kidney injury in some patients.

Calcium Channel Blockers

When used for rate control for chronic stable tachyarrhythmias, nondihydropyridine calcium channel blockers (eg, diltiazem, verapamil) may need to be continued in the perioperative setting. These benefits must be weighed against the risks of hypotension and side effects, such as constipation and orthostasis. Dihydropyridine calcium channel blockers (eg, amlodipine, felodipine) should be held if hypotension is anticipated or demonstrated.

Digoxin

Digoxin levels should be monitored during the postoperative period, particularly in the presence of fluctuating renal function or in patients with hypokalemia. Adverse effects of digoxin can been seen in older patients, even in those with serum levels within normal laboratory reference values; close monitoring for nausea, sedation, anorexia, and other signs of toxicity is necessary.

Loop Diuretics (Furosemide, Torsemide, Bumetanide)

Unlike some other cardiovascular medications, chronic diuretic therapy typically cannot be stopped indefinitely. Loop diuretics are usually held in the immediate preoperative and postoperative period, until perioperative blood loss and intravascular volume have stabilized.[36] Many older adults demonstrate diuretic-dependent urine production, and will remain oliguric, irrespective of intravascular volume status, until loop diuretics are resumed. Once resumed, close attention to renal function, weight, and pulmonary symptoms is necessary to ensure adequate dosing and tolerance.

Aldosterone Antagonists (Spironolactone, Eplerenone)

No studies indicate a short-term benefit of continuing aldosterone antagonists or any harm associated with abrupt discontinuation. Aldosterone antagonists can interfere with renal compensatory mechanisms in the face of fluctuating intravascular volume status, and any use should be accompanied by routine electrolyte monitoring and evaluation for hemodynamic and metabolic stability.

Antiplatelet Agents and Anticoagulants

No high-quality trials have quantified the risks and benefits of various anticoagulation strategies in the prevention of cardiac thromboembolic disease in the postoperative setting. Current guidelines[21] are based on limited observational data and expert opinion, and are not specific for many frail, older patients who have experienced a fragility fracture. In general, aspirin for secondary prevention of coronary artery disease can be resumed in patients without significant ongoing blood loss in the postoperative period. The bleeding risks of acutely resuming more potent antiplatelet agents (eg, clopidogrel) or using full-dose anticoagulation (eg, heparin, vitamin K antagonists, novel anticoagulants) must be weighed carefully against the benefit of using these drugs in the short term.

SUMMARY

Cardiovascular comorbidities and complications are common among older adults with fragility fractures. Postoperative care should be attentive to these conditions, and should anticipate the common issues of hypotension, fluctuating intravascular volume, arrhythmia, and heart failure. Most postoperative care plans should be guided by geriatric principles, including a focus on symptom control, avoidance of polypharmacy, and optimization of volume status. Many chronic medications may need to be temporarily held or dose-adjusted to produce optimal outcomes.

REFERENCES

1. Cheitlin MD. Cardiovascular physiology-changes with aging. Am J Geriatr Cardiol 2003;12(1):9–13.
2. Reich DL, Hossain S, Krol M, et al. Predictors of hypotension after the induction of general anesthesia. Anesth Analg 2005;101(3):622–8.
3. Desborough JP. The stress response to trauma and surgery. Br J Anaesth 2000; 85:109–17.
4. Lane N, Allen K. Hyponatremia after orthopedic surgery. BMJ 1999;318:1363–4.
5. Marsland D, Colvin PL, Mears SC, et al. How to optimize patients for geriatric fracture surgery. Osteoporos Int 2010;21(Suppl 4):S535–46.
6. Bettelli G. Anaesthesia for the elderly outpatient. Current Opinion in Anaesthesiology 2010;23(6):726–31.
7. Ekstein M, Gavish D, Ezri T, et al. Monitored anaesthesia care in elderly. Guidelines and recommendations. Drugs Aging 2008;25:477–500.
8. Geyskes GG, Boer P, Dorhout E. Clonidine withdrawal. Mechanism and frequency of rebound hypertension. British Journal of Clinical Pharmacology 1979;7(1):55–62.
9. Ross PJ, Lewis MJ, Sheridan DJ, et al. Adrenergic hypersensitivity after beta-blocker withdrawal. Br Heart J 1981;45:637–42.
10. Omae T, Kanmura Y. Management of postoperative atrial fibrillation. J Anesth 2012;26(3):429–37.
11. Ahmed A. Clinical manifestations, diagnostic assessment, and etiology of heart failure in older adults. Clin Geriatr Med 2007;23:11–30.
12. Samala RV, Navas V, Saluke E, et al. Heart failure in frail, older patients: We can do 'MORE'. Cleve Clin J Med 2011;78(12):837–45.
13. O'Hanlon R, O'Shea P, Ledwidge M. The biologic variability of B-type natriuretic peptide and N-terminal pro-B type natriuretic peptide in stable heart failure patients. J Card Fail 2007;13(1):50–5.
14. Wu AH. Serial testing of B-type natriuretic peptide and NTpro-BNP for monitoring therapy of heart failure: the role of biologic variation in the interpretation of results. Am Heart J 2006;152(5):828–34.
15. Prevention of pulmonary embolism and deep vein thrombosis with low dose aspirin: Pulmonary Embolism Prevention (PEP) trial. Lancet 2000;355(9212): 1295–302.
16. Friedman SM, Mendelson DA, Bingham KW, et al. Impact of a comanaged geriatric center on short-term hip fracture outcomes. Ann Intern Med 2009;169(18): 1712–7.
17. Huddleston JM, Gullerud RE, Smither F, et al. Myocardial infarction after hip fracture repair: a population-based study. J Am Geriatr Soc 2012;60:2020–6.
18. Tanindi A, Cemri M. Troponin elevation in conditions other than acute coronary syndromes. Vasc Health Risk Manag 2011;7:597–603.
19. Dunkelgrun M, Boersma E, Schouten O, et al. Bisoprolol and fluvastatin for the reduction of perioperative cardiac mortality and myocardial infraction in intermediate-risk patients undergoing noncardiovascular surgery: a randomized controlled trial (DECREASE-IV). Ann Surg 2009;249(6):921–6.
20. Ausset S, Minville V, Marquis C, et al. Postoperative myocardial damages after hip fracture repair are frequent and associated with a poor cardiac outcome: a three-hospital study. Age Ageing 2009;38:473–6.
21. Douketis JD, Spyropoulos AC, Spencer FA, et al. Perioperative management of antithrombotic therapy. Chest 2012;141(Suppl 2):e326S–50S.

22. Yang H, Raymer K, Butler R, et al. The effects of perioperative beta-blockade: results of the Metoprolol after Vascular Surgery (MaVS) study, a randomized controlled trial. Am Heart J 2006;152(5):983–90.
23. Juul AB, Wetterslev J, Gluud C, et al. Effect of perioperative beta blockade in patients with diabetes undergoing major non-cardiac surgery: randomized placebo controlled, blinded multicenter trial. BMJ 2006;332(7556):1482.
24. Brady AR, Gibbs JS, Greenhalgh RM, et al. Perioperative beta-blockade (POBBLE) for patients undergoing infrarenal vascular surgery: results of a randomized double-blind controlled trial. J Vasc Surg 2005;41(4):602–9.
25. Devereaux PJ, Yang H, Yusef S, et al. Effects of extended-release metoprolol succinate in patients undergoing non-cardiac surgery (POISE trial): a randomised controlled trial. Lancet 2008;371(9627):1839–47.
26. Beattie WS, Wijeysundera DN, Karkouti K, et al. Acute surgical anemia influences the cardioprotective effects of beta-blockade: a single-center, propensity-matched cohort study. Anesthesiology 2010;112(1):25–33.
27. Fleischmann KE, Beckman JA, Buller CE, et al. 2009 ACCF/AHA focused update on perioperative beta blockade: a report of the American College of Cardiology Foundation/American Heart Association Task Force on Practice Guidelines. Circulation 2009;120(21):2123–51.
28. Bouri S, Shun-Shin MJ, Cole GD, et al. Meta-analysis of secure randomized controlled trials of β-blockade to prevent perioperative death in non-cardiac surgery. Heart 2014;100:456–64.
29. Friedman SM, Mendelson DA, Kates SL, et al. Geriatric co-management of proximal femur fractures: total quality management and protocol-driven care result in better outcomes for a frail patient population. J Am Geriatr Soc 2008;56:1349–56.
30. Ishikawa S, Griesdale D, Lohser J. Acute kidney injury after lung resection surgery: incidence and perioperative risk factors. Anesth Analg 2012;114:1256–62.
31. Cittanova ML, Zubicki A, Savu C, et al. The chronic inhibition of angiotensin-converting enzyme impairs postoperative renal function. Anesth Analg 2001;93:1111–5.
32. Arora P, Rajagopalam S, Ranjan R, et al. Preoperative use of angiotensin-converting enzyme inhibitors/angiotensin receptor blockers is associated with increased risk for acute kidney injury after cardiovascular surgery. Clin J Am Soc Nephrol 2008;3(5):1266–73.
33. Onuigbo MA. Reno-prevention vs. reno-protection: a critical re-appraisal of the evidence-base from the large RAAS blockade trials after ONTARGET—a call for more circumspection. QJM 2009;102(3):155–67.
34. Garg R, Yusuf S, Bussmann WD, et al. Overview of randomized trials of angio-tensi-converting enzyme inhibitors on mortality and morbidity in patients with heart failure. JAMA 1995;273(18):1450–6.
35. Strippoli GF, Craig M, Deeks JJ, et al. Effects of angiotensin converting enzyme inhibitors and angiotensin II receptor antagonists on mortality and renal outcomes in diabetic nephropathy: systematic review. BMJ 2004;329(7470):828.
36. Golob AL, Julka R. Perioperative Medication Management. In: Wong CJ, Hamlin NP, editors. From The Perioperative Medicine Consult Handbook. New York: Springer Science and Business Media; 2013.

Transitions of Care and Rehabilitation After Fragility Fractures

Michelle Eslami, MD[a],*, Hong-Phuc Tran, MD[b]

KEYWORDS

- Rehabilitation • Skilled nursing facility (SNF) • Inpatient rehabilitation facility (IRF)
- Transitions in care • Transitional care • Home health • Medicare • Fragility fracture

KEY POINTS

- Transitions in care are a vulnerable time for patients in which unintended errors may occur; understanding the potential risks and taking proactive measures to prevent these risks can greatly improve patient safety and outcome.
- Rehabilitation (rehab) can be done in a variety of settings; most common locations are home (via home health care), skilled nursing facilities (SNFs, commonly pronounced "sniffs"), and inpatient rehab facilities (IRFs), commonly called *acute rehab*.
- In the United States, reimbursement for rehab at home, SNFs, and IRFs for patients 65 and older is typically paid through Medicare Part A. SNFs and IRFs are reimbursed via bundled payment. Physician services (which are not part of this bundled payment) can be billed separately through Medicare Part B. Supplemental insurance may provide varying degrees of additional coverage.
- Medical management includes pain management, pressure sore prevention, thromboprophylaxis, nutrition, and delirium prevention.
- Rehab goals of patients (or of patients' families and caregivers)—particularly for patients who are frail with multiple, complex comorbidities and cognitive deficits—may not match actual rehab outcomes; some patients may not return to their prior baseline function.
- Realistic goals and expectations for a patient's rehab outcome are important for improving the satisfaction of patients and their families and caregivers.

TRANSITIONS IN CARE

Transitions in care are areas of opportunities for improving patient safety and outcome. A transition in care occurs when patients go from home to hospital, hospital to SNF, and/or SNF to home. A transition is a vulnerable time for patients during which

Disclosures: The authors have no conflicts of interest to disclose.
[a] David Geffen School of Medicine at UCLA, 10945 Le Conte Avenue, Suite 2339, Los Angeles, CA 90095, USA; [b] UCLA Santa Monica - Geriatrics, 1245 16th Street, Suite 204, Santa Monica, CA 90404, USA
* Corresponding author.
E-mail address: MSEslami@mednet.ucla.edu

Clin Geriatr Med 30 (2014) 303–315
http://dx.doi.org/10.1016/j.cger.2014.01.017
0749-0690/14/$ – see front matter © 2014 Elsevier Inc. All rights reserved.

unintended errors may occur. For patients discharged from the hospital to a SNF for rehab, for instance, poorly implemented care transitions can lead to adverse events, patient and family dissatisfaction, unnecessary use of emergency room services, and avoidable rehospitalizations.[1,2]

Unintended errors may also occur, including the following:

- Medications inadvertently omitted or added to a patient's list
- Inaccurate medication dosages dispensed
- Discontinued medications accidentally resumed
- End dates for medications omitted on interfacility transfer orders

End dates (and start dates) of certain medications, in particular antibiotics, temporary diuretics, steroid taper, and short-term anticoagulation, must be included on interfacility transfer orders and discharge summaries to prevent adverse patient outcomes. Other potential risks in care transitions include the following:

- Failure to prepare timely discharge summaries
- Failure to include all pertinent information in the discharge summaries
- Failure to follow-up on important laboratory tests and studies pending at time of discharge
- Failure to arrange specialty follow-up appointments
- Failure to communicate the need for follow-up laboratory tests or studies
- Incomplete or no handoffs between physicians and/or nurses

Other potential risks when transferring patients from hospital to SNF concern logistics and also should be avoided. For instance, pharmacies are often off-site in SNFs. If a patient is discharged from the hospital in the late afternoon or evening, that patient invariably arrives at the SNF after the pharmacy is closed, thus may not receive necessary medication (eg, pain medication, antibiotic, or cardiac medication) until the following day.

Becoming aware of the potential risks in transitions and taking proactive steps to prevent those risks can improve patient safety and outcome. Standardizing elements of the discharge process may help reduce unintended errors. For example, using a discharge checklist of the critical elements for an optimal handoff can help prevent adverse events in care transitions.[1]

When transferring a patient from a hospital to a SNF, 3 components are necessary[3]:

- An interfacility transfer form, including discharge medications, discontinuation dates for short-term medications, and any dosage changes in all medications
- A discharge summary that includes a patient's baseline functional status, a list of important tests for which results are pending, and a list of necessary next steps, including physician follow-up appointments
- Verbal physician-to-physician sign-outs to ensure that all questions that the receiving physician has can be answered

Following these steps ensures a safer handoff and helps apprise the receiving physician of any important discussions that may have previously occurred among the patient, patient's family, and primary providers. Some of these discussions may have focused on the patient's advance directives and goals of care, which influence the receiving physician's management of the patient. Similarly, when a patient is ready for SNF discharge to home, the same steps and principles should be applied to ensure safe transition.

Several programs have been developed and evaluated to ensure safe care transitions to nursing homes and home.[4,5] The Care Transitions Program includes a personal health record, a discharge preparation checklist, and transition coaches who work with patients/caregivers prior to and after the transition to SNF or home.[3] In the Transitional Care Model, an advanced practice nurse bridges hospital and postdischarge care by providing continuity of care for patients with complex needs in both settings; this model has been shown to reduce hospital readmissions, lengthen the time between discharge and readmission for at-risk elders,[3] and reduce health care costs.[6]

Involvement of patients and their caregivers is critical for a successful care transition. The discharging health care provider should prepare patients and their caregivers for what to expect at the next care site and provide advice on how to contact a health care professional who is familiar with the patient if a patient's condition worsens.[2] Patients and their families and caregivers should have an opportunity to discuss their goals and preferences and have them incorporated in the care plan. Patients and caregivers may be helpful to the receiving health care provider by resolving medication discrepancies and facilitating communication across care sites (eg, relaying information about any needed follow-up appointments, laboratory tests, and studies).[2,3] Additionally, obtaining input from nursing staff, pharmacists (if available), and a patient's primary provider can facilitate safer care transitions.

TYPES OF REHABILITATION SETTINGS

There are different locations to which patients can go for rehab. Most common are home, SNFs, and IRFs (**Table 1**).

Rehab at home is usually provided through a home health agency. A home may be more than an apartment, house, or condominium where a patient resides. A home can also refer to an assisted living facility or a board and care home. Rehab services that are available through home health agencies include physical, occupational, and speech. Rehab at home is not as intensive as that in a SNF or IRF. Typically, home health rehab can be provided 1 to 3 times per week for 3 to 6 weeks and typically one-half hour to 1 hour at a time. The frequency of home health therapy visits may also be constrained by reimbursement barriers.

SNF rehab offers a greater intensity and variety of services than home health rehab. In SNFs, patients can typically get up to 2 hours of rehab daily, 5 to 7 days per week. Some SNFs offer rehab on the weekends whereas others do not. SNFs can differ in their equipment availability (eg, stationary bicycles, standing frames, and platform walkers) and available modalities for treating pain (eg, diathermy, electrical stimulation, and ultrasound). Physical, occupational, and speech therapies are typically available at all SNFs; a few SNF facilities may offer respiratory therapy.

SNFs provide 24-hour, daily coverage by licensed vocational nurses (LVNs) and daily coverage by registered nurses (RNs); the coverage provided by RNs usually is part time and depends on the number of patients at the facility (this number includes both rehab and long-term care patients). Other services available in SNFs include wound care and administration of intravenous antibiotics and tube feeds; although these skilled nursing services can also be provided by home health care, it is on a more limited basis because home health nurses are limited to once-daily visits due to reimbursement barriers. Hospitalized patients who are frailer, medically complex, and with multiple health needs may benefit from initially transitioning to SNF rehab before going home (with or without home health care after discharge).

IRFs offer a greater intensity of rehab and greater access to services than are provided at SNFs. IRFs offer intensive physical, occupational, and speech therapy as well as specialists in physical medicine, orthopedics, neurology, and psychiatry. To qualify

Table 1
Types of rehabilitation settings

	Home	Skilled Nursing Facility	Inpatient Rehabilitation Facility
Services available	PT, OT, ST	PT, OT, ST (sometimes RT)[a]	PT, OT, ST, RT Greater access to specialists, including physiatry, orthopedics, neurology, psychiatry
Intensity of rehab	1–3 Times per week for 3–6 wk (typically 1/2–1 h each time)[b]	5–7 Days per week, up to 2 h daily	At least 3 h daily
Nursing availability	Typically up to once-daily visits (depending on patient's needs [eg, wound care, IV antibiotic administration])	Daily 24-h coverage by LVNs 5–7 Days per week, typically part-time coverage by RNs	Daily 24-h coverage by RNs
Types of nursing services available	Wound care Antibiotic administration (typically only once daily) Tube feeds administration (typically once daily only)	Wound care Antibiotic administration (can do up to every 6 h, but usually up to every 8 h) Tube feeds administration	Wound care Antibiotic administration (can do up to every 6 h) Tube feeds administration
Frequency of physician visits	N/A (patients typically see their doctors in clinic)	Typically 1–2 times per week for rehab patients or less, depending on insurance coverage	Daily

Abbreviations: OT, occupational therapy; PT, physical therapy; RT, respiratory therapy; ST, speech therapy.
[a] SNFs can differ in the specialty services they offer. Some specialty services typically offered in SNFs include dentistry, optometry, podiatry, psychiatry, psychology. Less common specialty services offered in SNFs include ENT, dermatology, audiology, and physiatry.
[b] Frequency and duration of home health therapy covered depends on insurance coverage/reimbursement.

for an IRF, Centers for Medicare & Medicaid Services (CMS) guidelines require that a patient must need hospital level of care and intensive rehab. In IRFs, the focus is on patients with complex problems and high, premorbid functional baselines, such as younger stroke patients and victims of multiple traumatic injuries. Ideal candidates for IRFs are those who can tolerate a minimum of 3 hours of combined therapy (occupational, speech, and physical) daily, 5 to 7 days per week.[7] In IRFs, patients are seen by a physician almost daily, and interdisciplinary team (IDT) meetings are physician led; in contrast, in SNFs, a physician sees a rehab patient 1 to 2 times per week and IDT meetings do not require physician involvement.[7] Most of the nurses in IRFs are RNs whereas most of the nurses in SNFs are LVNs.[7] Overall, IRFs provide a higher level of service than can be provided in SNFs, leading to a lower readmission rate to general acute hospitals (9.5% vs 22%) and higher rate of patient discharge to the community (81.1% vs 45.5%).[7] Many elderly patients are more likely discharged from hospital to either home or SNFs for rehab because admission criteria for IRFs are stringent; furthermore, there has been a 54% decline in the number of IRFs since 1999 due to inadequate reimbursement and net negative margins to IRFs.[8] The prospective payment system (PPS) was designed to make no distinction between hospital-based SNFs (IRFs) and freestanding SNFs.[8]

REIMBURSEMENT FOR REHABILITATION

Many people over age 65 require some form of rehab from a home health agency, SNF, or IRF at some point. Because SNFs are one of the commonly used post–acute care settings for patients needing short-term rehab,[8,9] this section focuses primarily on reimbursement in the SNFs.

Unlike acute hospital services, a significant proportion of fees for SNF services are paid out of pocket by patients and/or their families (private pay). In addition to private pay, there are 5 other main sources of payment for SNF services: fee-for-service Medicare, Medicaid, managed care plans combining Medicare with other payment sources, private long-term care insurance, and private health insurance.

Medicare is a federal health insurance program for people ages 65 and older and for those under age 65 receiving Social Security disability benefits secondary to a chronic illness (eg, multiple sclerosis or HIV), with end-stage renal disease, or on hemodialysis or blindness (eg, glaucoma). It is administered by the CMS.[10] Qualification is based on age or disability, not on income or assets. Medicare is divided into parts that cover different types of medical services. SNF rehab is typically covered under Medicare Part A, which also covers services provided by general acute hospitals, long-term care hospitals, IRFs, hospices, and home health agencies (but not home support for basic activities of daily living). Patients in SNF rehab who are not covered under Medicare Part A still can receive coverage under Medicare Part B. Medicare Part B covers professional fees of physicians and physical, occupational, and speech therapists; additionally, Medicare Part B covers services of clinical social workers providing mental health services, psychologists, nurse practitioners, and physician assistants; laboratory tests; outpatient diagnostic procedures; and durable medical equipment (DME).[9]

Medicare covers 100% of the first 20 days of a SNF stay after a qualifying hospital stay. After that, patients are responsible for a 20% copayment from days 21 to 100. Medicare Advantage Plans, however, may offer different benefits. The daily copayment is indexed annually at one-eighth (12.5%) of the current Part A deductible[8]; for calendar year 2012, the copayment was $144.50 per day (**Table 2**).[8,11]

In order to qualify for Medicare Part A coverage for a SNF stay, patients must meet all the following criteria[8,11]:

- Hospitalization for at least 3 consecutive calendar days (midnights) in the 30 days immediately preceding the admission to a SNF (ie, inpatient admission to the hospital, not merely held for observation)
- Selected nursing home must be a Medicare-approved SNF
- A physician must certify that patient is medically benefiting from daily skilled care (ie, the services furnished can only be at a SNF)
- The reason for admission to SNF is a condition that was treated during the hospital stay

If a patient has multiple comorbidities, such as deconditioning, gait disorder, and generalized muscular weakness, or other conditions that were recognized during the SNF stay that required skilled services, each would qualify for SNF stay even though they might not be the primary diagnosis during the hospital stay.[8] CMS does not deny Medicare reimbursements to the SNF in these situations.[8]

| Table 2 |
| Medicare coverage in skilled nursing facility |

Skilled Nursing Facility Days	Medicare Covers	Patient and/or Family Pays
1–20	All eligible expenses	Nothing
21–100	All eligible expenses after patient pays daily copayment	Daily copayment[a]
100+	Nothing	Everything

This table applies to patients with Medicare Part A SNF coverage who had a qualifying hospital stay of at least 3 midnights. Medicare Part A covers 100 SNF days per benefit period, which starts on the first day that a patient uses hospital or SNF services under Medicare Part A. There is no limit to the number of benefit periods. Another 100 days of Medicare Part A SNF coverage can be regenerated after 60 days if a patient does not use any emergency room or acute hospital services during those 60 days. For a patient staying in a SNF, another benefit period of 100 days can be regenerated if no skilled services were used for 60 consecutive days and if the patient has a qualifying hospital stay of at least 3 midnights and which meets Medicare requirements.

[a] For calendar year 2012, the copayment was $144.50 per day. Medicare supplemental insurance (MedSup or Medigap) may cover some or all of Medicare's copayments and/or deductibles.

Data from Centers for Medicare & Medicaid Services. Medicare coverage of skilled nursing facilities. Available at: http://www.medicare.gov/Pubs/pdf/10153.pdf. Accessed September 8, 2013; and Med-Pac. Chapter 7: Skilled nursing facilities services. In: Report to the Congress: Medicare Payment Policy. 2012. Available at: http://www.medpac.gov/chapters/Mar12_Ch07.pdf. Accessed September 7, 2013.

Reimbursement for a patient's Medicare-covered SNF stay is bundled with a predetermined daily rate for each day of care, up to 100 days per benefit period (a benefit period begins on the day that a patient uses hospital or SNF services under Medicare Part A and is determined by different qualifying factors).[11] In the Balanced Budget Act of 1997, Congress mandated that most of the services (including rehab, medications, and laboratory tests) provided to patients in a Medicare-covered SNF stay be consolidated in a bundled PPS.[11] The PPS for SNF services started on July 1, 1998,[9] and uses the Minimum Data Set, a standardized patient assessment instrument, to calculate a Resource Utilization Group (RUG) for each Medicare beneficiary.[9,11] RUGs are case mix categories that differ from each other based on 3 main features—type of services provided (eg, number of minutes of physical/occupational/speech therapy a beneficiary has used or is expected to use or need for specialized feeding), complexity of patient's clinical condition, and an index of the patient's ability to perform basic activities of daily living.[9,11] Each RUG has a dollar amount associated with it.[9] For example, a RUG with a higher daily payment is assigned to a stroke patient needing temporary tube feeds and intensive rehab, whereas a RUG with a lower daily payment is assigned to a less medically complex patient who is getting SNF rehab for back pain (without fractures) after a mechanical fall. The daily rate paid to a SNF for each beneficiary is adjusted for geographic differences in area wage differences (labor costs), urban or rural facility locale, and a non–case mix component reflecting cost of room and board, linens, and administrative services.[8,9]

There are 53 RUGs that went into effect on January 1, 2006.[9] SNFs bill the Medicare Administrative Contractor for the consolidated services. During Medicare Part A–covered SNF stays, medical services (including rehab therapy, medications, and laboratory tests) and room and board are covered. When Medicare Part A benefits have been exhausted, then skilled SNF services are still covered by Medicare Part B, but room and board are not. Room-and-board expenses are covered by Medicaid only for patients who are dually eligible for Medicare-Medicaid or by private payment.

There are several services, however, that are excluded from bundled billing in the SNF. For patients covered under Medicare Part A, services excluded from bundled payment (eg, separately payable) include the following[8]:

- Physician's professional services
- Some dialysis-related services, including covered ambulance transportation services to dialysis centers
- Some ambulance services, including ambulance transfer from hospital to SNF, transport from SNF to home, transfers from SNF to specified types of emergency or intensive outpatient hospital services, and transfer to dialysis centers for dialysis services
- Erythropoietin for some dialysis patients
- Some chemotherapy drugs
- Some chemotherapy administration services
- Radioisotope services
- Customized prosthetic devices

For patients in SNF rehab who do not have Medicare Part A coverage, only therapy services are subject to consolidated billing.[8]

As people live longer and the geriatric population in the United States grows, there are more medically complex patients who need SNF rehab after discharge from the hospital. Although some chemotherapy drugs are excluded from bundled payment, expensive pain medications, psychotropic drugs, and certain expensive antibiotics are not. High-cost medications can result in a net loss of revenue for SNFs that care for patients with multiple comorbidities. In an attempt to fix this issue, in 2010, CMS revised the case mix categorization system (to RUG version IV) to shift program dollars away from therapy care and more toward care of medically complex patients.[9] Nonetheless, the current PPS continues to be a financial disincentive for SNFs to admit medically complex patients needing rehab; proposals for further revisions to the PPS have been made to improve the accuracy of payments.[9]

There is an important limitation to Medicare Part A coverage for SNF rehab. Although Medicare allows for a maximum of 100 days of SNF coverage per benefit period, only a small proportion of patients receiving Medicare actually use all 100 days.[11] The Medicare requirement that a patient is medically benefiting (ie, demonstrates continued improvement and would gain from further treatment) usually limits SNF coverage for rehab of most medical conditions. In 2010, the average number of Medicare-covered SNF days for a beneficiary was 27.1.[8]

If patients have exhausted Medicare coverage, either because of lack of benefit (eg, plateau in rehab in which patient demonstrates no significant functional gains) or because of reaching the maximum days of coverage, they typically are switched to Medicaid or private pay. Unfortunately, many patients and families have the erroneous belief that Medicare covers SNF services in the same way it covers hospital care; this can cause frustration and disappointment for patients and their families when patients have not yet reached their desired rehab goals but yet may need to pay out-of-pocket expenses for a longer SNF stay.

GOALS OF REHABILITATION

Assessment of a patient's rehab goals (and that of their families and caregivers) is important in creating an appropriate rehab program for the patient. Patients are evaluated by physical and occupational therapists (and speech therapists if needed) when they are enrolled for rehab through home health, SNF, or IRF. The therapists can then create an individualized care plan for patients with both short-term and long-term goals. The goal of rehab is to help patients achieve their prior premorbid functional baseline (or higher if possible), so that they can return to their prior living situation.

The rehab goals of patients may not match the goals that their families, caregivers, or medical providers have for them. For instance, a frail elderly patient with moderate to severe dementia, Parkinson disease, gait and balance disorder, osteoarthritis, and generalized weakness may desire a goal of being able to perform his/her own transfers (eg, in and out of bed/chair), grooming, and developing enough endurance to sit up long enough for meals. That patient's family/caregiver, however, may desire a different set of goals, such as having the patient able to perform his/her own lower body dressing, transfers to the restroom, toileting, and bathing. The family/caregiver may also desire the patient to walk a longer distance and at the community level (eg, outside the home). The patient's primary care provider may have a different goal, especially if the patient lives home alone and only has a part-time caregiver. The primary care provider may desire that the patient improves his/her safety awareness, balance, and gait in addition to the goals listed previously.

For patients who are frail with complex comorbidities and cognitive deficits, setting realistic expectations and appropriate short-term and long-term goals early in the rehab course is crucial to improving patient and family/caregiver satisfaction. The physical and occupational therapists can help determine the appropriate short-term and long-term goals.

COMMON MEDICAL ISSUES IN REHABILITATION

Many factors are involved in the rehab of a fragility fracture patient. Medical management includes pain management, pressure sore prevention, thromboprophylaxis, nutritional needs, and delirium prevention. Other issues that may arise include anemia, constipation, and urinary tract complications.

Within the first 30 days after hospitalization with a hip fracture, readmission rates from nursing home rehab are 14%, with pneumonia the most common reason. Certain comorbidities, such as fluid and electrolyte disorders, cardiac arrthymias, congestive heart failure, and chronic obstructive pulmonary disease, increase the risk of readmission.[12]

Pain Management

Pain management in the elderly can be complicated after a fragility fracture. There seems to be an age-related increase in pain thresholds and a tendency for older patients to underreport pain.[12] Cognitive impairment also can make pain assessment and treatment difficult. In general, pain intensity scales may be used. In patients with mild to moderate dementia, the 0-to-10 pain scale and verbal description scale have been found to have adequate (but not perfect) reliability and validity.[12] Control of postoperative pain is important in preventing delirium because higher pain at rest scores during the first 3 postoperative days and increased levels of pain are risk factors for the development of delirium.[12]

Unfortunately, little evidence exists regarding the best means of providing analgesia for the hip fracture population. When selecting narcotics for pain management, there is no difference in cognitive effects for fentanyl, morphine, and hydromorphone.[12] Merperidine is the only narcotic that has been associated with delirium; thus, it should be avoided. There is no difference in cognitive outcome between intravenous and epidural administration.[13]

Opiates themselves may induce delirium. Nonopioids, such as acetaminophen, may allow lower doses of opiates to be used and help prevent future side effects.[12] Good control of pain reduces delirium and improves patients' ability to participate in rehab.

Pressure Sore Prevention

Because a pressure sore can have a negative impact in the recovery of elderly patients with a fragility fracture, avoidance is the best approach. The prevalence of pressure sore after hip fracture is approximately 33%.[14] Many of these patients are transferred for rehab. Pressure sores can be painful and thus can interfere with a patient's rehab. Common sites include heels and sacrum. Pressure sores may take months to heal and often can result in complications, such as wound infection, additional surgery, or even death. Patients should be checked routinely at common sites, including the buttocks, heels, hips, and elbows, for blisters or redness that may indicate the beginning of a pressure sore. The treatment of pressure sores is based on the staging and involves relieving the pressure on the skin, débridement of any necrotic tissue, and frequent dressing changes. Pressure-reducing mattresses, frequent repositioning while in bed, and early ambulation also may be useful techniques.[14]

Thromboprophylaxis

Venous thromboembolism is common in patients with lower extremity fragility fractures and thromboprophylaxis is the standard of care. Early surgery and early immobilization have been shown to reduce the likelihood of thrombosis and should be instituted whenever possible.[15] Currently, there is no one accepted standard of prophylaxis. The American College of Chest Physicians recommends medications and/or devices, such as sequential pneumatic compression devices placed on the legs, which, however, is not readily available in the rehab setting. Pharmacologic means to prevent venous thrombosis include unfractionated heparin, low-molecular-weight heparin, warfarin, aspirin, direct thrombin inhibitors, and factor Xa inhibitors, the last 2 of which have been approved only for joint replacement thromboprophlaxis.[15]

Although heparins reduce the risk of venous thrombosis and embolism, they also can increase the incidence of bleeding at other sites. Low-molecular-weight heparins, such as enoxaparin or dalteparin, have been shown to provide effective prophylaxis of venous thrombosis after a hip fracture. Because the available evidence is based mostly on consensus from variety of organizations, the duration of therapy for low-molecular-weight heparin is usually continued for 28 to 35 days after surgery.[15]

Unfractionated heparin, used twice a day, has been effective. Aspirin has been shown effective post–joint replacement and may have a role in treatment of the hip fracture patient.[15] Warfarin is another agent sometimes used with a target international normalized ratio (INR) of 2.5. Bleeding complications can occur when the INR is greater than 3. Direct thrombin inhibitors (eg, dabigatran) and factor Xa inhibitors (eg, rivaroxaban) are 2 new classes of oral blood thinners. Currently, they are approved after joint replacement (hip/knee) surgery.[15] Further discussion of thromboprophylaxis in the acute setting is discussed in the article by Friedman and Uy elsewhere in this issue.

Nutrition

Nutrition is an essential part of rehab and recovery for elderly patients with a fracture. Proper nutrition allows for wound healing and, ultimately, better recovery. Malnutrition is also part of a geriatric syndrome, known as failure to thrive. A serum albumin less than 3 g/dL has been associated with poor outcomes after hip fracture.[16] Nutritional supplements used between or with meals have been effective in improving rehab, reducing pressure sores, and improving muscle strength. Oral nutrition supplementation (eg, Ensure or Sustical, 1–3 times a day between meals) may be beneficial in reducing postoperative complications in people with hip fractures. It has been shown to preserve body protein stores and reduce overall length of stay in the acute care setting.[16] Understanding patients' swallowing and feeding needs is important in the rehab setting because infections, such as pneumonia, are also possible post–fracture complications and a common reason for hospital readmission after a hip fracture.

Delirium

Delirium occurs in an estimated 11% to 30% of elderly general medicine patients and in as many as 61% of hip fracture patients. Despite its relevance, delirium is often misdiagnosed or unrecognized, particularly in the elderly. Delirium is a transient disorder characterized by difficulty with attention, thinking, memory, perception, cyclomotor behavior, and sleep-wake cycle. Delirium in hospitalized patients has been associated in increase of length of stay, risk complications, mortality, and institutionalization.[17] For further discussion of delirium in the inpatient setting, see the article by Javedan and Tulebaev elsewhere in this issue.

Delirium in patients with hip fracture can interfere with rehab activities and delay the return to weight-bearing activities. Prevention and appropriate treatment of delirium are important in the rehab setting. Once delirium has developed, there is little evidence that intervention can improve outcome. Thus, prevention is important. Patients whose delirium interferes with care may benefit from a low-dose neuroleptic.[14] This medication should be stopped as the delirium improves. All antipsychotics carry a black box warning for increased risk of arrhythmia and death in older people; thus, they should be closely monitored.

Other Medical Issues

Other issues that arise in patients with fragility fracture include constipation, urinary tract issues, and anemia. Constipation is especially common in patients who receive opioid analgesics. Cathartics, such as senna, may be helpful. Patients who have not had a bowel movement in 2 days should be treated with a gentle laxative.

Urinary catheters should be removed within 24 hours of surgery to prevent iatrogenic urinary tract infections. If voiding problems develop thereafter, intermittent catheterization can be done without increasing the rate of urinary tract infection.[18]

The optimal threshold for transfusion has been evaluated in a randomized clinical trial. This trial found similar outcomes in mortality, ambulatory status at 60 days, and cardiovascular events for postoperative hip fracture patients who received liberal transfusion maintaining a hemoglobin greater than 10 or symptomatic/restrictive transfusion for symptoms or when hemoglobin fell below 8.[19] It is reasonable to withhold transfusion in patients who have undergone surgery in the absence of symptoms of anemia or the absence of decline in hemoglobin even if they have underlying cardiovascular disease and cardiovascular risk factors. For further discussion of this topic, see the article by Carson and colleagues elsewhere in this issue.

OUTCOMES IN REHABILITATION

The goal of rehab after a fragility fracture is to restore patients to their preinjury status; 50% of elders who sustain a hip fracture never regain prefall level of function and 40% never recover their prefracture walking ability.[20,21] Currently, there is no consensus as to the best setting for rehab in patients with a fragility fracture. The recovery process after a fragility fracture needs to be assessed for each patient. It is influenced by several factors, including individual premorbid level of physical and mental function and the availability of social supports. The development of an individualized plan in this setting is to maximize independence, safety, and function (**Table 3**).

The IDT plays a key role.[13] The preparation for discharge needs to include a prescription for any DME, an assessment of the individual's home environment, and interventions as appropriate to facilitate a safe discharge. These may include home modification, DME, and appropriate support services such a caregiver.[13] Once an individual is transitioned to the community, rehab continues with in-home or ambulatory physical therapy.

SECONDARY PREVENTION IN REHABILITATION

Secondary prevention should be routinely initiated during patient rehab. The likelihood that osteoporosis is the predisposing factor for a patient's fragility fracture is high. Patients with hip fractures are at an increased risk for secondary fracture. The risk of a second fracture is greater in older patients.[22] It has been recommended that hip fracture patients maintain an adequate calcium intake (1200 mg/d) and vitamin D (400–800 IU/d). Treatment with vitamin D is recommended to reduce the fall risk in patients who have sustained a hip fracture. Vitamin D (2000 IU/d) may reduce the rate of hospital readmission after a hip fracture.[23] Bisphosphonates are considered the first-line drugs for treatment of osteoporosis. Bone density assessment is indicated to establish a baseline and to monitor response and is done after rehab stay. In a community-based study of women over age 65 with a recent hip fracture, only 13% were receiving adequate treatment of osteoporosis, defined by the National Osteoporosis Foundation.[24] The low rate of medical management may, in part, reflect life expectancy, because 6 months is needed to see the effectiveness of the bisphosphonates. General exercise reduces the risk of fall, and exercise programs that include a balance program are most effective. Extended exercise classes

Table 3 Goals of rehabilitation prevention	
Goals for Rehabilitation	**Outcomes**
Mobilization and early ambulation	• Avoids immobilization and bone loss • Improves bone healing quality and rate • Avoids pressure sore formation • Reduces risk of *venous thromboembolism*
Multidisciplinary rehab	• Improves body function • Early supported discharge • Evaluation of medical complications
Adequate balance training	• Reduces risk of falls • Reduces risk of a second fracture
Physical activity	• Reduces risk of falls • Increases muscle mass and strength • Increases bone mineral density
Nutrition	• Maintaining skin integrity, promoting wound healing, maintaining weight
Education and social measure	• Improvement in the ability to perform daily activities • Improves risk awareness • Speeds up mental and social recovery
Secondary prevention	• Osteoporosis evaluation and management

that focus on gait and balance training have been effective in reducing falls and may have a role in the secondary prevention of hip fractures.[25] For further discussion of secondary prevention of osteoporosis and falls, see the articles by Sale and colleagues & Demontiero and colleagues elsewhere in this issue, respectively.

REFERENCES

1. Halasyamani L, Kripalani S, Coleman E, et al. Transition of care for hospitalized elderly patients—Development of a discharge checklist for hospitalists. J Hosp Med 2006;1:354–60.
2. Coleman EA, Boult C. Improving the quality of transitional care for persons with complex care needs: position statement of the American Geriatrics Society Health Care Systems Committee. J Am Geriatr Soc 2003;51(4):556–7.
3. Reuben DB, Herr KA, Pacala JT, et al. Assessment and approach. In: Reuben DB, Herr KA, Pacala JT, et al, editors. Geriatrics at your fingertips. 15th edition. New York: American Geriatrics Society; 2013. p. 7–8.
4. Naylor MD, Brooten D, Campbell R, et al. Comprehensive discharge planning and home follow-up of hospitalized elders: a randomized clinical trial. JAMA 1999;281(7):613–20.
5. Coleman EA, Parry C, Chalmers S, et al. The care transitions intervention: results of a randomized controlled trial. Arch Intern Med 2006;166(17):1822–8.
6. Coleman EA. Falling through the cracks: challenges and opportunities for improving transitional care for persons with continuous complex care needs. J Am Geriatr Soc 2003;51(4):549–55.
7. American Hospital Association. Fact sheet: inpatient rehabilitation facilities. Available at: www.aha.org/content/12/12factsheet-irf.pdf. Accessed September 7, 2013.
8. Talga SR. Medicare's skilled nursing facility primer: benefit basics and issues. Congressional Research Service. 2012. Available at: http://greenbook. waysandmeans.house.gov/sites/greenbook.waysandmeans.house.gov/files/2012/ documents/R42401_gb.pdf. Accessed September 8, 2013.
9. Medicare Payment Advisory Commission (MedPac). Skilled nursing facility services payment system: Payment Basics. Available at: http://www.medpac.gov/ documents/MedPAC_Payment_Basics_08_SNF.pdf. Accessed September 7, 2013.
10. Centers for Medicare & Medicaid Services. Medicare program: general information. Available at: http://www.cms.gov/Medicare/Medicare-General-Information/ MedicareGenInfo/index.html. Accessed September 7, 2013.
11. Centers for Medicare & Medicaid Services. SNF consolicated billing: overview on skilled NursingFacilitySNF) ConsolidatedBilling. Available at: http://www.cms.gov/ Medicare/Billing/SNFConsolidatedBilling/index.html. Accessed September 7, 2013.
12. Abou-Setta AM, Beaupre LA, Rashiq S, et al. Comparative effectiveness of pain management interventions for hip fracture: a systematic review. Ann Intern Med 2011;155(4):234–45.
13. Bukata SV, Digiovanni BF, Friedman SM, et al. A guide to improving the care of patients with fragility fractures. Geriatr Orthop Surg Rehabil 2011;2(1): 5–37.
14. Beaupre LA, Jones CA, Saunders LD, et al. Best practices for elderly hip fracture patients. A systematic overview of the evidence. J Gen Intern Med 2005;20(11): 1019–25.

15. Falck-Ytter Y, Francis CW, Johanson NA, et al. Prevention of VTE in orthopedic surgery patients: Antithrombotic Therapy and Prevention of Thrombosis, 9th ed: American College of Chest Physicians Evidence-Based Clinical Practice Guidelines. Chest 2012;141(2 Suppl):e278S–325S.
16. Avenell A, Handoll HH. Nutritional supplementation for hip fracture aftercare in older people. Cochrane Database Syst Rev 2010 Jan 20;(1):CD001880.
17. Inouye SK. Delirium in older persons. N Engl J Med 2006;354(11):1157–65.
18. Skelly JM, Guyatt GH, Kalbfleisch R, et al. Management of urinary retention after surgical repair of hip fracture. CMAJ 1992;146(7):1185–9.
19. Carson JL, Terrin ML, Noveck H, et al. Liberal or restrictive transfusion in high-risk patients after hip surgery. N Engl J Med 2011;365(26):2453–62.
20. Haentjens P, Magaziner J, Colón-Emeric CS, et al. Meta-analysis: excess mortality after hip fracture among older women and men. Ann Intern Med 2010;152(6): 380–90.
21. French DD, Bass E, Bradham DD, et al. Rehospitalization after hip fracture: predictors and prognosis from a national veterans study. J Am Geriatr Soc 2008; 56(4):705–10.
22. Boockvar KS, Halm EA, Litke A, et al. Hospital readmissions after hospital discharge for hip fracture: surgical and nonsurgical causes and effect on outcomes. J Am Geriatr Soc 2003;51(3):399–403.
23. Grant AM, Avenell A, Campbell MK, et al. Oral vitamin D3 and calcium for secondary prevention of low-trauma fractures in elderly people (Randomised Evaluation of Calcium Or vitamin D, RECORD): a randomised placebo-controlled trial. Lancet 2005;365(9471):1621–8.
24. Bischoff Ferrari HA, Dawson-Hughes B, Platz A, et al. Effect of high-dosage cholecalciferol and extended physiotherapy on complications after hip fracture: a randomized controlled trial. Arch Intern Med 2010;170(9):813–20.
25. Bellantonio S, Fortinsky R, Prestwood K. How well are community-living women treated for osteoporosis after hip fracture? J Am Geriatr Soc 2001;49(9): 1197–204.

Secondary Prevention After an Osteoporosis-Related Fracture

An Overview

Joanna E.M. Sale, PhD[a,b],*, Dorcas Beaton, BScOT, PhD[a,b],
Earl Bogoch, MD, MSc, FRCSC[c,d]

KEYWORDS

- Fragility fracture • Postfracture secondary prevention • Fracture risk • Osteoporosis
- Interventions • Models of care

KEY POINTS

- Having a prior fracture is a major predictor of future fractures.
- There is strong evidence to support the rationale for postfracture secondary prevention programs.
- It is believed that a systems approach, with dedicated personnel, bone mineral density (BMD) testing within a program, or both, performs better whereas programs offering only education, awareness, and medication coverage are less effective.
- Gaps in care still exist despite the improvements demonstrated by postfracture secondary prevention programs; however, many barriers to care are modifiable.

BURDEN OF FRAGILITY FRACTURES

One in 2 women and 1 in 5 men have a fragility (sometimes referred to as a low trauma or osteoporotic) fracture after age 50.[1–3] The risk of fracture in a 1-year period for women over age 50 is higher than the risk of any cardiovascular disease event in that year.[4] Having a prior fracture, whether it is a confirmed fragility fracture[5–7] or not,[8–10] is a major predictor of future fracture,[5–10] especially in the first 5 years after the initial fracture.[8,10] According to one review, peri- and postmenopausal women with prior fractures had 2 times the risk of subsequent fractures compared with women with no prior fractures, and women with a preexisting vertebral fracture had

[a] Mobility Program Clinical Research Unit, Li Ka Shing Knowledge Institute, St. Michael's Hospital, 30 Bond Street, Toronto, Ontario M5B 1W8, Canada; [b] Institute of Health Policy, Management & Evaluation, University of Toronto, Suite 425, 155 College Street, Toronto, Ontario M5T 3M7, Canada; [c] Mobility Program, St. Michael's Hospital, 30 Bond Street, Toronto, Ontario M5B 1W8, Canada; [d] Department of Surgery, University of Toronto, 149 College Street, 5th Floor, Toronto, Ontario M5T 1P5, Canada
* Corresponding author. Mobility Program Clinical Research Unit, Li Ka Shing Knowledge Institute, St. Michael's Hospital, 30 Bond Street, Toronto, Ontario M5B 1W8, Canada.
E-mail address: salej@smh.ca

Clin Geriatr Med 30 (2014) 317–332
http://dx.doi.org/10.1016/j.cger.2014.01.009   **geriatric.theclinics.com**

4 times the risk of a subsequent vertebral fracture than those without prior fractures.[9] A subsequent fracture can be particularly devastating if it is a hip fracture. Individuals who subsequently sustain a hip fracture are at increased risk of death compared with individuals who do not refracture within 5 years of their index fracture.[11] Approximately 25% of patients who sustain a hip fracture die within 5 years[11] and only 50% of hip fracture patients regain their prefracture status as judged by the ability to walk and the need for aids at home.[12]

Fractures are associated with

- Increased mortality risk[11,13–15]: in the geriatric population, one study demonstrated that the presence of vertebral fractures and number of prevalent fractures at baseline both independently increased the mortality risk within a 3-year follow-up[16]
- Significant length of hospital stay[17,18]
- Disability-adjusted life years[19]
- Admission to extended care facilities and nursing homes[18]

Fracture patients at risk for future fracture pose a significant cost to the health care system:

- In Canada, the mean attributable cost in the first year after a hip fracture in patients ≥65 years is approximately $37,000 for women and $40,000 for men.[20]
- The economic impact of hip fractures alone in Canada is projected to rise to $2.4 billion annually by 2041.[21]
- Loss of mobility associated with hip fractures results in indirect costs to the health care system when factors, such as assistive devices, family support, and home care, are considered.[21,22]
- The cost of a second fracture in Medicare patients 50 years of age and older is estimated to be as much as $1.3 billion annually in the United States.[23]

THE EVIDENCE FOR PHARMACOLOGIC AND NONPHARMACOLOGIC AGENTS ON FRACTURE RISK REDUCTION

Evidence gained from rigorous study designs, such as randomized controlled trials, supports the use of both pharmacologic and nonpharmacologic agents in preventing fractures.

Pharmacologic Agents

Therapy for fracture risk reduction includes bisphosphonates (alendronate, etidronate, risedronate, and zoledronic acid), other antiresorptives (hormone therapy, raloxifene, calcitonin, and denosumab), and anabolic agents (teriparatide).[24]

According to one meta-analysis, alendronate and risedronate reduce the risk of fracture by approximately 25% to 50%.[25] Similar values for antifracture efficacy of other major pharmacologic treatments of osteoporosis (OP) are reviewed by Kanis and colleagues.[26]

Pharmacotherapy reduces risk but does not eliminate it. Approximately 23%[27] to 34%[28] of fragility fractures occur in patients who are on OP pharmacotherapy. These fractures do not necessarily occur because treatment has failed. Whether or not these fractures are due to other factors that could be influencing refracture risk requires further research.

Two systematic reviews on the efficacy of bisphosphonates for secondary prevention demonstrated absolute risk reductions ranging from 1% to 6%, depending on the type of fracture prevented.[29,30] There are few data, however, on the efficacy of pharmacotherapy in patients who have already had a low-trauma fracture, other than that of the vertebra or hip.[24] Treatment with antiresorptive medication after a vertebral fracture reduces the incidence of subsequent hip fractures by up to 60%.[31] Investigators have shown that once-yearly zoledronic acid is associated with reductions in subsequent clinical fractures in older persons who have had a recent hip fracture[32] and that risedronate reduces the risk of new vertebral fractures in those with a prior vertebral fracture.[33]

It has been shown that patients need to take antiresorptive medication for at least 6 months for fracture risk reduction to be realized.[34,35] In one study, the incidence of second hip fracture was 4.2% in patients with a medication possession ratio of more than 80% for 1 year after the hip fracture compared with 10.9% in patients with less than or equal to 80% medication possession ratio (where medication possession ratio was defined as the sum of days of supply of bisphosphonates divided by 365 days).[36] Although fractures in patients who have been on pharmacologic treatment for at least 1 year might be considered possible therapeutic failure, there are few data to support altering therapy for these patients.[37]

The safety considerations of OP pharmacotherapy are reviewed by Gates and colleagues[38]:

- Although no changes in medication dosages are recommended for elderly patients, elderly patients may be more sensitive to the medications, and they may experience more difficulty with administration, such as remembering to take the medication on an empty stomach.[38]
- Some adverse events common to patients who receive bisphosphonates (alendronate, risedronate, and ibandronate) are abdominal pain, diarrhea, and headaches.[38]
- One rare adverse event that has received much attention is osteonecrosis of the jaw, which has been reported with both oral and intravenous bisphosphonate therapy.[38,39]

Nonpharmacologic Agents, Including Supplements

Vitamin D supplementation is also associated with fracture reduction,[40,41] particularly when combined with adequate calcium intake.[42,43] A meta-analysis of randomized controlled trials demonstrated that combined vitamin D and calcium supplementation reduced the risk of hip fracture by 18% compared with no supplementation.[42] Data from a Women's Health Initiative clinical trial show mostly null or inconclusive health effects of calcium and vitamin D supplementation at recommended doses.[43] There seems to be insufficient evidence to support or refute the association between calcium and vitamin D supplementation and cardiovascular risk.[44]

Hip protector devices have also been shown to decrease the risk of hip fractures in nursing home residents and hospital inpatients.[45,46] In a bayesian meta-analysis, the mean odds of an elderly individual allocated to hip protector use sustaining 1 or more hip fractures was 0.40.[45] There is also evidence that exercise reduces the incidence of fractures, although the possibility of publication bias weakens the positive effect on overall fracture reduction.[47]

THE CONCEPT OF FRACTURE RISK IS REPLACING A DIAGNOSIS OF OP AND OSTEOPENIA

Since 1994, clinical practice guidelines worldwide have relied on a diagnosis of OP for bone health treatment recommendations.[48] A fundamental shift from a diagnosis of OP to absolute fracture risk has become a worldwide phenomenon, with tools such as the Fracture Risk Assessment Tool[49] translated and available across 19 countries.[50]

A recent systematic review identified 12 fracture risk assessment tools for women.[51] Between 1 and 31 risk factors were considered in the algorithms of these tools, with the most common risk factors including age, weight, prior fracture, BMD, and maternal/parental history of fracture.[51] Tools that are not gender-specific, for example, one developed by the Canadian Association of Radiologists and Osteoporosis Canada,[52] consider gender as a significant risk factor in its calculation of fracture risk. Many patients who are at high risk for future fracture (and/or who have had a fracture) have low bone density but do not have OP.[48,53]

CLINICAL PRACTICE GUIDELINES ACKNOWLEDGE THE NEED TO INTERVENE IN PATIENTS WHO ARE AT RISK FOR FUTURE FRACTURE

There has been a movement for clinical practice guidelines to recommend fracture risk assessment in advance of making treatment recommendations,[26,54,55] with some guidelines recommending pharmacotherapy for patients who are at high risk for future fracture.[54]

- According to the *2010 Clinical Practice Guidelines for the Diagnosis and Management of Osteoporosis in Canada*, all individuals 50 years of age and older who have had a hip or vertebral fragility fracture or who have had more than 1 fragility fracture are automatically considered high risk for future fracture and, therefore, have an indication for pharmacotherapy.[54]
- Patients with other nonvertebral, nonhip fractures may reach the high-risk threshold for pharmacotherapy depending on multiple factors in the risk assessment. The principle factors are old age, prevalent fragility fracture, low bone density, and female gender as well as prolonged corticosteroid therapy and rheumatoid arthritis.

THE INTRODUCTION OF POSTFRACTURE SECONDARY PREVENTION PROGRAMS

Despite the knowledge that prior fractures are a major predictor of future fractures,[5,8–10] it is well documented that fracture patients often do not undergo BMD testing or initiate bone health treatment after a fragility fracture.[15,56–60] For example, Papaioannou and colleagues[57] reported that the proportion of fracture patients who received an OP diagnostic test or physician diagnosis ranged from 1.7% to 50%. Given that approximately half of hip fracture patients have had a previous fragility fracture,[61,62] the rationale for targeting patients with an initial fragility fracture is strong. In order to prevent subsequent fractures, postfracture secondary programs, particularly in an orthopedic environment where fractures are referred for treatment, have been developed; published reports from these initiatives have been increasing in number since 2002.[63] In addition to capturing a majority of fracture patients, case findings from orthopedic environments are appealing because investigation rates with dual-energy x-ray absorptiometry (DXA) seem better for patients who are referred for assessment from these environments compared with those referred for assessment by general practitioners.[64]

THE SCOPE OF POSTFRACTURE SECONDARY PREVENTION PROGRAMS

Postfracture secondary prevention programs are currently established worldwide. Although most programs typically screen all fragility fracture patients over age 50, some have reported data on older adults, ages 65 and older.[65,66] The International Osteoporosis Foundation Capture the Fracture report describes several coordinator-based models of care that have a systematic approach to fragility fracture prevention in Australia, Canada, Singapore, the Netherlands, the United Kingdom, and the United States.[67] These programs include but are not limited to

- Fracture Liaison Services, established in Glasgow, Scotland, in 1999[68]
- Kaiser Permanente Healthy Bones Program, established in 2001 in Southern California[69]
- Osteoporosis Exemplary Care Program, established in Toronto, Canada, in 2002[28]
- Minimal Trauma Fracture Liaison service, established in Sydney, Australia, in 2005[70]
- Osteoporosis Patient Targeted and Integrated Management for Active Living, established in Singapore in 2008[71]

One of the larger coordinator-run programs currently operating is the Fracture Clinic Screening Program funded through the Ontario Osteoporosis Strategy in Ontario, Canada. Reports are just being published from this program that screens approximately 6000 fragility fracture patients annually.[72]

Although not predominantly coordinator based, the American Orthopaedic Association Own the Bone[73] operates in more than 800 sites in the United States. There is no single model used by the hospitals, medical centers, and private practice groups participating in Own the Bone.

The content of postfracture secondary prevention programs (both coordinator and noncoordinator based) varies considerably. Several investigators have classified postfracture secondary prevention programs based on common elements. In one systematic review, interventions were classified into 12 categories, ranging from programs where dedicated personnel screened and educated patients to more intense programs where treatment, and sometimes BMD testing, occurred within the program.[63] In this systematic review, a majority of interventions were coordinator based in that they had dedicated personnel to implement the intervention.[63] **Table 1** lists examples of two programs, one with dedicated personnel and one without such personnel.

In a more recent meta-analysis, Ganda and colleagues[76] described 4 models of interventions ranging in intensity: type A models were complex, involving many components and representing a coordinated approach to secondary fracture prevention with a fracture liaison coordinator central to this model of care; type D models were

Table 1
Description of two postfracture secondary prevention programs

Author, Year	Dedicated Staffing	Patient Education	Primary Care Physician Education	BMD Test Done Within Program	Treatment Prescribed Within Program
Davis et al,[74] 2007	No	General education	General education via the patient	No	No
Majumdar et al,[75] 2007	Yes	Patient-specific education, including BMD test results	Patient-specific education sent directly to physician	Yes	Yes

education-based, only including pamphlets, personal communication to the patient, or a patient-specific letter.

THE EFFECT OF POSTFRACTURE SECONDARY PREVENTION PROGRAMS
Reduction in Health Care Costs

The effects of postfracture secondary prevention programs on several outcomes have been reported. Some programs have been shown at least cost effective or even cost saving.[77–80]

Improved Investigation and Treatment Rates

According to several recent systematic reviews, these programs have had positive effects on BMD testing[63,76] and bone health treatment initiation.[63,76,81] Little and Eccles[81] showed that based on postintervention differences between the intervention and control groups of randomized controlled trials, a variety of interventions improved rates of BMD testing by 36% and OP pharmacotherapy by 20%. Based on a retrospective cohort study, one program that included education of geriatrics and rehabilitation teams seems to have improved new diagnoses of OP as well as initiation of bisphosphonate therapy among hospitalized patients admitted with hip fracture.[82]

Participation in Exercise

Recently, Chandran and colleagues[71] reported that at the end of 2 years, approximately 62% of patients screened through one such program reported exercising regularly.

Reduction in Refracture Rates

Few studies have reported refracture outcomes[83]; however, there is some evidence that postfracture secondary prevention programs are associated with a reduction in fractures.[70,84] Over a 4-year period, Lih and colleagues[70] reported that 4.1% of patients referred to an intervention program experienced a new fracture compared with 19.7% in the control group (those patients who elected to follow-up with their primary care physician). The intervention consisted of a standardized series of assessments and investigations, including a BMD test; patient-specific education; and initiation of treatment, including pharmacotherapy if indicated.[70] During a 6-year follow-up study, Astrand and colleagues[84] reported that 18% of patients screened through a program that included a DXA scan, a copy of the results, and advice to follow-up with their primary care physician reported a new fracture compared with 29% of those patients who were not screened.

What Makes a Program Effective?

Many of these programs are complex in nature, making it a challenge to identify the elements that make them successful or not. It is believed that initiatives adopting a systems approach, with dedicated personnel, BMD testing within the program, or both, perform better whereas programs offering only education, awareness, and medication coverage are less effective.[63] Similarly, based on their meta-analysis, Ganda and colleagues[76] showed a trend where higher-intensity interventions were associated with increased BMD testing and treatment initiation. The International Osteoporosis Foundation proposes that coordinator-based, postfracture models of care have successfully closed the secondary fracture prevention gap in many countries throughout the world.[85]

POTENTIAL REASONS FOR THESE GAPS IN BONE HEALTH STILL EXIST DESPITE POSTFRACTURE SECONDARY PREVENTION PROGRAMS

There are opportunities for improvement at several stages in postfracture bone secondary prevention, from identifying patients at risk for future fracture to promoting patients to follow treatment recommendations. For example:

- Chevalley and colleagues[86] reported that 72 patients were given recommendations for medication but only 45 patients were prescribed medication by their family physicians and only 30 patients were still on medication at 6 months.
- In Sale and colleagues'[63] systematic review, up to 71% of patients were investigated with BMD but <35% initiated pharmacotherapy. Studies included in that systematic review demonstrated that ≤50% of patients screened through postfracture secondary interventions were taking calcium and/or vitamin D.[74,87–89]
- Other reports have demonstrated that less than 50% of patients followed-up with their family physician as advised[90–92] and that 55% to 62% of patients declined offers of a free BMD test.[91,93]

A body of research is emerging to partially explain the gaps in postfracture secondary prevention. Most of this research has been conducted from the patient perspective and is based on qualitative studies. It is the authors' opinions that many of the barriers to secondary prevention uptake by patients are modifiable. Less research has been reported on barriers at the level of the health care system or health care providers.

Patients Do Not Connect Their Fragility Fracture to Underlying Bone Health

A major barrier to treatment initiation (pharmacologic and nonpharmacologic) is patients' failure to connect their fracture to bone health status,[72,94–98] even after patients have been screened through a postfracture secondary prevention program.[72,94,95] Beaton and colleagues[72] reported that only 11% of patients connected their fracture with bone health status after they had been screened and educated about bone health through a postfracture secondary prevention program. One reason for the disconnect may be communication around the term, *fragility fracture*. In one study, in patients screened through a postfracture initiative, fragility fracture was considered a misnomer by patients who perceived the fracture as a traumatic event, both emotionally and physically.[99]

Patients Are Unclear About Several Aspects of Their Care

Several studies have demonstrated that patients screened through a postfracture secondary prevention program were unclear about many aspects of their care, including BMD test results[94,95] and treatment recommendations.[94] For example, some patients have been found to consider evidence of compromised bone health neither accurate nor serious.[95] Many fracture patients also are still uncertain about some aspect of their recommended care after screening, such as recommended doses and duration of treatment.[94] It has been shown that knowledge of OP and perceived benefits of treatment predict initiation of OP pharmacotherapy in patients screened through such programs.[72]

Patients Are Concerned About Side Effects

One study demonstrated that some patients had a difficult time with the decision to take OP pharmacotherapy because they were concerned about perceived and actual side effects of the medication.[100] In one study, 36 of 283 patients with a bisphosphonate prescription reported side effects, and approximately half of these patients (n = 19) had discontinued the medication by 3 months due to the side effects.[101] Others have reported patient concerns about side effects that led to patients declining an offer of medication or discontinuing their medication.[102–104]

OP Pharmacotherapy Use Fluctuates

Several studies have indicated that OP medication use varies over time because patients may start, stop, and then restart medication.[100,105–107] Individuals 65 years and older who were high risk for future fracture and screened through a postfracture initiative indicated that they might be persuaded to start or stop pharmacotherapy depending several circumstances.[100] The investigators of that study concluded that health care providers should consistently check in with patients to determine if willingness to take OP pharmacotherapy has changed.[100] In another study, 13% of patients who were on OP pharmacotherapy at baseline had discontinued therapy within 6 months of screening.[27]

Programs that Target Primary Care Providers Alone Are Not Enough

A recent multicomponent intervention consisting of 1-on-1 educational visits targeting primary care physicians in rural Ontario, Canada, demonstrated no improvement in postfracture care for patients.[108] The investigators concluded that there is a need for more active interventions to promote evidence-based care in rural care settings and smaller hospitals.[108]

BMD Test Reports Underestimate Fracture Risk

One reason that fracture patients who are indicated for pharmacotherapy do not initiate treatment may be related to lack of appropriate identification through BMD testing. One study of patients screened through a postfracture initiative found that BMD test reports underestimated fracture risk because the reports failed to consider prevalent or prior fractures as risk factors in the fracture risk assessment.[109]

FUTURE RESEARCH DIRECTIONS IN POSTFRACTURE SECONDARY PREVENTION

Postfracture secondary prevention programs have had considerable positive effects on bone health. Despite these successes, there are several opportunities for improvement:

- There is a need for consistent information to be relayed to patients beyond the orthopedic environment so that health care providers can promote long-term adherence to treatment recommendations.[94]
- Because the concept of fracture risk is relatively new, health care providers need to be aware of revisions to clinical practice guidelines concerning bone health. For example, the classification of high risk for future fracture changed in Canada between 2002[110] and 2010[54] and this has had significant effects on indications for pharmacotherapy.
- Special populations may need interventions tailored to their specific needs. Elderly patients who have had a hip fracture are especially vulnerable to not receiving postfracture secondary prevention. These patients are likely to present with dementia or cognitive impairment[111,112] both of which have been associated with lower prescriptions for OP pharmacotherapy.[113] Hip fracture patients are also likely to present with multiple comorbidities[111,114] and multiple comorbidities are also associated with decreased persistence with nonpharmacologic[115] and pharmacologic OP therapy.[116]

One challenge in developing postfracture secondary prevention programs is finding the highest-risk patients where they are likely concentrated (for example, hip fracture patients in orthopedic wards) and ensure that at least these highest-risk patients receive appropriate intervention. This is the most cost-effective activity when resources are limited.[69] Determining which patients are at high risk for future fracture needs to be considered because fracture risk varies from country to country.[117]

Secondary fracture prevention programs can be developed in stages. The program can start by targeting high-risk fractures, such as hip fractures, then expanded to target other fragility fracture patients if resources, the environment (eg, fracture clinic), and a well-organized health system are available.[69,118] If an efficient electronic health record is at the core of the health system, much of the screening can be done electronically. In some countries, there may be no fracture clinics and it may be difficult to find concentrations of fragility fracture patients in multiple centers and offices.

From a methodological perspective, the evidence base for the effect of postfracture secondary interventions needs to be developed further. For example, key outcomes, such as refracture rates and intervention costs, need to be reported[83] and comparisons among programs conducted with the same indicators (numerators and denominators). Currently, comparisons are difficult due to heterogeneous standards in reporting,[119] suggesting that there is a need to standardize data collection and selection of indicators used for reporting. It has been shown that reporting for antiresorptive medication initiation alone is problematic.[119]

SUMMARY

- Adults who have had a fragility fracture should be assessed for fracture risk and treated for bone health if indicated.
- Postfracture secondary prevention programs that aim to improve bone health after a fracture exist worldwide and programs that are coordinator based are endorsed by the International Osteoporosis Foundation.
- Opportunities to improve the success of these programs include facilitating patients' understanding of bone health recommendations and the connection between their fracture and bone health.
- Future research should aim to improve identification and screening of elderly patients, promote long-term adherence by patients to treatment recommendations, and standardize data collection and reporting from these programs.

REFERENCES

1. Kanis JA, Johnell O, Oden A, et al. Long-term risk of osteoporotic fracture in Malmo. Osteoporos Int 2000;11:669–74.
2. Johnell O, Kanis J. Epidemiology of osteoporotic fractures. Osteoporos Int 2005; 16(Suppl 2):S3–7.
3. van Staa TP, Dennison EM, Leufkens HG, et al. Epidemiology of fractures in England and Wales. Bone 2001;29:517–22.
4. Cauley JA, Wampler NS, Barnhart JM, et al. Incidence of fractures compared to cardiovascular disease and breast cancer: the women's health intitiative observational study. Osteoporos Int 2008;19:1717–23.
5. Langsetmo L, Goltzman D, Kovacs CS, et al, CaMos Research Group. Repeat low-trauma fractures occur frequently among men and women who have osteopenic bone mineral density. J Bone Miner Res 2009;24:1515–22.
6. Center JR, Bliuc D, Nguyen TV, et al. Risk of subsequent fracture after low-trauma fracture in men and women. JAMA 2007;297:387–94.

7. Kanis JA, Johnell O, De LC, et al. A meta-analysis of previous fracture and subsequent fracture risk. Bone 2004;35:375–82. http://dx.doi.org/10.1016/j.bone.2004.03.024. pii:S8756328204001309.
8. van Geel TA, Geusens PP, Nagtzaam IF, et al. Risk factors for clinical fractures among postmenopausal women: a 10-year prospective study. Menopause Int 2007;13:110–5.
9. Klotzbuecher CM, Ross PD, Landsman PB, et al. Patients with prior fractures have an increased risk of future fractures: a summary of the literature and statistical synthesis. J Bone Miner Res 2000;15:721–39.
10. van Geel TA, van Helden S, Geusens PP, et al. Clinical subsequent fractures cluster in time after first fractures. Ann Rheum Dis 2009;68:99–102.
11. Ioannidis G, Papaioannou A, Hopman WM, et al. Relation between fractures and mortality: results from the Canadian Multicentre Osteoporosis Study. CMAJ 2009;181:265–71.
12. Sernbo I, Johnell O. Consequences of a hip fracture: a prospective study over 1 year. Osteoporos Int 1993;3:148–53.
13. Center JR, Nguyen TV, Schneider D, et al. Mortality after all major types of osteoporotic fracture in men and women: an observational study. Lancet 1999;353:878–82.
14. Bliuc D, Nguyen ND, Milch VE, et al. Mortality risk associated with low-trauma osteoporotic fracture and subsequent fracture in men and women. JAMA 2009;301:513–21.
15. Rabenda V, Vanoverloop J, Fabri V, et al. Low incidence of anti-osteoporosis treatment after hip fracture. J Bone Joint Surg Am 2008;90:2142–8.
16. van der Jagt-Willems HC, Vis M, Tulner CR, et al. Mortality and incident vertebral fractures after 3 years of follow-up among geriatric patients. Osteoporos Int 2013;24:1713–9.
17. Papaioannou A, Adachi JD, Parkinson W, et al. Lengthy hospitalization associated with vertebral fractures despite control for comorbid conditions. Osteoporos Int 2001;12:870–4.
18. Haentjens P, Lamraski G, Boonen S. Costs and consequences of hip fracture occurrence in old age: an economic perspective. Disabil Rehabil 2005;27:1129–41.
19. Johnell O, Kanis JA. An estimate of the worldwide prevalence and disability associated with osteoporotic fractures. Osteoporos Int 2006;17:1726–33.
20. Nikitovic M, Wodchis WP, Krahn MD, et al. Direct health-care costs attributed to hip fractures among seniors: a matched cohort study. Osteoporos Int 2013;24:659–69.
21. Wiktorowicz ME, Goeree R, Papaioannou A, et al. Economic implications of hip fracture: health service use, institutional care and cost in Canada. Osteoporos Int 2001;12:271–8.
22. Keene GS, Parker MJ, Pryor GA. Mortality and morbidity after hip fractures. BMJ 1993;307:1248–50.
23. Song X, Shi N, Badamgarav E, et al. Cost burden of second fracture in the US Health Sytem. Bone 2011. http://dx.doi.org/10.1016/j.bone.2010.12.021.
24. Papaioannou A, Morin S, Cheung AM, et al, for the Scientific Advisory Council of Osteoporosis Canada. Clinical practice guidelines for the diagnosis and management of osteoporosis in Canada. Background Technical Report 2010;1–228.
25. Cranney A, Guyatt G, Griffith L, et al, The Osteoporosis Methodology Group aTORAG. IX: summary of meta-analyses of therapies for postmenopausal osteoporosis. Endocr Rev 2002;23:570–8.
26. Kanis JA, McCloskey EV, Johansson H, et al, Scientific Advisory Board of the European Society for Clinical and Economic Aspects of Osteoporosis and Osteoarthritis

(ESCEO) and the Committee of Scientific Advisors of the International Osteoporosis Foundation (IOF). European guidance for the diagnosis and management of osteoporosis in postmenopausal women. Osteoporos Int 2013;24:23–57.

27. Sale JE, Beaton DE, Elliot-Gibson VI, et al. A post-fracture initiative to improve osteoporosis management in a community hospital in Ontario. J Bone Joint Surg Am 2010;92:1973–80.

28. Bogoch ER, Elliot-Gibson V, Beaton DE, et al. Effective initiation of osteoporosis diagnosis and treatment for patients with a fragility fracture in an orthopaedic environment. J Bone Joint Surg Am 2006;88(1):25–34.

29. Wells GA, Cranney A, Peterson J, et al. Alendronate for the primary and secondary prevention of osteoporotic fractures in postmenopausal women. Cochrane Database Syst Rev 2008;(1):CD001155.

30. Wells GA, Cranney A, Peterson J, et al. Risedronate for the primary and secondary prevention of osteoporotic fractures in postmenopausal women. Cochrane Database Syst Rev 2008;(1):CD004523.

31. McClung MR, Geusens P, Miller PD, et al, for the Hip Intervention Program Study Group. Effects of risedronate on the risk of hip fracture in elderly women. N Engl J Med 2001;344:333–40.

32. Lyles KA, Colon-Emeric CS, Mazaziner JS, et al, for the HORIZON Recurrent Fracture Trial. Zoledronic acid and clinical fractures and mortality after hip fracture. N Engl J Med 2007;357:1799–809.

33. Kanis JA, Barton IP, Johnell O. Risedronate decreases fracture risk in patients selected solely on the basis of prior vertebral fracture. Osteoporos Int 2005; 16:475–82.

34. Gallagher AM, Rietbrock S, Olsen M. Fracture outcomes related to persistence and compliance with oral bisphosphonates. J Bone Miner Res 2008;23:1569–75.

35. Harrington JT, Ste-Marie LG, Brandi ML, et al. Risedronate rapidly reduces the risk of nonvertebral fractures in women with postmenopausal osteoporosis. Calcif Tissue Int 2004;74:129–35.

36. Lee YK, Ha YC, Yoon BH, et al. Incidence of second hip fracture and compliant use of bisphosphonate. Osteoporos Int 2013;24:2099–104.

37. Carey JJ. What is a 'failure' of bisphosphonate therapy for osteoporosis? Cleve Clin J Med 2005;72:1033–9.

38. Gates BJ, Sonnett TE, DuVall CA, et al. Review of osteoporosis pharmacotherapy for geriatric patients. Am J Geriatr Pharmacother 2009;7:293–323.

39. Sambrook PN, Chen JS, Simpson JM, et al. Impact of adverse news media on prescriptions for osteoporosis: effect on fractures and mortality. Med J Aust 2010;193:154–6.

40. Bischoff-Ferrari HA, Willett WC, Wong JB, et al. Prevention of nonvertebral factures with oral vitamin D and dose dependency: a meta-analysis of randomized controlled trials. Arch Intern Med 2009;169:551–61.

41. Bischoff-Ferrari HA, Willett WC, Wong JB, et al. Fracture prevention with vitamin D supplementation: a meta-analysis of randomized controlled trials. JAMA 2005; 293:2257–64.

42. Boonen S, Lips P, Bouillon R, et al. Need for additional calcium to reduce the risk of hip fracture with vitamin D supplementation: evidence from a comparative metaanalysis of randomized controlled trials. J Clin Endocrinol Metab 2007; 92:1415–23.

43. Prentice RL, Pettinger MB, Jackson RD, et al. Health risks and benefits from calcium and vitamin D supplementation: women's health initiative clinical trial and cohort study. Osteoporos Int 2013;24:567–80.

44. Abrahamsen B, Sahota O. Do calcium plus vitamin D supplements increase cardiovascular risk? Insuffcient evidence is available to support or refute the association. BMJ 2011;342:d2080.

45. Sawka AM, Boulos P, Beattie K, et al. Hip protectors decrease hip fracture in elderly nursing home residents: a Bayesian meta-analysis. J Clin Epidemiol 2007;60:336–44.

46. Oliver D, Connelly JB, Victor CR, et al. Strategies to prevent falls and fractures in hospitals and care homes and effect of cognitive impairment: systematic review and metaanalysis. Br Med J 2006;334:82–7.

47. Kemmler W, Haberle L, von Stengel S. Effects of exercise on fracture reduction in older adults. Osteoporos Int 2013;24:1937–50.

48. Leslie WD, Siminoski K, Brown JP. Comparative effects of densitometric and absolute fracture risk classification systems on projected intervention rates in postmenopausal women. J Clin Densitom 2007;10:124–31.

49. Kanis JA, Oden A, Johansson H, et al. FRAX and it's applications to clinical practice. Bone 2009;44:734–43.

50. Bogoch ER, Cheung AM, Elliot-Gibson VI, et al. Preventing the second hip fracture: addressing osteoporosis in hip fracture patients. In: Waddell JP, editor. Fractures of the proximal femur. Maryland Heights (MO): Elsevier; 2010. p. 243–61.

51. Rubin KH, Friis-Holmberg T, Hermann AP, et al. Risk assessment tools to identify women with increased risk of osteoporotic fracture: complexity or simplicity? A systematic review. J Bone Miner Res 2013;28:1701–17.

52. Leslie WD, Berger C, Langsetmo L, et al, Canadian Multicentre Osteoporosis Study Research Group. Construction and validation of a simplified fracture risk assessment tool for Canadian women and men: results from the CaMos and Manitoba cohorts. Osteoporos Int 2011;22:1873–83.

53. Cranney A, Jamal SA, Tsang JF, et al. Low bone mineral density and fracture burden in postmenopausal women. CMAJ 2007;177:575–80.

54. Papaioannou A, Leslie WD, Morin S, et al, Scientific Advisory Council of Osteoporosis Canada. 2010 Clinical practice guidelines for the diagnosis and management of osteoporosis in Canada. Can Med Assoc J 2010;182:1864–73.

55. Compston J, Bowring C, Cooper A, et al. Diagnosis and management of osteoporosis in postmenopausal women and older men in the UK: National Osteoporosis Guideline Group (NOGG) update 2013. Maturitas 2013. http://dx.doi.org/10.1016/j.maturitas.2013.05.013.

56. Giangregorio L, Papaioannou A, Cranney A, et al. Fragility fractures and the osteoporosis care gap: an international phenomenon. Semin Arthritis Rheum 2006;35:293–305.

57. Papaioannou A, Giangregorio L, Kvern B, et al. The osteoporosis care gap in Canada [Review]. BMC Musculoskelet Disord 2004;5(1):11.

58. Elliot-Gibson V, Bogoch ER, Jamal SA, et al. Practice patterns in the diagnosis and treatment of osteoporosis after a fragility fracture: a systematic review [Review]. Osteoporos Int 2004;15(10):767–78.

59. Hooven F, Gehlbach SH, Pekow P, et al. Follow-up treatment for osteoporosis after fracture. Osteoporos Int 2005;16:301.

60. Leslie WD, Giangregorio LM, Yogendran M, et al. A population-based analysis of the post-fracture care gap 1996-2008: the situation is not improving. Osteoporos Int 2012;23:1623–9.

61. Edwards BJ, Bunta AD, Simonelli C, et al. Prior fractures are common in patients with subsequent hip fractures. Clin Orthop Relat Res 2007;461:226–30.

62. Port L, Center J, Briffa NK, et al. Osteoporotic fracture: missed opportunity for intervention. Osteoporos Int 2003;14:780–4.
63. Sale JE, Beaton D, Posen J, et al. Systematic review on interventions to improve osteoporosis investigation and treatment in fragility fracture patients. Osteoporos Int 2011;22:2067–82.
64. Queally JM, Kiernan C, Shaikh M, et al. Initiation of osteoporosis assessment in the fracture clinic results in improved osteoporosis management: a randomised controlled trial. Osteoporos Int 2013;24:1089–94.
65. Inderjeeth CA, Glennon DA, Poland KE, et al. A multimodal intervention to improve fragility fracture management in patients presenting to emergency departments. Med J Aust 2010;193:149–53.
66. Langridge CR, McQuillian C, Watson WS, et al. Refracture following fracture liaison service assessment illustrates the requirement for integrated falls and fracture services. Calcif Tissue Int 2007;81(2):85–91.
67. Akesson K, Mitchell P. Capture the fracture: a global campaign to break the fragility fracture cycle. International Osteoporosis Foundation report. Switzerland: Nyon; 2012. p. 1–28.
68. McLellan AR, Gallacher SJ, Fraser M, et al. The fracture liaison service: success of a program for the evaluation and management of patients with osteoporotic fracture. Osteoporos Int 2003;14(12):1028–34.
69. Dell R. Fracture prevention in Kaiser Permanente Southern California. Osteoporos Int 2011;22:S457–60.
70. Lih A, Nandapalan H, Kim M, et al. Targeted intervention reduces refracture rates in patients with incident non-vertebral osteoporotic fractures: a 4-year prospective controlled study. Osteoporos Int 2011;22:849 58. http://dx.doi.org/10.1007/s00198-010-1477-x.
71. Chandran M, Tan MZ, Cheen M, et al. Secondary prevention of osteoporotic fractures - an "OPTIMAL" model of care from Singapore. Osteoporos Int 2013. http://dx.doi.org/10.1007/s00198-013-2368-8.
72. Beaton D, Dyer S, Jiang D, et al. Factors influencing the pharmacological management of osteoporosis after a fragility fracture: results from the Ontario Osteoporosis Strategy's Fracture Clinic Screening Program. Osteoporos Int 2013. http://dx.doi.org/10.1007/s00198-013-2430-6.
73. Tosi LL, Gliklich R, Kannan K, et al. The American Orthopaedic Association's "own the bone" initiative to prevent secondary fractures. J Bone Joint Surg Am 2008;90(1):163–73.
74. Davis JC, Guy P, Ashe MC, et al. HipWatch: osteoporosis investigation and treatment after a hip fracture: a 6-month randomized controlled trial. J Gerontol A Biol Sci Med Sci 2007;62(8):888–91.
75. Majumdar SR, Beaupre LA, Harley CH, et al. Use of a case manager to improve osteoporosis treatment after hip fracture: results of a randomized controlled trial. Arch Intern Med 2007;167(19):2110–5.
76. Ganda KP, Chen JS, Speerin R, et al. Models of care for the secondary prevention of osteoporotic fractures: a systematic review and meta-analysis. Osteoporos Int 2013;24:393–406.
77. Cooper MS, Palmer AJ, Seibel MJ. Cost-effectiveness of the Concord Minimal Trauma Fracture Liaison service, a prospective, controlled fracture prevention study. Osteoporos Int 2012;23:97–107.
78. Majumdar S, Lier DA, Beaupre LA, et al. Osteoporosis case manager for patients with hip fractures: results of a cost-effectiveness analysis conducted alongside a randomized trial. Arch Intern Med 2009;169:25–31.

79. Majumdar SR, Johnson JA, Lier DA, et al. Persistence, reproducibility, and cost-effectiveness of an intervention to improve the quality of osteoporosis care after a fracture of the wrist: results of a controlled trial. Osteoporos Int 2007;18(3): 261–70.
80. Sander B, Elliot-Gibson V, Beaton DE, et al. A coordinator program in post-fracture management of osteoporosis improves outcomes and saves costs. J Bone Joint Surg Am 2008;90:1197–205.
81. Little EA, Eccles MP. A systematic review of the effectiveness of interventions to improve post-fracture investigation and management of patients at risk of osteoporosis. Implement Sci 2010;5:80.
82. Haaland DA, Cohen DR, Kennedy CC, et al. Closing the osteoporosis care gap - increased osteoporosis awareness among geriatrics and rehabilitation teams. BMC Geriatr 2009;9:28–36.
83. Sale JE, Beaton D, Posen J, et al. Key outcomes are not usually reported in published fracture secondary prevention programs - results of a systematic review. Arch Orthop Trauma Surg 2013. http://dx.doi.org/10.1007/s00402-011-1442-y.
84. Astrand J, Nilsson J, Thorngren KG. Screening for osteoporosis reduced new fracture incidence by almost half: a 6-year follow-up of 592 patients from an osteoporosis screening program. Acta Orthop 2012;33:665.
85. Marsh D, Akesson K, Beaton D, et al, the IOF CSA Fracture Working Group. Coordinator-based systems for secondary prevention in fragility fracture patients. Osteoporos Int 2011;22:2051–65.
86. Chevalley T, Hoffmeyer P, Bonjour JP, et al. An osteoporosis clinical pathway for the medical management of patients with low-trauma fracture. Osteoporos Int 2002;13:450–5.
87. Majumdar SR, Johnson JA, McAlister FA, et al. Multifaceted intervention to improve diagnosis and treatment of osteoporosis in patients with recent wrist fracture: a randomized controlled trial. CMAJ 2008;178(5): 569–75.
88. Majumdar SR, Rowe BH, Folk D, et al. A controlled trial to increase detection and treatment of osteoporosis in older patients with a wrist fracture. Ann Intern Med 2004;141(5):366–73.
89. Hawker G, Ridout R, Ricupero M, et al. The impact of a simple fracture clinic intervention in improving the diagnosis and treatment of osteoporosis in fragility fracture patients. Osteoporos Int 2003;14(2):171–8.
90. Ho C, Cranney A, Campbell A. Measuring the impact of pharmacist intervention: results of patient education about osteoporosis after fragility fracture. Can J Hosp Pharm 2006;59:184–93.
91. Bliuc D, Eisman JA, Center JR. A randomized study of two different information-based interventions on the management of osteoporosis in minimal and moderate trauma fractures. Osteoporos Int 2006;17(9):1309–17.
92. Gardner MJ, Brophy RH, Demetrakopoulos D, et al. Interventions to improve osteoporosis treatment following hip fracture. A prospective, randomized trial [see comment]. J Bone Joint Surg Am 2005;87(1):3–7.
93. Harrington JT, Barash HL, Day S, et al. Redesigning the care of fragility fracture patients to improve osteoporosis management: a health care improvement project. Arthritis Rheum 2005;53(2):198–204.
94. Sale JE, Beaton DE, Sujic R, et al. "If it was osteoporosis, I would have really hurt myself". Ambiguity about osteoporosis and osteoporosis care despite a screening program to educate fracture patients. J Eval Clin Pract 2010;16: 590–6.

95. Sale JE, Beaton D, Fraenkel L, et al. The BMD muddle: the disconnect between bone densitometry results and perception of bone health. J Clin Densitom 2010; 13:370–8.
96. Meadows LM, Mrkonjic LA, Petersen KM, et al. After the fall: women's views of fractures in relation to bone health at midlife. Womens Health 2004;39:47–62.
97. Meadows LM, Mrkonjic LA. Breaking–bad news: women's experiences of fractures at midlife. Can J Public Health 2003;94:427–30.
98. Giangregorio L, Dolovich L, Cranney A, et al. Osteoporosis risk perceptions among pateints who have sustained a fragility fracture. Patient Educ Couns 2009;74:213–20.
99. Sale JE, Gignac M, Hawker G, et al. Patients reject the concept of fragility fracture - a new understanding based on fracture patients' communication. Osteoporos Int 2012;23:2829–34.
100. Sale J, Gignac M, Hawker G, et al. Decision to take osteoporosis medication in patients who have had a fracture and are 'high' risk for future fracture. BMC Musculoskelet Disord 2011;12:92.
101. Blonk MC, Erdtsieck RJ, Wernekinck MG, et al. The fracture and osteoporosis clinic: 1-year results and 3-month compliance. Bone 2007;40(6):1643–9.
102. Miki RA, Oetgen ME, Kirk J, et al. Orthopaedic management improves the rate of early osteoporosis treatment after hip fracture. A randomized clinical trial. J Bone Joint Surg Am 2008;90:2353.
103. Che M, Ettinger B, Liang J, et al. Outcomes of a disease-management program for patients with recent osteoporotic fracture. Osteoporos Int 2006;17(6):847–54.
104. Laslett LL, Whitham JN, Gibb C, et al. Improving diagnosis and treatment of osteoporosis: evaluation of a clinical pathway for low trauma fractures. Arch Osteoporos 2007;2(1–2):1–6.
105. Brookhart MA, Avorn J, Katz JN, et al. Gaps in treatment among users of osteoporosis medications: the dynamics of noncompliance. Am J Med 2007;120:251–6.
106. Weiss TW, McHorney CA. Osteoporosis medication profile preference: results from the PREFER-US study. Health Expect 2007;10:211–23.
107. Melo M, Qiu F, Sykora K, et al. Persistence with bisphosphonate therapy in older people. J Am Geriatr Soc 2006;54:1015–6.
108. Jaglal SB, Hawker G, Bansod V, et al. A demonstration project of a multi-component educational intervention to improve integrated post-fracture osteoporosis care in five rural communities in Ontario, Canada. Osteoporos Int 2009;20:265–74. http://dx.doi.org/10.1007/s00198-008-0654-7.
109. Sale JE, Frankel L, Inrig T, et al. BMD reporting underestimates fracture risk in Ontario. Fragility Fracture Network Global Congress. 2013.
110. Brown JP, Josse RG, Scientific Advisory Council of the Osteoporosis Society of Canada. 2002 clinical practice guidelines for the diagnosis and management of osteoporosis in Canada. CMAJ 2002;167:S1–34.
111. Gruber-Baldini AL, Zimmerman S, Morrison S, et al. Cognitive impairment in hip fracture patients: timing of detection and longitudinal follow-up. J Am Geriatr Soc 2003;51:1227–36.
112. Mauck KF, Cuddihy MT, Trousdale RT, et al. The decision to accept treatment for osteoporosis following hip fracture: exploring the woman's perspective using a stage-of-change model. Osteoporos Int 2002;13:560–4.
113. Jones G, Warr S, Francis E, et al. The effect of a fracture protocol on hospital prescriptions after minimal trauma fractured neck of the femur: a retrospective audit. Osteoporos Int 2005;16:1277–80.

114. Morrish DW, Beaupre LA, Bell NR, et al. Facilitated bone mineral density testing versus hospital-based case management to improve osteoporosis treatment for hip fracture patients: additional results from a randomized trial. Arthritis Rheum 2009;61:209–15.
115. Giusti A, Barone A, Razzano M, et al. Persistence with calcium and vitamin D in elderly patients after hip fracture. J Bone Miner Metab 2009;27:95–100.
116. Solomon DH, Avorn J, Katz JN, et al. Compliance with osteoporosis medications. Arch Intern Med 2005;165:2414–9.
117. Siris E, Delmas PD. Assessment of 10-year absolute fracture risk: a new paradigm with worldwide application. Osteoporos Int 2008;19:1–2.
118. Akesson K, Marsh D, Mitchell PJ, et al, IOF Fracture Working Group. Capture the fracture: a best practice framework and global campaign to break the fragility fracture cycle. Osteoporos Int 2013. http://dx.doi.org/10.1007/s00198-013-2348-z.
119. Sale JE, Beaton D, Posen J, et al. Medication initiation rates are not directly comparable across secondary fracture prevention programs: reporting standards based on a systematic review. J Clin Epidemiol 2013;66:379–85.

Postoperative Prevention of Falls in Older Adults with Fragility Fractures

Oddom Demontiero, MBBS, FRACP[a,b],
Piumali Gunawardene, MBBS, FRACP[a,b],
Gustavo Duque, MD, PhD, FRACP[a,b,c],*

KEYWORDS

- Falls • Sarcopenia • Falls prevention • Fragility fracture • Postoperative care
- Falls risk assessment • Older adults • Secondary prevention of falls

KEY POINTS

- Falls and fractures are interconnected, with patients suffering a fragility fracture being at high risk of falls, especially during the postoperative period.
- Patients at higher risk of falls should be identified either at admission or during the immediate postoperative period.
- A comprehensive falls prevention plan should be established in postfracture patients. This plan should be multicomponent and directed to correct as many risk factors as possible.
- Any falls prevention plan initiated during the postoperative period should be continued as an outpatient, with appropriate multidisciplinary intervention in the community.

INTRODUCTION

Falls are associated with significant morbidity and disability in the older population. The risk of falling increases rapidly with age,[1] with one-third of people aged 65 years and older falling each year[2] and with half of such cases being recurrent.[3] Furthermore, the risk increases exponentially with the number of risk factors; 1-year risk of falling

Funding Sources: Rebecca Cooper Foundation, Nepean Medical Research Foundation (O. Demontiero); Nepean Medical Research Foundation (P. Gunawardene); NHMRC, Nepean Medical Research Foundation, Amgen, Novartis Pharma, Eli Lilly, and Merck (G. Duque).
Conflicts of Interest: None (O. Demontiero & P. Gunawardene); Consultant and speaker for Novartis, Amgen, and Procter & Gamble (G. Duque).
a Department of Geriatric Medicine, Nepean Hospital, PO Box 63, Penrith, New South Wales 2750, Australia; b Ageing Bone Research Program, Sydney Medical School Nepean, The University of Sydney, Penrith, New South Wales, Australia; c Division of Geriatric Medicine, Sydney Medical School Nepean, The University of Sydney, PO Box 63, Penrith, New South Wales 2750, Australia
* Corresponding author. Ageing Bone Research Program, Sydney Medical School Nepean, PO Box 63, Penrith, New South Wales 2750, Australia.
E-mail address: gustavo.duque@sydney.edu.au

Clin Geriatr Med 30 (2014) 333–347
http://dx.doi.org/10.1016/j.cger.2014.01.018
0749-0690/14/$ – see front matter © 2014 Elsevier Inc. All rights reserved.

Case

Mrs J was an 82-year-old white woman admitted into the hospital with a right hip fracture after falling over a lamp cord in her single-level, carpeted home. She was diagnosed with 2 vertebral fractures in her lumbar spine (L1-L2) 2 years previously. She also reported 5 falls within the last year, 2 at the shopping center and 3 at home. The falls were asymptomatic and the patient was able to stand up afterward without assistance. No falls-related trauma was reported until the current presentation. She had a hysterectomy at age 45 years for fibroids; the ovaries were not removed. She experienced menopause at age 53 years and had not taken hormone therapy. She was taking a β-blocker (metoprolol), diuretic (furosemide), and benzodiazepine (lorazepam). Her dietary calcium intake was consistent, at about 250 mg daily. She did not smoke. She did not engage in regular weight-bearing exercise. The patient was 152.5 cm (5′ 0″) and she weighed 47.5 kg (105 lb). Her height had decreased 1.5 cm over the previous 3 years. Chemistry profile, thyroid studies, urinalysis, and complete blood count were normal.

The patient was assessed by the orthogeriatrics team and was taken to surgery within the first 24 hours after fracture. Her immediate postoperative (24 hour) period was good; however, the patient was confused at day 3 and was diagnosed with delirium. No evident cause of the delirium was found. Management was started with haloperidol at low dose. On day 5 postoperatively, the patient left her bed to go to the toilet by herself. Ten minutes later, the nursing staff found the patient lying on the ground with a bleeding laceration in her forehead and complaining of back pain. A computed tomography scan of her brain showed no intracranial bleeding, but a radiograph of her spine showed a new vertebral crushing in L3. The patient was still in delirium, with poor oral intake.

Three days later, the patient had significantly improved. Her oral intake was better and her delirium had resolved. Haloperidol was discontinued. The interdisciplinary team recommended transferring her to one of the orthorehabilitation beds. One week after being transferred, and while receiving physical therapy, the patient suffered a new asymptomatic fall, this time witnessed and without associated trauma. Two weeks after fracture, the patient was discharged back home, with a home visit by an occupational therapist scheduled within 2 weeks after discharge. The patient was also scheduled to have a follow-up at the local falls and fractures clinic.

---

doubles with each additional factor, starting from 8% with none, and reaching 78% with 4 risk factors.[4]

Several established risk factors for falls have been described both in community[2,4] and hospital settings,[5,6] with some of these risk factors increasing fracture risk as well.[7] Although only 1% to 5% of falls result in fractures,[8] hip fractures occur almost always secondary to falls[9,10] and are associated with significant morbidity, a median survival of around 2 years, and substantial inpatient and residential care costs.[11,12] Furthermore, although both bone-related and fall-related risk factors predict hip fractures,[13] fall-related risk factors are more prevalent than bone-related risk factors in patients with recent clinical fractures,[14] and falling tendency is the more important predictor of fragility fractures in the older population.[15] In patients with any recent clinical fractures, the incidence of falling again within 3 months ranges from 11%[16] to 15%,[17] with a falls rate of 1.5 to 3.5 falls per patient year.[17,18] After hip fractures, studies[19–22] showed that between 18% and 53% fall again within 2 to 6 months after subacute rehabilitation. Another study[23] showed that within 12 months, up to 56% of people fall again at least once, and 28% fall more than once, resulting in a new fracture in 12% of cases and a second hip fracture in 5% of cases. Only 1 earlier study did not find a significant increase in the falls incidence rate among patients with hip fractures compared with age-matched and gender-matched controls at 6 to 12 months after fracture.[24] However, this hip fracture cohort was noted to be less mobile and inferior on overall functional parameters compared with the control group.

Data on risk of falls after hip fractures are lacking. One study reported the overall risk of falling to be 6.4 per 1000 patient-days after any clinical fractures.[18] Nevertheless, abundant evidence suggests that falls and fractures result in dramatic health, social, and psychological consequences. Therefore, it is not surprising that the focus in fracture prevention has shifted from osteoporosis toward fall prevention,[25] at least in the older population. In addition, because of the complex cause of falls, risk should be addressed along the continuum of care of aging adults. Thus, in the context of the patient described earlier, the hospital offers a good setting for secondary falls prevention, including early identification of falls risk and prevention of associated injuries in the postoperative period. In-hospital interventions (preoperative and postoperative) should include multifactorial assessments and interventions, which should continue during inpatient rehabilitation, complemented with individualized interventions tailored to the identification of intrinsic and extrinsic risk factors. This program should be continued as an outpatient, with the combination of a suitable exercise program in the community, multidisciplinary intervention plan, and follow-up at a specialized falls and fractures clinic.

RISK FACTORS FOR FALLS

Several risk factors for falls in community-dwelling adults have been previously identified (**Box 1**),[9] with some of these having stronger association with falling than others.[4] In Mrs J's case, she was identified as at high risk of recurrent falls on admission based on her gender, age older than 80 years, orthostatic hypotension from antihypertensive medication, benzodiazepine medication, and, most importantly, 5 falls in the previous 12 months. Another risk factor that is often overlooked is fear of falling, which can be severely debilitating and create additional risks of falling through self-protective immobility.[26]

Furthermore, several risk factors have been identified during the immediate preoperative and transoperative periods, which also predict postoperative falling and injurious falls, some up to 1 year (**Box 2**).[23,27,28] Based on her preoperative history of

---

Box 1
Independent risk factors for falls in the community setting with associated relative risk and odds ratio[a]

Previous falls	1.9–6.6
Balance impairment	1.2–2.4
Decreased muscle strength	2.2–2.6
Visual impairment	1.5–2.3
Polypharmacy (>4 medications) or psychoactive drugs	1.1–2.4
Gait impairment or walking difficulty	1.2–2.2
Depression	1.5–2.8
Dizziness or orthostatic hypotension	2.0[a]
Functional limitations	1.5–6.2
Age >80 years	1.1–1.3
Female sex	2.1–3.9
Low body mass index	1.5–1.8
Urinary incontinence	1.3–1.8
Cognitive impairment	2.8[a]
Arthritis	1.2–1.9
Diabetes	3.8[a]
Pain	1.7[a]

[a] Indicates odds ratio.

Box 2
Preoperative and transoperative risk factors for recurrent falls in the general postoperative period. Those factors in bold have the higher relative risk for new falls

Preoperative

Anemia

American Society of Anesthesiologists score ≥3

Congestive heart failure

Continuous peripheral nerve blocks

Functional dependence

Higher preoperative Geriatric Depression Scale scores

History of falling

Lower albumin level

Male gender

Need for an emergency surgery

Nocturnal incontinence

Nutritional status

Older age

Poorer quality of life

Transoperative

Increased transfusion requirement

Longer surgical time

falling, having a fractured hip, old age, and having continuous peripheral nerve blocks for postoperative analgesia, Mrs J would be at high risk of recurrent falls during her postoperative period, and therefore, a more comprehensive intervention plan for falls prevention should be designed in this case.

Early in the postoperative period, Mrs J would be at greater risk of falls because of her acute illnesses and complications such as delirium. Postoperative delirium in the first few days after surgery is common, with incidence in various postoperative settings ranging from 4% up to 65% of cases after hip surgery.[29–31] An observational study of inpatient falls in various acute surgical settings, including orthopedics, reported the main precipitants of postoperative falls to be delirium (43%), disability (34%), and environmental factors (13%).[32] Furthermore, a delirium during admission is one of the most important independent risk factors for failure to return to prefracture level of mobility.[33]

Adverse effects of medications can also contribute to falls, because hospitalization often leads to increased complexity of medication regimens for older patients. Polypharmacy is well known to be associated with falls, with individual classes of medication being associated with high fall risk in both community and inpatient settings (Box 3).[3–6,34–37] Of these medications, psychotropic drugs have the most robust association with delirium.[38] It is not certain whether the use of haloperidol with Mrs J contributed to her fall, because it was prescribed to ameliorate her delirium.

The other potential contributing factor to Mrs J falling on day 5 is her prolonged immobilization. Older adults can lose significant muscle mass and strength in only a few days of bed rest. Inactivity and bed rest cause muscle shortening and changes

---

Box 3
Specific medication classes associated with falls and reported relative risk and odds ratio[a]

Anticonvulsants[3–6,35,a]	1.9–2.2
Antidepressants[3–6,35,a]	1.2–1.7
Antihypertensive medications[4,6,35,a]	1.3–2.4
Benzodiazepines[3–5,35,36]	1.4–2.2
Polypharmacy[3]	1.7–2.7
Psychotropics[3,5,6,35,a]	0.4–2.3
Tranquilizers[a]	1.5[a]
β-Blockers[35]	1.0[a]
Diuretics[6,35,a]	0.8–1.1
Antiparkinsonians[6,a]	1.7[a]

[a] Indicates odds ratio.

---

in periarticular and cartilaginous joint structures, which contribute to limitation of mobility and thus predispose to falls. The most significant change in loss of muscle strength takes place during the first week of immobilization.[39] Loss of muscle strength from immobility can occur at 1% or more per day in younger adults and is likely to be higher in older adults.[40] This phenomenon is highlighted by the fact that weakness in certain muscle groups has been shown to predict falls after hip surgery. Pils and colleagues[18] showed that although deficits in hip range of movement were more pronounced in fallers compared with nonfallers, the only predictor for falls among all the functional deficits studied was a hip abduction-adduction deficit of the nonoperated side. More recently, Yau and colleagues[41] reported that the presence of knee extensor and flexor weakness soon after hip surgery increased the risk of falling by nearly 5-fold.

Another important factor to recognize is that most falls occur in the context of patients being acutely unwell, being in an unfamiliar environment, and in some cases, not being adequately supervised by hospital staff. This situation typically occurs with agitated delirious patients or impulsive patients with dementia. The environmental circumstances in which Mrs J fell are typical and are consistent with various studies reported in the literature (summarized in see **Box 4**).[42–44] Although a consistent relationship between fall incidents, staffing levels, and patient case mix is lacking,[45] intuitively, understaffed units in which delays in responding to patients' needs are commonplace would almost inevitably experience an increase in falls.

Box 4
Environmental circumstances of inpatients falls

- Falls happened when patients were trying to undertake a task without supervision
- Falls occurred mainly from the bed or as patients made their way to bathrooms and from a chair
- Most falls were unwitnessed
- More than half of the falls occurred in and around the bed unit area when patients were transferring to and from the bed
- Nurses were not physically present with the patient at time of most falls
- One-third of the falls occurred in the bathroom/toilet when patients tried to stand up unassisted after using the toilet or shower
- Patient behaviors (unaware of inability to mobilize/transfer independently, removing O_2, attempting to stand on wet floor, unwilling or unable to use the call bell)

During subacute rehabilitation, similar risk factors responsible for falls in the community setting also contribute to falls in the rehabilitation setting (**Box 5**).[6] After hip fractures, specifically, several studies again showed that recurrent falls are associated with the less mobile and less active patients,[18] higher number of chronic diseases and medications, higher prefracture disability, chronic heart failure, and lower vitamin D levels, handgrip strength, and quality of life. Similar to patients without hip fracture in the community, the use of a rollator frame (rolling walker) and nocturnal urinary incontinence are also associated with falls.[28] The measures of impairment before hip fracture (disability, poor vitamin D status, and a more sedentary lifestyle), combined with strength and balance impairments persistent after surgery, identified the most vulnerable individuals, who would go on to suffer injurious falls again.[23] Hip abductor weakness had the strongest relationship with fall-related injuries risk.[23]

As mentioned earlier, the incidence of recurrent falls among patients with hip fracture is high, even after successful rehabilitation. The risks associated with these falls resemble those in the population without hip fracture. Studies varying in lengths of follow-up from 3 months to 2 years reported significant risks to be age, female sex, difficulties in activities of daily living, orthostatic hypotension and polypharmacy[17,46] more handicap, lower ABC (activities-specific balance confidence) and falls efficacy score,[20] worry over further falls,[19,46] previous falls and poor performance with the 5-m TUG (timed up and go) test, timed 10-m walk, and turn 180 test.[47]

RISK ASSESSMENT

Several scales have been proposed to identify patients at risk of falling across various settings. However, only 3 nursing assessment tools have been validated in multiple studies across different populations, which include postoperative inpatients. These tools are the Morse Fall Scale (MFS),[48] St Thomas's Risk Assessment Tool in Falling Elderly Inpatients (STRATIFY),[49] and the Hendrich Fall Risk Model (HFRM).[50,51]

Several systematic reviews have compared these 3 tools,[5,52–54] and whereas some confirmed the usefulness of the MFS, HFRM, and STRATIFY tools, others found them to show relatively low pooled specificity and sensitivity and even lower positive predictive value.[55–57] One meta-analysis concluded that the MFS and STRATIFY were comparable in accuracy with nurses' clinical judgment.[58] In addition, these tools generally fail to adequately take into account extrinsic factors, and thus, selecting the appropriate tool is complicated by the lack of agreement of sensitivity and specificity thresholds. In addition, the validities of these tools are specific to particular study settings

Box 5	
Risk factors for falls in rehabilitation settings and reported relative risk and odds ratio[a]	
Age ≥71 y	2.2[a]
Vertigo	5.3[a]
Stroke	2.7[a]
Functional impairment	1.7[a]
Delirium/cognitive impairment	3.8–5.2
Previous falls	1.8–2.1
Sleep disturbance	2.4[a]
Carpet floor	8.3[a]
Visual/hearing impairment	1.2–1.5
Use of a wheel chair	1.2[a]

[a] Indicates odds ratio.

and populations, making it difficult to generalize their use in practice, which has led most investigators to recommend a combination of risk assessment tools to identify patients at risk in the in-hospital setting. Overall, the MFS has the highest sensitivity, whereas the STRATIFY tool has the highest specificity, leaving the HFRM as the tool of choice only when a more comprehensive assessment is required.[59] Because of the myriad risk factors for falls, the variability in the assessment tools, and because a fall event tends to be multifactorial, we recommend assessing patients in a continuum of care, as shown in **Box 6**.

The baseline falls risk and any risk factors for delirium and functional decline should be evaluated on admission. The subsequent assessment and care plan should involve a multidisciplinary team responsible for preventing new in-hospital episodes. This team should also identify all potential risk factors for subsequent falls, integrating a fracture risk assessment tool within the equation. Once the patient is out of hospital,

---

Box 6
Postoperative assessment of falls risk in older adults with fragility fractures

Inpatient

- On admission
  - Preexisting falls risk factors (see **Box 1**)
  - Risk factors identified during the preoperative assessment (see **Box 2**)
  - Identification of risk for delirium (see **Box 3**)
  - Medications (see **Box 4**)
- Postoperative
  - Confusion assessment method + early detection of delirium
  - Identification of transoperative risk factors (see **Box 2**)
  - Functional decline/deconditioning
  - Analgesia/sedation
  - Environmental factors (see **Box 5**)

Outpatient

- Assessment for:
  - Nutritional risk
  - Depression
  - Visual impairment
  - Hearing impairment
  - Fear of falling
  - Polypharmacy
- Bone health assessment (risk factors for fracture + densitometry by dual-energy X-ray absorptiometry scan)
- Cognitive assessment
- Functional assessment
- Gait and balance assessment (see **Table 1**)
- Blood tests: vitamin D, parathyroid hormone, electrolytes, albumin, hemoglobin, renal and thyroid function

multifaceted evaluation should continue, with a view to implementing targeted multi-component interventions, for which several reliable scales are available (**Table 1**),[52] as part of an effective falls prevention program.

STRATEGIES FOR SECONDARY PREVENTION OF FALLS
Postoperative Inpatients

Mortality is significantly increased after hip fracture, and functional recovery is limited to less than 50%. About 25% of patients reside in long-term care facilities for a year or more after fracture, and the impact of hip fracture on health-related quality of life is considerable and long lasting.[12] Thus, preventing the next fracture is of highest priority and requires an integrated coordinated approach from admission to discharge to prevent falls. This suggested approach is summarized in **Box 7**.

As mentioned earlier, reducing falls in the acute phase should focus on preventing deconditioning and delirium, ensuring a safe environment for the patient, and encouraging early mobilization. One of the main causes of prolonged immobilization after hip surgery is poorly controlled postoperative pain. Undertreated pain limits early rehabilitation, increases time in bed, and has been associated with prolonged hospital stays and more complications. Pain should be well controlled both at rest and during physical therapy by providing analgesics before painful events (such as dressing or wound healing), and before physical activity.[15,23,60,61] Efficacy and side effects of prescribed analgesics should be monitored on a regular basis,[18,24] including the use of pain scales,[18,60,61] in particular, in patients with (or at risk of) delirium.

Another reversible cause of poor physical performance, and poor functional recovery, is severe anemia.[62] The prevalence of postoperative anemia may be as high as 51% to 87%,[19] and factors such as repeated phlebotomy and hemodilution from intravenous fluids may be attributable. However, a meta-analysis of 6 randomized controlled trials[63] showed that although oral or intravenous iron was effective in raising the hemoglobin level at 6 weeks after hip fracture, there was no difference in clinical outcomes, including length of stay, postoperative complications, or infections. More recently, a randomized trial of a liberal versus restrictive transfusion strategy after hip fracture (routine transfusion for hemoglobin <10 g/dL vs transfusion for symptomatic anemia only)[64] showed no between-group differences in 60-day mortality, ambulatory ability, or cardiovascular outcomes. Although there is evidence that recommends transfusion at a higher cutoff point (see the article by Carson and colleagues elsewhere in this issue), we recommend a regular strategy of transfusion in symptomatic or high-risk patients with hemoglobin levels less than 8 g/dL.

Table 1
Commonly used fall risk assessment tools in older persons

	Berg Balance Test (%)	Elderly Fall Screening Test (%)	Dynamic Gait Index (%)	Timed Get Up and Go[a] (%)	Tinetti Performance Oriented Mobility (%)
Sensitivity	77	93	85	87	80
Specificity	86	78	38	87	74

[a] Performed at discharge with a cutoff point of 24 seconds significantly predicted falls over a 6-month follow-up period.[21]

Data from Kristensen MT, Foss NB, Kehlet H. Timed "Up & Go" test as a predictor of falls within 6 months after hip fracture surgery. Phys Ther 2007;87:24–30.

Box 7
Postoperative interventions to prevent new falls in older adults with fragility fractures

Inpatient

- On admission
  - Assessment by the orthogeriatrics team
  - Delirium prevention
  - Hydration
  - Medication review
  - Optimization of analgesia and sedation
- Postoperative
  - Close nursing supervision
  - Early mobilization/physical therapy
  - Geriatric consultation
  - Nutrition and hydration
  - Regular analgesia
  - Transfusion (if hemoglobin level <8 g/dL)
  - Treatment of delirium (if present)

Outpatient

- Follow up at falls and fractures clinic
- Multifactorial prevention program[74–76]
  - Correction of vision and hearing impairment
  - Education on falls prevention
  - Exercise program: balance and strength
  - Fracture prevention: osteoporosis treatment
  - Home visit by an occupational therapist + environmental modification
  - Medication review
  - Protein supplements (if at nutritional risk)
  - Vitamin D supplementation

Nutritional support (postoperative oral or nasogastric protein and micronutrient supplements) is another important component of postoperative care, although there is no evidence that it reduces falls or improves mortality or disability. However, a Cochrane[65] review did report a trend toward reduction in a composite outcome of mortality or medical complications after hip fracture. Furthermore, given that delirium, pressure sores, and prolonged hospital stay are major common complications in frail patients and that nutritional intervention may contribute to patients suffering fewer days with delirium, fewer pressure sores, and shorter hospitalization,[66] we recommend nutritional assessment as part of routine care.

The most common and most challenging postoperative complication is delirium, which is comprehensively revised in another article by Javedan and Tulebaev elsewhere in this issue. Delirium is associated with lower functional recovery 1 year after fracture[33] and higher mortality,[67] and therefore, prevention is of utmost priority. One study[68] found that geriatrics consultation reduced delirium by more than one-third and reduced severe delirium by more than one-half. Another randomized control trial showed that a team applying comprehensive geriatric assessment, management, and rehabilitation halved the duration of delirium, and this result was associated with shorter hospitalization and fewer complications, such as pressure sores, urinary tract infections, nutritional complications, sleeping problems, and falls.[69]

However, given that available evidence for the best way to prevent falls in hospitals favors multifaceted programs, the same approach would be effective in the population with hip fracture. A randomized controlled trial by Stenvaal and colleagues[70] using multidisciplinary multifactorial assessment and intervention reported a reduction of falls and fall-related injuries in patients with femoral neck fractures. Patients aged 70 years or older with femoral neck fracture were randomized to postoperative care in a geriatric ward with a special intervention program or to conventional care in an orthopedic ward. The intervention ward was a geriatric unit specializing in geriatric orthopedic patients. The staff worked in teams (allied health and geriatricians), applying individual care planning and measures to prevent, detect, and treat postoperative complications such as falls, delirium, pain and decubitus ulcers, optimizing nutrition and rehabilitation based on functional retraining, with special focus on falls risk factors. The fall incidence was significantly lower in the intervention group (incidence rate ratio [IRR] 0.38; 95% confidence interval [CI] 0.20–0.76; $P = .006$) and among patients with dementia (IRR 0.07; 95% CI 0.01–0.57; $P = .013$). The difference in fall risk, expressed as time lapse to first fall, was also significantly lower in the intervention group (IRR 0.41; 95% CI 0.20–0.82; $P = .012$). There were in total 3 minor or moderate injuries in the intervention group compared with 15 in the control group. Furthermore, a meta-analysis[71] reported that orthogeriatric collaboration was associated with a significant reduction of in-hospital mortality, long-term mortality, and length of stay, particularly in the shared care model. However, it remains to be known whether applying comprehensive geriatric assessment and intervention during the in-hospital acute phase improves important clinical outcomes in the short-term (1 and 4 months postoperatively) and long-term (12 months postoperatively). A randomized controlled trial[72,73] addressing this question has recently been completed, and the results are eagerly awaited.

The current evidence supports multicomponent interventions to reduce hospital falls, including the immediate postoperative setting (see **Box 7**). These interventions involve a set of preoperative and postoperative assessments and multidisciplinary interventions. Mrs J's case shows a combination of risk factors that should have been identified and targeted on admission. Being a strange environment for the patient, the hospital setting should be adapted to prevent new episodes in patients at high risk of falls. In addition to delirium prevention, medication review and early mobilization, patients at high risk of falls should be regularly monitored by the nursing and medical staff. Because of the association between falls and fractures, an appropriate concomitant fracture care and prevention program should be implemented in high-risk patients optimally during the immediate postoperative period while the patient is still in the hospital.

Postoperative Outpatients

Considering that there are not specific recommendations for fall prevention in the postfracture setting, it would be reasonable to apply the general recommendations that have been validated in the general postacute setting. A recent meta-analysis concluded that fall prevention exercise programs, home safety interventions, vitamin D supplementation in people with low vitamin D levels, and individually targeted multifactorial interventions were associated with lower fall rates in community-dwelling people. The components are described in **Box 7**.

Although these interventions could be implemented in general clinical practice, high-risk patients should be assessed and a care plan should be implemented at a more specialized setting such as a falls prevention clinic, if available. These clinics have been defined as "… specialist multidisciplinary services, which focus on the assessment and management of clients with falls, mobility and balance problems. Clinics commonly provide time limited, specialist intervention to the client and advice and referral to mainstream services for ongoing management. They provide education and training to clients, to carers, and to health professionals."[74]

Overall, these programs offer a comprehensive assessment and varied interventions focused on falls prevention in older persons, which have been shown to be effective in improving functional performance, reducing fear of falling and decreasing the incidence of new falls.[75] However, few of these falls prevention clinics take into consideration bone health assessment. Until 2000, it was a common practice not to include any assessment to evaluate osteoporosis risk or to perform bone mineral density in falls prevention trials. As a consequence, osteoporosis risk assessment was not considered as part of a major falls prevention guideline.[76]

In 2001, the National Health Service in the United Kingdom established the National Service Framework for Older People, a comprehensive strategy to ensure fair, high-quality, integrated health and social care services for older people. The National Service Framework set out standards for specialized and integrated falls services to improve care and treatment of those who have fallen and, for the first time, included interventions to prevent and treat osteoporosis in those at high risk. After implementation of these guidelines, there was an increasing understanding of the natural association between falls and fractures, and thus, incorporating a routine bone health assessment as part of a comprehensive assessment for falls and fractures risk in older persons was proposed.[77] However, little operational guidance was provided until a review and clinical guideline undertaken by the National Health Service policy body, the National Institute for Health and Clinical Excellence (NICE), was published in 2004.[78] In those guidelines, NICE suggested that specialist falls services should be operationally linked to bone health (osteoporosis) services and recommended that an osteoporosis risk assessment should be an essential element of a comprehensive falls assessment.[78] Since the release of these guidelines, the number of falls clinics that integrates a bone health component has increased exponentially, particularly at university hospitals.[79–81] The effectiveness of these combined clinics in secondary prevention of falls and fractures in older persons is a subject of intense research.

SUMMARY

In this article, the current evidence is reviewed on the postoperative prevention of falls in older persons after suffering a fragility fracture. Assessment of falls risk should be a common practice during the preoperative and postoperative periods. In the preoperative period, falls risk assessment should be focused on history of previous falls, presence of risk factors, and prediction of postoperative delirium. The immediate postoperative period should focus on prevention and treatment of delirium, close patient supervision, appropriate hydration and transfusion (if required), proper use of medications, and early rehabilitation and mobilization. Secondary prevention of falls in the postdischarge period should involve the identification of risk factors and targeted multifactorial interventions, which should also include interventions for fracture prevention and osteoporosis treatment.

REFERENCES

1. Amador L, Loera J. Preventing postoperative falls in the older adult. J Am Coll Surg 2007;204(3):447–53.
2. Tinetti M, Speechley M, Ginter S. Risk factors for falls among elderly persons living in the community. N Engl J Med 1988;319:1701–7.
3. Tinetti M, Kumar C. The patient who falls: "it's always a trade-off". JAMA 2010; 303(3):258–66.
4. Deandrea S, Lucenteforte E, Bravi F, et al. Risk factors for falls in community-dwelling older people: a systematic review and meta-analysis. Epidemiology 2010;21(5):658–68.
5. Oliver D, Daly F, Martin F, et al. Risk factors and risk assessment tools for falls in hospital in-patients: a systematic review. Age Ageing 2004;33(2):122–30.
6. Vieira E, Freund-Heritage R, Costa BD. Risk factors for geriatric patient falls in rehabilitation hospital settings: a systematic review. Clin Rehabil 2011;25(9): 788–99.
7. Kannus P, Sievänen H, Palvanen M, et al. Prevention of falls and consequent injuries in elderly people. Lancet 2005;366(9500):1885–93.
8. Tinetti M. Clinical practice. Preventing falls in elderly persons. N Engl J Med 2003;348(1):42–9.
9. Abolhassani F, Moayyeri A, Naghavi M, et al. Incidence and characteristics of falls leading to hip fracture in Iranian population. Bone 2006;39(2):408–13.
10. Cummings S, Kelsey J, Nevitt M, et al. Epidemiology of osteoporosis and osteoporotic fractures. Epidemiol Rev 1985;7(2):178–208.
11. Boonen S, Autier P, Barette M, et al. Functional outcome and quality of life following hip fracture in elderly women: a prospective controlled study. Osteoporos Int 2004;15(2):87–94.
12. von Friesendorff M, Besjakov J, Åkesson K. Long-term survival and fracture risk after hip fracture: a 22-year follow-up in women. J Bone Miner Res 2008;23(11): 1832–41.
13. Nguyen N, Pongchaiyakul C, Center J, et al. Identification of high-risk individuals for hip fracture: a 14-year prospective study. J Bone Miner Res 2005;20: 1921–8.
14. van Helden S, van Geel AC, Geusens PP, et al. Bone and fall-related fracture risks in women and men with a recent clinical fracture. J Bone Joint Surg Am 2008;90(2):241–8.
15. Garrdsell P, Johnell O, Nilsson BE, et al. The predictive value of fracture, disease, and falling tendency for fragility fractures in women. Calcif Tissue Int 1989;45:327–30.
16. Rucker D, Rowe BH, Johnson JA, et al. Educational intervention to reduce falls and fear of falling in patients after fragility fracture: results of a controlled pilot study. Prev Med 2006;42:316–9.
17. van Helden S, Wyers CE, Dagnelie PC, et al. Risk of falling in patients with a recent fracture. BMC Musculoskelet Disord 2007;8:55.
18. Pils K, Meisner W, Haas W, et al. Risk assessment after hip fracture: check the "healthy" leg! Z Gerontol Geriatr 2011;44:375–80.
19. McKee KJ, Orbell S, Austin CA, et al. Fear of falling, falls efficacy, and health outcomes in older people following hip fracture. Disabil Rehabil 2002;24(6):327–33.
20. Whitehead C, Miller M, Crotty M. Falls in community-dwelling older persons following hip fracture: impact on self-efficacy, balance and handicap. Clin Rehabil 2003;17:899–906.

21. Kristensen MT, Foss NB, Kehlet H. Timed 'Up & Go' test as a predictor of falls within 6 months after hip fracture surgery. Phys Ther 2007;87:24–30.
22. Shumway-Cook A, Ciol MA, Gruber W, et al. Incidence of and risk factors for falls following hip fracture in community-dwelling older adults. Phys Ther 2005;85:648–55.
23. Lloyd BD, Williamson DA, Singh NA, et al. Recurrent and injurious falls in the year following hip fracture: a prospective study of incidence and risk factors from the sarcopenia and hip fracture study. J Gerontol A Biol Sci Med Sci 2009;64(5):599–609.
24. Hall SE, Williams JA, Griddle RA. A prospective study of falls following hip fracture in community dwelling older adults. Australas J Ageing 2001;20(2):73–8.
25. Jarvinen T, Sievanen H, Khan K, et al. Shifting the focus in fracture prevention from osteoporosis to falls. BMJ 2008;336(7636):124–6.
26. Walker J, Howland J. Falls and fear of falling among elderly persons living in the community: occupational therapy interventions. Am J Occup Ther 1991;45(2):119–22.
27. Swinkels A, Newman J, Allain T. A prospective observational study of falling before and after knee replacement surgery. Age Ageing 2009;38(2):175–81.
28. Pils K, Neumann F, Meisner W, et al. Predictors of falls in elderly people during rehabilitation after hip fracture–who is at risk of a second one? Z Gerontol Geriatr 2003;36:16–22.
29. Inouye S, van Dyck CH, Alessi C, et al. Clarifying confusion: the confusion assessment method: a new method for detection of delirium. Ann Intern Med 1990;113:941–9.
30. Damuleviciene G, Lesauskaite V, Macijauskiene J. Postoperative cognitive dysfunction of older surgical patients. Medicina (Kaunas) 2010;46(3):169–75.
31. Rudolph J, Marcantonio E. Review articles: postoperative delirium: acute change with long-term implications. Anesth Analg 2011;112:1202–11.
32. Shurch C, Robinson T, Angles E, et al. Postoperative falls in the acute hospital setting: characteristics, risk factors, and outcomes in males. Am J Surg 2011; 201:197–202.
33. Vochteloo A, Moerman S, Tuinebreijer W, et al. More than half of hip fracture patients do not regain mobility in the first postoperative year. Geriatr Gerontol Int 2013;13(2):334–41.
34. Wierenga P, Buurman B, Parlevliet J, et al. Association between acute geriatric syndromes and medication-related hospital admissions. Drugs Aging 2012; 29(8):691–9.
35. Frazier S. Health outcomes and polypharmacy in elderly individuals: an integrated literature review. J Gerontol Nurs 2005;31:4–11.
36. Ziere G, Dieleman J, Hofman A, et al. Polypharmacy and falls in the middle age and elderly population. Br J Clin Pharmacol 2006;61:218–23.
37. Lamis RL, Kramer JS, Hale L, et al. Fall risk associated with inpatient medications. Am J Health Syst Pharm 2012;69:1888–94.
38. Dasgupta M, Dumbrell A. Preoperative risk assessment for delirium after noncardiac surgery: a systematic review. J Am Geriatr Soc 2006;54:1578–89.
39. Appell H. Muscular atrophy following immobilisation. A review. Sports Med 1990;10(1):42–58.
40. Hamers J, Gulpers M, Strik W. Use of physical restraints with cognitively impaired nursing home residents. J Adv Nurs 2004;45(3):246–51.
41. Yau DT, Chung RC, Pang MY. Knee muscle strength and visual acuity are the most important modifiable predictors of falls in patients after hip fracture surgery: a prospective study. Calcif Tissue Int 2013;92:287–95.

42. Johnson M, George A, Tran DT. Analysis of falls incidents: nurse and patient preventive behaviours. Int J Nurs Pract 2011;17(1):60–6.
43. Lovallo C, Rolandi S, Rossetti A, et al. Accidental falls in hospital inpatients: evaluation of sensitivity and specificity of two risk assessment tools. J Adv Nurs 2010;66(3):690–6.
44. Krauss M, Nguyen S, Dunagan W, et al. Circumstances of patient falls and injuries in 9 hospitals in a midwestern healthcare system. Infect Control Hosp Epidemiol 2007;28(5):544–50.
45. Dunton N, Gajewski B, Taunton R, et al. Nurse staffing and patient falls on acute care hospital units. Nurs Outlook 2004;52:53–9.
46. Sherrington C, Lord SR. Increased prevalence of fall risk factors in older people following hip fracture. Gerontology 1998;44:340–4.
47. Morris R, Harwood RH, Baker R, et al. A comparison of different balance tests in the prediction of falls in older women with vertebral fractures: a cohort study. Age Ageing 2007;36:78–83.
48. Morse J, Black C, Kberle O, et al. A prospective study to identify the fall-prone patient. Soc Sci Med 1989;28(1):81–6.
49. Oliver D, Britton M, Seed P, et al. Development and evaluation of evidence based risk assessment tool (STRATIFY) to predict which elderly inpatients will fall: case control and cohort studies. BMJ 1997;315(7115):1049–53.
50. Hendrich A, Nyphis A, Kippenbrock T, et al. Hospital falls: development of a predictive model for clinical practice. Appl Nurs Res 1995;8:129–39.
51. Hendrich A, Bender P, Nyhuis A. Validation of the Hendrich II Fall Risk Model: a large concurrent case/control study of hospitalized patients. Appl Nurs Res 2003;16(1):9–21.
52. Perell K, Nelson A, Goldman R, et al. Fall risk assessment measures: an analytic review. J Gerontol A Biol Sci Med Sci 2001;56(12):M761–6.
53. Myers H. Hospital fall risk assessment tools: a critique of the literature. Int J Nurs Pract 2003;9:223–35.
54. Scott V, Votova K, Scanlan A, et al. Multifactorial and functional mobility assessment tools for fall risk among older adults in community, home-support, long-term and acute care settings. Age Ageing 2007;36(2):130–9.
55. Oliver D, Papaionnou A, Giangregorio L, et al. A systematic review and meta-analysis of studies using the STRATIFY tool for prediction of falls in hospital patients: how well does it work? Age Ageing 2008;37(6):1–7.
56. Vassallo M, Stockdale R, Sharma J, et al. A comparative study of the use of four fall risk assessment tools on acute medical wards. J Am Geriatr Soc 2005;53(6):1034–8.
57. Schwendimann R, Geest SD, Milisen K. Evaluation of the Morse Falls Scale in hospitalised patients. Age Ageing 2006;35(3):311–3.
58. Haines T, Bennell K, Osborne R, et al. A new instrument for targeting falls prevention interventions was accurate and clinically applicable in a hospital setting. J Clin Epidemiol 2006;59:168–75.
59. Cumbler E, Simpson J, Rosenthal L, et al. Inpatient falls: defining the problem and identifying possible solutions. Part I: an evidence-based review. Neurohospitalist 2013;3(3):135–43.
60. Peeters G, van Schoor NM, Lips P. Fall risk: the clinical relevance of falls and how to integrate fall risk with fracture risk. Best Pract Res Clin Rheumatol 2009;23:797–804.
61. van Helden S, Cals J, Kessels F, et al. Risk of new clinical fractures within 2 years following a fracture. Osteoporos Int 2006;17:348–54.
62. Vochteloo A, Borger van der Burg BL, Mertens B, et al. Outcome in hip fracture patients related to anemia at admission and allogeneic blood transfusion: an

analysis of 1262 surgically treated patients. BMC Musculoskelet Disord 2011; 12:262.

63. Yang Y, Li H, Li B, et al. Efficacy and safety of iron supplementation for the elderly patients undergoing hip or knee surgery: a meta-analysis of randomized controlled trials. J Surg Res 2011;171:e201–7.

64. Carson J, Terrin M, Noveck H, et al. Liberal or restrictive transfusion in high-risk patients after hip surgery. N Engl J Med 2011;365:2453–62.

65. Avenell A, Handoll H. Nutritional supplementation for hip fracture aftercare in older people. Cochrane Database Syst Rev 2006;(4):CD001880.

66. Olofsson B, Stenvall M, Lundström M, et al. Malnutrition in hip fracture patients: an intervention study. J Clin Nurs 2007;16:2027–38.

67. Lee K, Ha Y, Lee Y, et al. Frequency, risk factors, and prognosis of prolonged delirium in elderly patients after hip fracture surgery. Clin Orthop Relat Res 2011;469:2612–20.

68. Marcantonio E, Flacker J, Wright R, et al. Reducing delirium after hip fracture: a randomized trial. J Am Geriatr Soc 2001;49(5):516–22.

69. Lundström M, Olofsson B, Stenvall M, et al. Postoperative delirium in old patients with femoral neck fracture: a randomized intervention study. Aging Clin Exp Res 2007;19(3):178–86.

70. Stenvall M, Olofsson B, Lundström M, et al. A multidisciplinary, multifactorial intervention program reduces postoperative falls and injuries after femoral neck fracture. Osteoporos Int 2007;18(2):167–75.

71. Adunsky A, Lusky A, Arad M, et al. A comparative study of rehabilitation outcomes of elderly hip fracture patients: the advantage of a comprehensive orthogeriatric approach. J Gerontol A Biol Sci Med Sci 2003;58A(6):542–7.

72. Sletvold O, Helbostad JL, Thingstad P, et al. Effect of in-hospital comprehensive geriatric assessment (CGA) in older people with hip fracture. The protocol of the Trondheim Hip Fracture Trial. BMC Geriatr 2011;11:18.

73. Robertson M, Gillespie L. Fall prevention in community-dwelling older adults. JAMA 2013;309(13):1406–7.

74. Hill K, Smith R, Schwarz J. Falls clinics in Australia: a survey of current practice, and recommendations for future development. Aust Health Rev 2001;24(4):163–74.

75. Hill K, Moore K, Dorevitch M, et al. Effectiveness of falls clinics: an evaluation of outcomes and client adherence to recommended interventions. J Am Geriatr Soc 2008;56(4):600–8.

76. Feder G, Cryer C, Donovan S, et al. Guidelines for the prevention of falls in people over 65. BMJ 2000;321(7267):1007–11.

77. Close J, McMurdo M. Falls and bone health services for older people. Age Ageing 2003;32(5):494–6.

78. National Institute for Health and Clinical Excellence. Clinical Guideline 21: Falls. The Assessment and Prevention of Falls in Older People. London: National Institute for Health and Clinical Excellence; 2004. Accessed March 10, 2014. Available at: http://www.nice.org.uk/nicemedia/pdf/CG021NICEguideline.pdf.

79. Sze P, Cheung W, Lam P, et al. The efficacy of a multidisciplinary falls prevention clinic with an extended step-down community program. Arch Phys Med Rehabil 2008;89(7):1329–34.

80. Gomez F, Curcio C, Suriyaarachchi P, et al. Differing approaches to falls and fracture prevention between Australia and Colombia. Clin Interv Aging 2013;8:61–7.

81. Schoon Y, Hoogsteen-Osssewaarde M, Scheffer A, et al. Comparison of different strategies of referral to a fall clinic: how to achieve an optimal case mix? J Nutr Health Aging 2011;15(2):140–5.

Atypical Femur Fractures

Wakenda Tyler, MD, MPH[a],*, Susan Bukata, MD[b],
Regis O'Keefe, MD, PhD[a]

KEYWORDS

- Hip fractures • Femur fractures • Atypical • Bisphosphonates • Osteoporosis

KEY POINTS

- Atypical femur fractures have an extremely low incidence and make up a very small subset of femur fractures.
- The fractures are associated with bisphosphonate use but can occur in patients without exposure to bisphosphonates.
- Increasing duration of bisphosphonate use has been associated with increased the risk of an atypical femur fracture.
- Other medications or conditions can increase the risk of an atypical femur fracture, including diabetes, glucocorticosteroid, and proton pump inhibitors.
- Among patients with atypical femur fractures, 30% have bilateral involvement that is located in the same anatomic location on both femurs.
- Risk of an atypical femur fracture is reduced by 70% in the first year after cessation of a bisphosphonate.
- Treatment of patients with atypical femur fractures includes discontinuation of bisphosphonates, normalization of serum calcium and vitamin D levels, activity modification, and possible surgery for complete fractures or those at risk for progression to complete fracture.

INTRODUCTION

Atypical fractures that occur in the subtrochanteric region of the femur represent a unique group of fractures that occur in patients with osteoporosis or other systemic or local metabolic conditions of bone. These fractures have a distinct radiographic pattern and clinical presentation that distinguishes them from other more prevalent types of femur fractures occurring in the subtrochanteric region and along the femoral shaft. Atypical fractures have been associated with bisphosphonate use over the past decade, but they can occur in patients who are naive to treatment with bisphosphonates.[1]

[a] Department of Orthopaedic Surgery, University of Rochester, 601 Elmwood Avenue, Box 665, Rochester, NY 14642, USA; [b] Department of Orthopaedic Surgery, University of California, Los Angeles, Los Angeles, California, USA
* Corresponding author.
E-mail address: Wakenda_Tyler@URMC.Rochester.edu

Clin Geriatr Med 30 (2014) 349–359
http://dx.doi.org/10.1016/j.cger.2014.01.010
0749-0690/14/$ – see front matter © 2014 Elsevier Inc. All rights reserved.

Atypical fractures generally present as either complete or evolving transverse fractures of the subtrochanteric femur region. Patients often present with an associated stress response of the bone in the lateral cortex, which can be seen on a radiograph as a thickening (beaking) of the lateral cortex at the site of the fracture (**Fig. 1**). The fractures are transverse or short oblique fractures with minimal comminution or fragmentation at the fracture site (see **Fig. 2** for nonatypical/standard femur fracture). Approximately 70% of patients have a prodrome of thigh pain prior to development of a complete fracture. When these fractures occur in the setting of bisphosphonate use, it is generally after greater than 5 years of continuous use of the drug. For reasons that are not clear, the distribution of fractures tends to be shifted toward a younger (55–70 years of age) population of elderly patients on bisphosphonates.[1,2] The incidence is also higher in the Asian women.[2] The pathophysiology of these fractures and their association with antiresorptive medications for osteoporosis is still being fully elucidated, although understanding of mechanisms at work is gaining.

This article discusses understanding to date of the clinical presentation, epidemiology, pathophysiology, and management of atypical femur fractures.

CLINICAL PRESENTATION

Atypical femur fractures represent a spectrum of a disease entity. These fractures are thought to evolve slowly over time, usually starting out as stress reactions, then forming incomplete laterally based fractures and ultimately complete fractures with displacement. This slow evolution means that patients can present at any point along the spectrum. A typical patient who presents with an atypical femur fracture is a woman over age 40 who in most cases may have other risk factors for osteoporosis. Glucorticosteroid and proton pump inhibitor use in addition to bisphosphonate use was found in higher incidence among patients who presented with atypical fractures.[1] Other chronic disease entities have also been associated with atypical fracture formation, including rheumatoid arthritis and renal disease.[1] One atypical femur fracture was

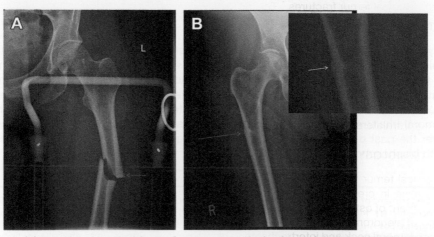

Fig. 1. (A) Completed atypical femur fracture. Note the beaking of the lateral cortex (*arrow*) and short oblique nature of the fracture. There is also minimal comminution noted. (B) Incomplete atypical femur fracture. Note the lateral cortex beaking (*arrow*). Also note the black line that represents the incomplete/nondisplaced fracture of the lateral cortex (*inset, white arrow*).

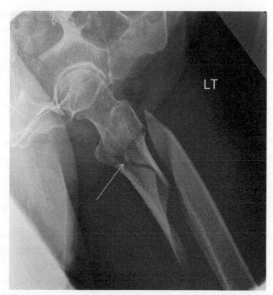

Fig. 2. Nonatypical femur fracture. Note the very long oblique pattern of this fracture. Also note the greater degree of comminution seen (*white arrow*). These are typically higher-energy injuries when seen.

also reported in the FREEDOM extension trial for denosumab, another potent antiresorptive treatment of osteoporosis with a mechanism of action that is different from bisphosphonates.[3]

In the setting of complete fractures, incomplete fractures, or early stress reactions, patients frequently reports a several-month history of thigh or groin pain often made worse with increasing activity but which can be present at rest as well. This prodromal onset of pain before presentation has been reported in as many as 70% of patients with atypical femur fractures.[1] The symptoms may be gradual in onset and often present for several months. Early atypical fractures may also have no clinical symptoms but have radiographic evidence of the development of an atypical fracture. Complete fractures are frequently displaced at the time of presentation and are most commonly associated with no trauma or very low-energy trauma, such as a fall from a standing height. Approximately one-third of patients present with bilateral symptoms and/or findings on radiograph consistent with bilateral femur involvement.[1] All patients with evidence of an evolving or complete atypical fracture should have a radiograph of the contralateral femur.

EPIDEMIOLOGY AND PATHOPHYSIOLOGY

Atypical femur fractures have gained attention over the past decade because of the increase in prevalence, particularly among women who take bisphosphonates for treatment of osteoporosis. Epidemiology reports have shown that since the introduction of alendronate in 1996 and the initiation of widespread use of bisphosphonates, both femoral neck and intertrochanteric hip fracture incidence have sharply declined.[4] The incidence of subtrochanteric femur fractures, however, has either remained stable or increased during this same time period.[1,4] More specifically, there has been a rise in the reporting of fractures that ultimately came to be defined as atypical femur fractures. Because atypical femur fractures are a subclassification of femur fractures, this observation was based on careful scrutiny of the radiographic images since the initial description of this unique fracture pattern.[5]

Incidence of atypical femur fracture is extremely low.

- Fewer than 1% of all femur and hip fractures in patients with osteoporosis are considered atypical fractures.[6,7]
- For patients on bisphosphonates, the incidence of an atypical femur fracture is less than 2/100,000 person-years for those who are on bisphosphonates less than 2 years.[7]
- The risk goes up to 113/100,000 person-years for those on bisphosphonates for longer than 9 years.[7]
- To place that into perspective, estimates for fragility fracture rates (distal radius, spine, and hip) in patients older than age 85 are as high as 5000–8200/100,000.[8]
- Estimates suggest that for a reduction of 100 typical femoral neck or intertrochanteric fractures during this time there was an increase of 1 subtrochanteric fracture.[9]

The studies are unable to define whether these additional subtrochateric fractures are standard fragility fractures (see **Fig. 2**) or atypical fractures (see **Fig. 1**). The trend of an increasing incidence and relative risk of developing an atypical femur fracture with increasing time of exposure to bisphosphonates has been seen in several large studies both in the United States and abroad.[6,7,10] The risk of an atypical fracture declines by approximately 70% with each year after bisphosphonate withdrawal.[6] This latter discovery suggests that there is recovery of normal bone metabolism with time after discontinuation of use of bisphosphonates.

Despite their low incidence, atypical femur fractures in the setting of bisphosphonate use have raised concerns among clinicians about the amount of time patients should be treated with bisphosphonates. There is still a 33-times greater likelihood of developing an atypical femur fracture in patients who are treated with bisphosphonates compared with similar-aged patients not exposed to bisphosphonates.[6] More importantly, these fractures can be difficult to treat once they develop, can have prolonged healing periods, and can go on to form nonunions. Because of this, preventing these fractures from developing initially and going on to complete fracture is ideal. In 2010, the Food and Drug Administration (FDA) issued an advisory describing an increased incidence of atypical femur fracture in patients with sustained bisphosphonate use and recommending consideration of discontinuation after 3 to 5 years of use.[11]

The pathophysiology of atypical femur fractures is still being elucidated. One proposed mechanism is that these fractures occur due to suppression of bone turnover and remodeling, which ultimately leads to brittle failure of the bone.[1,12] The skeleton is constantly undergoing stresses that result in microscopic damage to the bone matrix. Normally, these areas of microdamage undergo rapid remodeling with osteoclast-mediated resorption of the injured bone and subsequent formation of new bone. Conditions that suppress osteoclast activity are thought to potentially impair normal remodeling, leading to accumulation and extension of areas of microdamage of bone and eventual catastrophic fracture of the bone.

Consistent with this hypothesis, atypical femur fractures typically originate as microstress cracks in an area of the femur with maximum tensile strain. The lateral cortex of the human femur is under high tensile forces due to the bending moment at that site. Under normal remodeling conditions, the coupled activity of both the bone-resorbing cell (osteoclast) and the bone-forming cell (osteoblast) allow for these microcracks to be repaired and remodeled into normal cortical and trabecular bone. The human skeleton is undergoing constant remodeling throughout life. This remodeling and repair process that takes place requires the 2 cell types to work in conjunction with each other. Both cells produce cytokines that influence the other cell's activity. If 1 cell is not properly functioning, it can alter the activity of the other cell.

Bisphosphonates work by inhibiting osteoclastic bone resorption. Although osteoclastic bone remodeling occurs throughout the skeleton, the activation frequency of osteoclast-mediated bone remodeling is concentrated in areas of injury. The end result is that the normal remodeling process that occurs at the site of microfracture is inhibited. Several studies that have looked at bone biopsies of patients on long-term bisphosphonate treatment have shown that there is a decrease in both osteoclast and osteoblast cells within the bone.[1] Patients with atypical femur fractures maintain the capacity to produce both endosteal and periosteal callus and bone, as evidenced by the cortical thickening or beaking that is often seen on plain radiograph. Intracortical repair is suppressed, however, thereby preventing complete fracture healing. This results from abnormal bone being laid down by the osteoblasts and improper remodeling of this bone by both the osteoclasts and osteoblasts. The bone in the area remains brittle with insufficient healing. Moreover, the increased blood flow that results from the body's attempt to heal the fracture increases the delivery of more bisphosphonates to the area.[1] This may further uncouple the activity of the osteoclasts and osteoblasts.

There is evidence suggesting that bone geometry may play a role in the development of atypical femur fractures. A few studies have shown differences in mechanical and anatomic axis between the femur and the tibia as well as greater radius of curvature in the femurs of patients who go on to develop either stress fractures or atypical femur fractures.[13,14] These studies suggest that patient-specific biomechanical factors as well as biology related to bone turnover and cellular function may be working in combination to initiate the development of atypical femur fractures. Additional study is needed to fully understand the etiology and pathogenesis of atypical femur fractures. A better understanding of these processes will improve prevention, detection, and treatment of these fractures in the future.

EVALUATION AND WORK-UP OF PATIENTS

A patient suspected of an atypical femur fracture based on either clinical presentation (prodromal symptoms, history of bisphosphonate use, and so forth) or radiographic criteria should have a complete metabolic bone laboratory panel performed (Table 1). A 25-hydroxyvitamin D level and a calcium level are essential to determine if a patient has the adequate vitamin and mineral elements needed for fracture healing and bone remodeling. The other laboratory results are important for determining the amount of bone suppression that may be present and to rule out other common metabolic disorders that could influence bone healing and remodeling.

All patients suspected of an atypical femur fracture should have bilateral full-length femur films. Approximately one-third of patients have both sides involved. Plain radiograph is the best way to assess if a fracture pattern fits that of an atypical femur fracture. Atypical femur fracture is located below the lesser trochanter and above the supracondylar region of the distal femur. It has a short oblique pattern that originates in the lateral cortex. The fracture may be complete (through both cortices) or incomplete (involving only the lateral cortex). An incomplete fracture with periosteal bone formation that causes lateral cortical thickening and beaking with a linear lucent line through the lateral cortex is at particularly high risk for fracture. The appearance of

Table 1
Laboratory tests in patients suspected of atypical femur fractures

Laboratory	Reference Range	Purpose
25-Hydroxyvitamin D	30–74 ng/mL	Deficiency can greatly inhibit bone healing and should be replenished if low.
Calcium	8.5–10.2 mg/dL	If low, should get ionized calcium and again replete to allow for adequate reserves for bone healing.
PTH (intact PTH)	10–55 pg/mL	High or low levels may indicate hyper- or hypoparathyroidism, which could lead to increased fracture risk.
Urine N-telopeptide	<25 nM BCE/mM (low) >80 nM BCE/mM (high)	These values vary depending on pre- and postmenopausal status and often have a large range. Also impacted by presence of fracture. A very low number indicates excessive bone remodeling suppression. High levels may be seen in high turnover states, such as Paget disease or poorly controlled osteoporosis.
Bone-specific alkaline phosphotase	≤22 µg/L (for adults)	This is an age-dependent level and can be higher in children. Elevated levels in adults may indicate abnormally increased bone turnover.
Osteocalcin	9–42 ng/mL (adult levels)	Increased in states of high bone turnover and low in states of bone turnover suppression. Is produced by the osteoblast cell and is released into the blood stream on bone remodeling by osteoclasts.
Basic metabolic panel	Variable	Should be obtained if concern for renal dysfunction is suspected. Renal failure can greatly influence metabolic activity of bone and affect all of the above laboratory results.

Abbreviation: BCE, bone collagen equivalent.

the linear lucent area of bone resorption in the lateral cortex is frequently referred to as "the dreaded black line." MRI and CT scans may be helpful if trying to determine if the cortical thickening that is present on plain film is associated with an incomplete fracture or not. The incomplete fracture line can be difficult to see on plain film alone. MRI shows a cortical line and surrounding edema within the cortex and adjacent marrow space. A CT scan with thin cuts through the area of interest may also show a fracture line. If a fracture line is absent, this should be considered an early stress reaction for an evolving atypical femur fracture. It is sometimes necessary to obtain a bone scan to confirm the presence of an evolving atypical femur fracture. The bone scan shows a discretely hot area at the lateral cortex. Bone scan is less specific for distinguishing between an early cortical reaction or stress reaction versus the more-advanced lateral cortex fracture but is still a helpful test for diagnosing an early presentation of an evolving atypical fracture.

Table 2 lists the major and minor radiographic and clinical criteria established by an American Society for Bone and Mineral Research task force on atypical femur fractures as criteria for defining these fractures in patients. These criteria are a guide to

Table 2
Major and minor criteria for determining presence of an atypical femur fracture

Major Criteria	Minor Criteria
Fracture is associated with minimal or no trauma.	Generalized increase in cortical thickness of the femoral diaphysis.
Fracture line originates at lateral cortex and is substantially transverse in its orientation, although it may become oblique as it progresses medially.	Unilateral or bilateral prodromal symptoms, such as dull or aching pain in the groin or thigh.
Complete fractures extend through both cortices and may include a medial spike; incomplete fractures only involve the lateral cortex.	Bilateral; incomplete or complete femoral diaphysis fractures.
The fracture is noncomminuted or minimally comminuted.	Delayed fracture healing.
Localized endosteal or periosteal thickening of the lateral cortex is present at the fracture site (beaking or flaring).	—

Modified from Shane E, Burr D, Abrahamsen B, et al. Atypical subtrochanteric and diaphyseal femoral fractures: second report of a task force of the American Society for Bone and Mineral Research. J Bone Miner Res 2014;29(1):1 23.

determine the presence of an atypical femur fracture; 4 of 5 major criteria must be present. None of the minor criteria is required but they are sometimes also present in patients presenting with atypical femur fractures.[1]

Although these guidelines are helpful in determining when patients may have an atypical femur fracture, good clinical judgment on the part of a provider is paramount. Although these fractures are uncommon, their detection is critical, because the presence of an atypical femur fracture may greatly alter the future care.

MANAGEMENT OF PATIENTS WITH ATYPICAL FEMUR FRACTURE

Management goals for patients with atypical femur fractures are to restore function, reduce pain, and facilitate fracture healing of the fracture. Complete atypical fractures are associated with delayed healing and an increased rate of additional surgery.[15] Atypical femur fractures can result in prolonged loss of function and pain and even permanent disability. Therefore, it is ideal to identify the presence of an atypical fracture prior to complete fracture formation.

Table 3 summarizes the management of patients with atypical femur fractures.

In patients who present with an early stress response or incomplete fracture, all antiresorptive osteoporosis therapy should be stopped. Calcium and vitamin D levels should be restored to normal with oral supplementation. Patients should be maintained on dosing of vitamin D and calcium that maintain levels in the normal range. 25-Vitamin D should be above 30 ng/mL and a level of up 50 ng/mL should be considered for patients with atypical femur fractures.[16] It is imperative that other metabolic conditions be ruled out as the cause of the fracture. This can be done by obtaining the laboratory tests listed in **Table 1**.

For patients with an early stress response and mild to moderate pain or patients with an incomplete fracture and no pain, nonoperative management should be considered. This generally includes modification of activity and, in many cases, the use of a crutch with limitations in weight bearing. Activity limitations may be continued for 3 to

Table 3
Management of patients with atypical femur fractures

Type of Atypical Fracture	Presence of Pain	Management
Stress response	Yes or no	• Discontinue bisphosphonate use • Metabolic bone turnover laboratory tests • Calcium and vitamin D supplementation • Activity modification • Consider PTH if no healing at 3 mo
Incomplete fracture	No	• Discontinue bisphosphonate use • Metabolic bone turnover laboratory tests • Calcium and vitamin D supplementation • Activity modification • Consider PTH if no healing at 3 mo • Consider surgery if no healing at 3–6 mo
Incomplete fracture	Yes	• Discontinue bisphosphonate use • Metabolic bone turnover laboratory tests • Calcium and vitamin D supplementation • Surgical intervention • Consider PTH if fracture still present at 6 mo postoperatively or other risk factors for nonhealing (if not already being used to treat osteoporosis)
Complete fracture	—	• Discontinue bisphosphonate use • Metabolic bone turnover laboratory tests • Calcium and vitamin D supplementation • Surgical intervention • Consider PTH if fracture still present at 6 mo postoperatively or other risk factors for nonhealing (if not already being used to treat osteoporosis) • Monitor closely for delayed healing

4 months until healing is noted or symptoms improve. It is currently controversial as to whether these patients should also be treated with the bone anabolic agent, parathyroid hormone (PTH) 1-34 (teriparatide). There are anecdotal case reports of decreased time to healing and reduced need for further surgical intervention in patients with atypical fractures treated with PTH 1-34.[17,18] The analyses with larger patient populations, however, have not shown a significant improvement in outcomes in patients with atypical fractures treated with PTH 1-34.[1] It may be likely that a small subset of these patients achieve a beneficial outcome from use of PTH 1-34. The authors' current recommendations are consideration of PTH 1-34 therapy if there is a failure of healing after 3 months of activity modification and nutritional supplementation. Patients with incomplete fractures but no pain who continue to have radiographic evidence of nonhealing of the fracture (persistent edema on MRI or presence of a fracture line on plain film) for 3 to 6 months after initiation of nonoperative management, should be considered for surgery. These patients are at risk for progression to a complete fracture.

Patients with radiographic evidence of an incomplete fracture and pain are at very high risk for progression to a complete fracture. These patients should be strongly considered for surgical intervention. The surgical intervention of choice in most cases is intramedullary nail fixation of the femur (**Fig. 3**). In general, long nails are preferred over short nails because they protect the entire length of the femur and do not leave a site of increased stress at the end of a short intramedullary device. Intramedullary

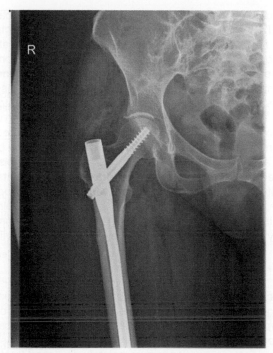

Fig. 3. Intramedullary nail of atypical fracture. The nail acts as an internal splint to prevent further fracture. It also acts as a load-sharing device to offload the tension stresses that are occurring at the fracture sight.

nails require small incisions and less soft tissue dissection than plate fixation. Furthermore, the use of intramedullary reaming during placement of the nail can stimulate an endosteal bone surface and further stimulates the healing process. These patients should also receive the same careful medical management as patients treated nonoperatively.

Patients who present with complete fractures should be treated with surgical stabilization of the fracture. As in the case of an incomplete fracture, intramedullary nail fixation with an intramedullary device that spans the length of the femur is the most appropriate treatment. The complexity of the fracture and other unforeseen problems may require modification of this surgical plan. These patients should receive the same medical work-up and management as other patients with atypical femur fractures. Atypical fractures should be closely monitored for delayed healing or complications from surgery. The use of PTH 1-34 in this patient population may be beneficial but remains investigational at this point. PTH 1-34 therapy can be considered in patients who are suspected to be at high risk for nonunion and it can also be used as an alternative treatment of patients' underlying osteoporosis, because they should no longer be considered candidates for bisphosphonate treatment of their osteoporosis.

MANAGEMENT OF PATIENTS WITHOUT ATYPICAL FRACTURES ON LONG-TERM BISPHOSPHONATES

There has been a great deal of concern among practitioners who care for patients with osteoporosis about whether long-term use of bisphosphonates is safe in light of the newer findings regarding risk of atypical fracture formation. Atypical fractures are a very rare entity. The reduced relative risk of a hip or spine fracture from use of bisphosphonates far outweighs the risk of developing an atypical femur fracture. Currently, the recommendation from the FDA is that discontinuation of bisphosphonates should be considered after 3 to 5 years of continued use of the drug for osteoporosis.[11] At the authors' institutions, if a patient has been on a bisphosphonate for more than 5 years consecutively, metabolic bone turnover laboratory tests are obtained, as listed in **Table 1**. If a patient shows significant suppression of bone turnover, then a bisphosphonate holiday for 6 months to 2 years is considered. Bone turnover laboratory tests are checked every 6 months to a year to see if the bone is regaining normal turnover activity. When normal turnover returns, the bisphosphonate is frequently restarted at that time. During the holiday period, patients are maintained on calcium and vitamin D. Depending on the severity of their osteoporosis and prior history of fracture, PTH therapy as an alternative treatment of their osteoporosis is often considered in patients on a bone holiday. Patients with mild osteoporosis often do not require any pharmacologic treatment beyond calcium and vitamin D.

SUMMARY

Atypical femur fractures are a rare but serious event that has an increased incidence in the setting of long-term bisphosphonate use. Other factors can increase the risk of developing an atypical femur fracture, including use of glucocorticosteroids and proton pump inhibitors. Atypical femur fractures present as a disease spectrum that evolves from an early stress reaction to a completely displaced fracture. Early detection of the stress response prior to completion of the fracture prevents significant morbidity and mortality. Patients frequently present with a prodrome of pain in the thigh or groin area prior to detection of the fracture. Full-length femur films of both femurs should be obtained as well as any other imaging modalities that may be necessary to fully detect the presence of a fracture line. The presence of lateral cortex beaking or localized thickening of the lateral cortex is highly suggestive of the presence of an atypical femur fracture. Patients suspected of an atypical femur fracture should stop all antiresorptive osteoporosis medications and have a full laboratory work-up for bone turnover status and to rule out other underlying metabolic conditions that could be contributing to the process. Calcium and vitamin D deficiencies should be corrected. Surgery is indicated in any patient who is thought to have a complete fracture or is at high risk for developing a complete fracture. The use of crutches with either non–weight bearing or partial weight bearing can be used for other patients not at imminent risk of fracture to facilitate the healing process. These fractures may take 3 to 6 months to fully heal and require patience on the part of caregiver and patient.

Atypical fractures are a phenomenon that is new in the field of osteoporosis care. A much greater understanding of the risk factors, pathophysiology, and etiology of this condition is still necessary. As this information is gathered by the medical and scientific communities, clinicians caring for patients with osteoporosis should be aware of this entity and the morbidity it can create. There is a strong correlation with length of exposure to bisphosphonates and development of an atypical fracture. Therefore, vigilance should be maintained for any symptoms or signs of a developing atypical femur fracture in patents on bisphosphonates for extended periods of time. As understanding of this disease entity moves forward, which subset of patients may be at increased risk for development of these fractures and what ways may be available to prevent and treat them may be better determined.

REFERENCES

1. Shane E, Burr D, Abrahamsen B, et al. Atypical subtrochanteric and diaphyseal femoral fractures: second report of a task force of the American society for bone and mineral research. J Bone Miner Res 2014;29(1):1–23.
2. Donnelly E, Saleh A, Unnanuntana A, et al. Atypical femoral fractures: epidemiology, etiology, and patient management. Curr Opin Support Palliat Care 2012; 6(3):348–54.
3. Bone HG, Chapurlat R, Brandi ML, et al. The effect of 3 or 6 years of denosumab exposure in women with postmenopausal osteoporosis: results from the FREEDOM extension. J Clin Endocrinol Metab 2013;98(11):4483–92.
4. Nieves JW, Bilezikian JP, Lane JM, et al. Fragility fractures of the hip and femur: incidence and patient characteristics. Osteoporos Int 2010;21(3):399–408.
5. Goh SK, Yang KY, Koh JS, et al. Subtrochanteric insufficiency fractures in patients on alendronate therapy: a caution. J Bone Joint Surg Br 2007;89(3):349–53.
6. Schilcher J, Michaelsson K, Aspenberg P. Bisphosphonate use and atypical fractures of the femoral shaft. N Engl J Med 2011;364(18):1728–37.
7. Dell RM, Adams AL, Greene DF, et al. Incidence of atypical nontraumatic diaphyseal fractures of the femur. J Bone Miner Res 2012;27(12):2544–50.
8. Boonen S, Ferrari S, Miller PD, et al. Postmenopausal osteoporosis treatment with antiresorptives: effects of discontinuation or long-term continuation on bone turnover and fracture risk–a perspective. J Bone Miner Res 2012;27(5):963–74.
9. Wang Z, Bhattacharyya T. Trends in incidence of subtrochanteric fragility fractures and bisphosphonate use among the US elderly, 1996–2007. J Bone Miner Res 2011;26(3):553–60.
10. Gedmintas L, Solomon DH, Kim SC. Bisphosphonates and risk of subtrochanteric, femoral shaft, and atypical femur fracture: a systematic review and meta-analysis. J Bone Miner Res 2013;28(8):1729–37.
11. U.S. Food and Drug Administration Website. FDA drug safety communication: ongoing safety review of oral bisphosphonates and atypical subtrochanteric femur fractures. Published March 10, 2010. Available at: www.fda.gov. Accessed October 15, 2013.
12. Compston J. Pathophysiology of atypical femoral fractures and osteonecrosis of the jaw. Osteoporos Int 2011;22(12):2951–61.
13. Crossley K, Bennell KL, Wrigley T, et al. Ground reaction forces, bone characteristics, and tibial stress fracture in male runners. Med Sci Sports Exerc 1999;31(8): 1088–93.
14. Sasaki S, Miyakoshi N, Hongo M, et al. Low-energy diaphyseal femoral fractures associated with bisphosphonate use and severe curved femur: a case series. J Bone Miner Metab 2012;30(5):561–7.
15. Weil YA, Rivkin G, Safran O, et al. The outcome of surgically treated femur fractures associated with long-term bisphosphonate use. J Trauma 2011;71(1):186–90.
16. Lamberg-Allardt C, Brustad M, Meyer HE, et al. Vitamin D - a systematic literature review for the 5th edition of the Nordic Nutrition Recommendations. Food Nutr Res 2013;57. http://dx.doi.org/10.3402/fnr.v57i0.22671.
17. Ettinger B, San Martin J, Crans G, et al. Differential effects of teriparatide on BMD after treatment with raloxifene or alendronate. J Bone Miner Res 2004;19(5):745–51.
18. Gomberg SJ, Wustrack RL, Napoli N, et al. Teriparatide, vitamin D, and calcium healed bilateral subtrochanteric stress fractures in a postmenopausal woman with a 13-year history of continuous alendronate therapy. J Clin Endocrinol Metab 2011;96(6):1627–32.

Fragility Fractures Requiring Special Consideration
Vertebral Fractures

Christian Kammerlander, MD, PD[a],*, Michael Zegg, MD[a],
Rene Schmid, MD, PD[a], Markus Gosch, MD[b], Thomas J. Luger, MD[c],
Michael Blauth, MD[a]

KEYWORDS

- Fracture treatment • Elderly • Osteoporotic fracture • Vertebral fracture
- Augmented instrumentation • Comorbidities • Odontoid fracture

KEY POINTS

- The incidence of osteoporotic vertebral compression fractures (VCFs) is steadily increasing, although many VCFs in the elderly remain undiagnosed.
- The comorbid conditions of the elderly, and especially their underlying osteoporosis, are the main factors that make the management of these types of fractures difficult.
- There is still an ongoing discussion as to whether odontoid fractures should be managed operatively or conservatively.
- Early mobilization is the key for improved outcome of patients with thoracolumbar fractures; surgical stabilization, including the use of bone cement, may be helpful in achieving this goal, although there is ongoing debate on the efficacy of this approach.

INTRODUCTION
Epidemiology

Advanced age and osteoporosis have been identified as the 2 main risk factors for vertebral fractures[1–3]; hence, vertebral compression fractures (VCFs) in the thoracolumbar spine as well as fractures of the cervical spine increase with the aging of the population.

Osteoporosis causes more than 8.9 million fractures annually worldwide (approximately 1000 per hour).[4] VCFs are the most common manifestation of osteoporosis. In geriatric patients with osteoporosis, the probability of suffering from VCF is high.

None of the authors has a conflict of interest regarding the topics discussed in this article.
^a Department for Trauma Surgery and Sports Medicine, Medical University of Innsbruck, Anichstrasse 35, 6020 Innsbruck, Austria; ^b Department of Acute Geriatrics, State Hospital Hochzirl, Austria; ^c Department of Anaesthesia and Intensive Care, Medical University of Innsbruck, Anichstrasse 35, 6020 Innsbruck, Austria
* Corresponding author. Department for Trauma Surgery and Sports Medicine, Medical University of Innsbruck, Anichstraße 35, Innsbruck 6020, Austria.
E-mail address: christian.kammerlander@uki.at

Clin Geriatr Med 30 (2014) 361–372
http://dx.doi.org/10.1016/j.cger.2014.01.011
0749-0690/14/$ – see front matter © 2014 Elsevier Inc. All rights reserved.

geriatric.theclinics.com

The number of annually new osteoporotic vertebral fractures is 214,000 in America, 490,000 in Europe, 253,000 in South-East Asia, 405,000 in Western Pacific, including Japan and China, and 12,000 in Africa.[4] The estimated costs of osteoporotic fractures were reported to be 37 billion euros in 2010, whereas vertebral fractures counted for 1.8 billion euros,[5] and in the United States, total costs, including prevalent fractures, exceeded 19 billion dollars.[6] In Europe, the incidence of a new vertebral fracture at the age 50 to 79 years is 1.1% per year in women and 0.6% per year in men. Furthermore, the incidence of fracture increases with age in both women and men, with a prevalence of 50% in a geriatric population.[7–9] The estimated number of unreported cases is probably higher, given that many VCFs do not come to medical attention; only one-fourth to one-third of vertebral fractures are clinically diagnosed.[10–13] Because of decreasing bone density in geriatric patients, the risk of developing a VCF increases approximately 2 times for every standard deviation lower than average vertebral bone density.[14]

Because of demographic changes, the prevalence of cervical spine injuries in the elderly is expected to increase progressively in Europe and North America. Although the incidence of neck injury in individuals younger than 65 years is declining, it is constant or increasing for the elderly after a minor trauma.[15,16] Moreover, upper cervical spine injuries are the most common.[16–18]

Challenge: Geriatric Patient

Comorbidities

A similarly severe injury in elderly patients leads to inferior clinical outcome with higher mortality compared with younger patients.[19–22] The presence of comorbidities complicates recovery after trauma. More than 50% of elderly trauma patients have underlying hypertension and more than 30% have heart disease.[23] Moreover diabetes, previous cerebrovascular events, chronic obstructive pulmonary disease, dementia, arrhythmias, and endocrine disorders are each identified in more than 10% of the geriatric trauma population.[23] Because of the impaired health of elderly patients at baseline, they are at increased risk of certain types of trauma and in-hospital complications after any trauma.[24] Vertebral fractures after a simple fall are associated with increased risk of death, because of preexisting comorbidities.[25,26] In elderly patients with chronic lung disease, a vertebral collapse with subsequent thoracal kyphosis leads to further loss of vital capacity and resulting breathlessness. Medical treatment, including oral steroids, induces further loss of bone mass and thereby increases the fracture risk.[12]

Interdisciplinary management of geriatric patients with fracture is crucial to ensure quality, prevent complications, and (depending on the patient's individual needs) optimization of concurrent medication. Over the last decade, there have been several studies showing the advantages of an interdisciplinary approach to fragility fractures, which was originally championed by the British Orthopedic Association.[27–33]

Osteoporosis

Vertebral fractures are the most common manifestation of osteoporosis. Bone density of the vertebral column decreases steadily with age, and women have lost almost half of their bone mass by the time they reach their 80s.[34] About 50% of men and women with symptomatic vertebral fractures have evidence of osteoporosis on densitometry, and a further 40% have osteopenia.[35,36] Identification of the individual fracture risk and determination of who should receive a specific antiosteoporotic medication are the main goals when evaluating patients for osteoporosis. Detecting osteoporosis after diagnosed VCF in the elderly is crucial for further treatment determination. The gold standard for measuring bone mineral density is the dual-energy radiograph absorptiometry.[37]

Bone density is reported as a T score, in which osteoporosis is defined as a T score less than −2.5 and osteopenia is defined as a T score between −1 and −2.5, according to the World Health Organization criteria.[38] In 2011, Schreiber and colleagues[39] reported that Hounsfield units obtained from clinical computed tomography (CT) scans that are made for other purposes provide an alternative method of determining regional bone mineral density. The information could be applied to fracture risk assessment, diagnosis of osteoporosis, and early initiation of needed treatment.[39] In any case, the primary treatment target for patients with osteoporosis should be prevention of fractures.[40]

Disability

A recent review[41] showed that VCFs detected or undetected can lead to numerous complications, causing disability of the geriatric patient. Strong pain at the beginning followed by continuous low back pain, increasing thoracic kyphosis, impaired pulmonary function, fatigue, early satiety and weight loss, increasing osteoporosis caused by inactivity, deep vein thrombosis, low self-esteem, and emotional and social problems are the main complications causing disability, and therefore, these patients are more likely to be admitted to a nursing home. Rarely occurring damage to the spinal cord or the cauda equina may induce weakness, loss of sensation of the lower extremities, or even bowel or bladder incontinence.[26,34] Different studies have reported mortality between 15% and 35% after a cervical spine injury in geriatric patients.[42–47] In another study,[42] group disability occurred especially after immobilization of these patients. Lower respiratory tract infection, dysphagia, deep vein thrombosis, pulmonary embolism, and subsequent falls have been reported, causing prolonged stays in supportive care units.

Treatment goals

Geriatric patients suffering from spine fractures are in need of particular attendance by health care professionals. Achieving status quo ante is the overall goal. The clinical diagnostics, a multidisciplinary medical treatment, the standardized handling of complications, and early mobilization are keys in handling geriatric patients with spinal fractures.

SPECIAL CONSIDERATIONS
Cervical Spine Fractures

Simple falls, considered as a low energy mechanism, are the main cause for cervical spine fractures in the elderly, whereas high energy trauma such as motor vehicle collisions ranks first in the younger population. A minor trauma in the elderly can cause serious spinal cord damage and neurologic deficit, which is strongly associated with high mortality and limited potential for recovery.[47–50] A swelling of the prevertebral soft tissue is seen in conventional radiographs in 83% of patients with injuries to the upper cervical spine and in 60% of patients with injuries to the lower cervical spine. Upper cervical spine fractures predominate in elderly patients, because of degenerative osseous changes in almost all patients.[51,52] Therefore, we have to distinguish between fractures of the upper cervical spine and the lower cervical spine.

Upper cervical spine fractures C1-C2

Because of degenerative osseous changes in the cervical spine in the elderly with sometimes spontaneous fusion of the lower cervical spine, the C1-C2 motion segment becomes the most mobile portion of the cervical spine, predisposing the atlantoaxial segment to be injured after low energy trauma.[15,52,53] Odontoid fractures are the most frequent fractures of the cervical spine in persons aged 65 years and older[16,18,45,48,52–54] and are classified as previously described by Anderson and D'Alonzo.[55] In geriatric patients, the type II fracture dislocation of the odontoid is most frequent.[43,54] There is still no agreement on the best medical treatment of these fractures in the elderly. Conservative treatment by immobilization over several weeks using a halo vest or a rigid collar is accepted; nonetheless, a high incidence of complications is associated with the halo device,[56–58] and sole external immobilization is associated with a high risk of nonunion.[44,45,59] Lateral flexion-extension radiographs uncover instability in initially undisplaced odontoid fractures, although these examinations should be made with care under observation. Primary internal fixation is recommended in unstable odontoid fractures.[43] Surgical treatment of odontoid fractures in the elderly with anterior screw fixation shows good functional results and high fusion rates, with relatively low complication rates.[60] A high rate of fracture union and good functional results are also reported after posterior fusion of C1 and C2 in the elderly.[61,62]

Lower cervical spine C3-C7

Acute mortality in geriatric patients with subaxial injuries is equal to patients with odontoid fractures. There are no large trials dealing specifically with lower cervical spine fractures, because of their rare incidence in geriatric patients. Treatment strategies are equal to younger patients, considering the comorbidities in the elderly, including osteoporosis.[51]

Thoracic and Lumbar Spine

When symptomatic, patients with VCFs present with sudden incipient, focal back pain. Because of the vertebral bodies supporting 80% of the weight of the body,[63] back pain is typically worse when sitting up or standing and decreases when lying down. Usually, lateral thoracic and lumbar spine radiographs are sufficient to identify VCFs.[64] Incidentally discovered VCFs in elderly patients who undergo radiographs for other indications should be reported and treated by means of an osteoporosis assessment and treatment to reduce the risk of further fractures.[65] Basic radiologic classification of VCFs is performed by describing the vertebral shape. So, wedge, biconcave, and compression fractures can be distinguished; wedge fractures are most frequent.[66] Several qualitative and quantitative methods to define VCFs have been developed; the semiquantitative fracture assessment method developed by Genant and colleagues[67,68] is widely accepted. Further imaging options are helical CT and magnetic resonance imaging (MRI). Helical CT is recommended for accurate assessment of spinal canal compromise and for accurate classification of the fracture, whereas MRI is recommended for determining the level and extent of spinal cord or nerve roots injury and for judging fracture age.

Treatment of diagnosed VCFs in the elderly poses many challenges, yet no widely accepted guidelines for the best management of this injury in this sensitive patient population have been reported. As pointed out earlier, rapid mobilization is crucial when dealing with geriatric patients. With surgery on the one and conservative treatment on the other hand, 2 treatment options are available. Yet, when dealing with the individual geriatric patient, choice of treatment often proves to be difficult, considering the complexity of each individual case, and so no general consensus in the literature can be found.[10,12,34,41,69]

Conservative treatment includes adequate pain medication, allowing early mobilization after short rest. However, avoiding adverse effects and achieving sufficient pain relief often proves to be challenging in elderly patients, who are particularly susceptible.[12] Several oral pain medications, including opioids, are available for acute pain management. When used as first line-therapy in younger adults, nonsteroidal antiin-flammatory drugs (NSAIDs) reduce opiate requirements and concomitant opiate-related adverse effects of sedation, confusion, and nausea; however, NSAIDs are usually avoided in the elderly because of risks of cardiovascular events (stroke, heart attack, accelerated hypertension, and heart failure), bleeding, delirium, and renal fail-ure. With opioids and muscle relaxants, sufficient pain relief may be achieved, but potential side effects including reduced gastrointestinal motility, urinary retention, reduced respiratory drive, cognitive deficits with loss of balance, increasing falls, abuse, and dependency are formidable.[34,69,70]

Besides typical and adjuvant pain medications, the treatment of osteoporosis may also reduce pain,[69] because patients treated with bisphosphonates have improved and sustained pain relief and better physical condition at the end of treatment with clodronate or pamidronate.[71–73] Furthermore, patients treated with teriparatide show reduced risk of new or increasing back pain.[74,75] Calcitonin was recently removed from the market in Europe, because of concerns regarding cancer with long-term use.[76]

Only 1 study is available describing treatment with a special orthesis in patients with osteoporotic VCFs. Patients wearing this orthesis for a 6-month period after sustaining the fracture had less pain and better quality of life than the control group without orthesis. However, the use of bracing is still largely opinion based.[69,77]

Mobilization with rehabilitation, physiotherapy, and exercise programs is important in conservative management of geriatric patients with VCFs. The main goals of reha-bilitation are prevention of falls, reduction of kyphosis, enhancing axial muscle strength, and providing correct spine alignment.[69] Physiotherapy provides pain relief and improvement of physical function.[78] Moreover, different exercise programs such as spinal extensor strengthening or proprioceptive training lead to increasing bone density, reduced risk for VCFs, and reduction of kyphotic deformity. Also, patients performing home exercise show improvement in quality of life.[79–82]

Acute pain after a new VCF should normally resolve over a period of 6 to 12 weeks.[83] Hence, operative treatment should be considered in patients suffering from ongoing resistant pain beyond this period or strong pain interfering with mobilization during the first days despite adequate conservative pain management. If follow-up radio-graphs show fracture progression with increasing kyphosis, surgical stabilization should be considered as well. In fractures affecting the spinal cord with neurologic compromise, surgical decompression and fixation may be appropriate.[34]

Several surgical options are available for the management of painful osteoporotic fractures. Vertebral cement augmentation is 1 possible operative treatment option to achieve pain improvement and to prevent fracture progression.[84] The most popular minimally invasive techniques for performing vertebral augmentation are vertebro-plasty and kyphoplasty. In 1984, the vertebroplasty was introduced by Galibert and colleagues,[85] and since then, it has been performed to treat VCFs. Vertebroplasty is a minimally invasive image-guided procedure that involves the percutaneous injection of a polymethylmethacrylate (PMMA) cement into the fractured vertebral body.[86,87] Pain relief may occur by stabilizing the fracture and preventing further vertebral collapse.[88] As a second possible vertebral augmentation technique, balloon kypho-plasty was first performed in 1998, adding an additional step before cement injection by placing an inflatable balloon tamp in the fractured vertebral body. Kyphoplasty involves the initial inflation of the balloon tamp that creates a low-resistance cavity within the vertebral body, into which cement is injected subsequently.[86] Kyphoplasty can reverse spinal deformity by height restoration of the vertebral body by 50% to 70%, with a segmental kyphosis reduction of 6° to 10°.[87,89,90] In addition to pain relief, kyphoplasty can prevent the pulmonary and gastrointestinal complications associated with severe kyphosis.[90] After vertebral augmentation of VCFs in elderly patients, pain relief may occur within 24 hours, and overall reported complication rates are particularly low in osteoporotic VCFs (<4%).[84,91,92] Two large open-label randomized controlled trials have shown efficacy for vertebroplasty and kyphoplasty, respectively, over best conservative medical management.[93,94] Nonetheless, much debate about efficacy of vertebral augmentation has remained ever since 2 small double-blind randomized controlled trials were published in the *New England Journal of Medicine* in 2009.[95,96] In these 2 trials, comparing vertebroplasty with sham procedure rather than with conservative medical treatment, no benefit with respect to pain, functional disability, or quality of life could be identified between the 2 groups. The investigators of these 2 trials suggested that reported benefits of vertebroplasty in previous trials were secondary to a procedural placebo effect.[97,98] Although about 300 articles have been published annually on vertebral augmentation in the last 5 years, the debate about these minimally invasive techniques continues, and further randomized controlled trials are required to improve the strength of evidence available to assess these procedures.

In a subgroup of geriatric patients with osteoporotic vertebral fractures, vertebral augmentation is not approved or sufficient and so different operative techniques are required.[99,100] Thus, it is not possible to perform vertebral augmentation in completely collapsed vertebral bodies or to achieve height restoration or kyphosis improvement in old fractures with posttraumatic kyphosis. Furthermore, risk of cement extrusion into the spinal canal is greatly increased if the posterior wall of the vertebral body is fractured. An absolute contraindication is bony retropulsion with neurologic compromise, because augmentation could worsen the condition.[34] Hence, other operative treatment options are indicated in these special cases. Because clinical trials have shown reduced rates of screw loosening in the osteoporotic vertebral bone after cement augmentation of the pedicle screws,[101,102] augmented dorsal instrumentation is performed as a possible technique.[99]

SUMMARY

With aging of the population, the number of osteoporotic vertebral fractures is increasing, and the economic burden is evident. VCFs tend to remain underdiagnosed. The overall treatment goal is the remobilization of the patient as soon as possible to prevent medical complications. The treatment of these fractures is complicated, because of the comorbid conditions of elderly patients; this means their medical problems on one hand and the underlying osteoporosis on the other hand. The latter leads to subsequent malalignment of the weakened bone and impedes fracture fixation. The treatment of osteoporotic vertebral fractures is widely empirical, because standardized and accepted treatment evidence-based concepts are missing for certain fracture types. As in other osteoporotic fractures in the elderly, the key for good outcome may be a combination of interdisciplinary treatment approaches and adapted surgical procedures.

REFERENCES

1. van der Klift M, de Laet CE, McCloskey EV, et al. Risk factors for incident vertebral fractures in men and women: the Rotterdam Study. J Bone Miner Res 2004; 19(7):1172–80.
2. Black DM, Arden NK, Palermo L, et al. Prevalent vertebral deformities predict hip fractures and new vertebral deformities but not wrist fractures. Study of

Osteoporotic Fractures Research Group. J Bone Miner Res 1999;14(5): 821–8.
3. Gertzbein SD, Khoury D, Bullington A, et al. Thoracic and lumbar fractures associated with skiing and snowboarding injuries according to the AO Comprehensive Classification. Am J Sports Med 2012;40(8):1750–4.
4. Johnell O, Kanis JA. An estimate of the worldwide prevalence and disability associated with osteoporotic fractures. Osteoporos Int 2006;17(12):1726–33.
5. Hernlund E, Svedbom A, Ivergard M, et al. Osteoporosis in the European Union: medical management, epidemiology and economic burden: a report prepared in collaboration with the International Osteoporosis Foundation (IOF) and the European Federation of Pharmaceutical Industry Associations (EFPIA). Arch Osteoporos 2013;8(1–2):136.
6. Burge R, Dawson-Hughes B, Solomon DH, et al. Incidence and economic burden of osteoporosis-related fractures in the United States, 2005-2025. J Bone Miner Res 2007;22(3):465–75.
7. Felsenberg D, Silman AJ, Lunt M, et al. Incidence of vertebral fracture in Europe: results from the European Prospective Osteoporosis Study (EPOS). J Bone Miner Res 2002;17(4):716–24.
8. Melton LJ 3rd, Kan SH, Frye MA, et al. Epidemiology of vertebral fractures in women. Am J Epidemiol 1989;129(5):1000–11.
9. Cooper C, O'Neill T, Silman A. The epidemiology of vertebral fractures. European Vertebral Osteoporosis Study Group. Bone 1993;14(Suppl 1):S89–97.
10. Ensrud KE, Schousboe JT. Clinical practice. Vertebral fractures. N Engl J Med 2011;364(17):1634–42.
11. Fink HA, Milavetz DL, Palermo L, et al. What proportion of incident radiographic vertebral deformities is clinically diagnosed and vice versa? J Bone Miner Res 2005;20(7):1216–22.
12. Francis RM, Baillie SP, Chuck AJ, et al. Acute and long-term management of patients with vertebral fractures. QJM 2004;97(2):63–74.
13. Cooper C. Epidemiology and public health impact of osteoporosis. Baillieres Clin Rheumatol 1993;7(3):459–77.
14. Marshall D, Johnell O, Wedel H. Meta-analysis of how well measures of bone mineral density predict occurrence of osteoporotic fractures. BMJ 1996; 312(7041):1254–9.
15. Malik SA, Murphy M, Connolly P, et al. Evaluation of morbidity, mortality and outcome following cervical spine injuries in elderly patients. Eur Spine J 2008; 17(4):585–91.
16. Brolin K. Neck injuries among the elderly in Sweden. Inj Control Saf Promot 2003;10(3):155–64.
17. Ryan MD, Henderson JJ. The epidemiology of fractures and fracture-dislocations of the cervical spine. Injury 1992;23(1):38–40.
18. Weller SJ, Malek AM, Rossitch E Jr. Cervical spine fractures in the elderly. Surg Neurol 1997;47(3):274–80 [discussion: 280–71].
19. Levy DB, Hanlon DP, Townsend RN. Geriatric trauma. Clin Geriatr Med 1993; 9(3):601–20.
20. Morris JA Jr, MacKenzie EJ, Edelstein SL. The effect of preexisting conditions on mortality in trauma patients. JAMA 1990;263(14):1942–6.
21. Schwab CW, Kauder DR. Trauma in the geriatric patient. Arch Surg 1992;127(6): 701–6.
22. Smith DP, Enderson BL, Maull KI. Trauma in the elderly: determinants of outcome. South Med J 1990;83(2):171–7.

23. Thompson HJ, McCormick WC, Kagan SH. Traumatic brain injury in older adults: epidemiology, outcomes, and future implications. J Am Geriatr Soc 2006;54(10):1590–5.

24. Bonne S, Schuerer DJ. Trauma in the older adult: epidemiology and evolving geriatric trauma principles. Clin Geriatr Med 2013;29(1):137–50.

25. Karlsson MK, Magnusson H, von Schewelov T, et al. Prevention of falls in the elderly–a review. Osteoporos Int 2013;24(3):747–62.

26. Ensrud KE, Thompson DE, Cauley JA, et al. Prevalent vertebral deformities predict mortality and hospitalization in older women with low bone mass. Fracture Intervention Trial Research Group. J Am Geriatr Soc 2000;48(3):241–9.

27. Kates SL, O'Malley N, Friedman SM, et al. Barriers to implementation of an organized geriatric fracture program. Geriatr Orthop Surg Rehabil 2012;3(1):8–16.

28. Kates SL, Mendelson DA, Friedman SM. The value of an organized fracture program for the elderly: early results. J Orthop Trauma 2011;25(4):233–7.

29. Kates SL, Mendelson DA, Friedman SM. Co-managed care for fragility hip fractures (Rochester model). Osteoporos Int 2010;21(Suppl 4):S621–5.

30. Friedman S, Mendelson D, Kates S, et al. Geriatric co-management of proximal femur fractures: total quality management and protocol-driven care result in better outcomes for a frail patient population. J Am Geriatr Soc 2008;56(7): 1349–56.

31. Friedman SM, Mendelson DA, Bingham KW, et al. Impact of a comanaged Geriatric Fracture Center on short-term hip fracture outcomes. Arch Intern Med 2009;169(18):1712–7.

32. Kammerlander C, Gosch M, Blauth M, et al. The Tyrolean Geriatric Fracture Center: an orthogeriatric co-management model. Z Gerontol Geriatr 2011;44(6): 363–7.

33. Kammerlander C, Roth T, Friedman SM, et al. Ortho-geriatric service–a literature review comparing different models. Osteoporos Int 2010;21(Suppl 4):S637–46.

34. Wong CC, McGirt MJ. Vertebral compression fractures: a review of current management and multimodal therapy. J Multidiscip Healthc 2013;6:205–14.

35. Scane AC, Francis RM, Sutcliffe AM, et al. Case-control study of the pathogenesis and sequelae of symptomatic vertebral fractures in men. Osteoporos Int 1999;9(1):91–7.

36. Selby PL, Davies M, Adams JE. Do men and women fracture bones at similar bone densities? Osteoporos Int 2000;11(2):153–7.

37. Slemenda CW, Hui SL, Longcope C, et al. Predictors of bone mass in perimenopausal women. A prospective study of clinical data using photon absorptiometry. Ann Intern Med 1990;112(2):96–101.

38. Kanis JA. Assessment of fracture risk and its application to screening for postmenopausal osteoporosis: synopsis of a WHO report. WHO Study Group. Osteoporos Int 1994;4(6):368–81.

39. Schreiber JJ, Anderson PA, Rosas HG, et al. Hounsfield units for assessing bone mineral density and strength: a tool for osteoporosis management. J Bone Joint Surg Am 2011;93(11):1057–63.

40. NIH Consensus Development Panel on Osteoporosis Prevention, Diagnosis, and Therapy. Osteoporosis prevention, diagnosis, and therapy. JAMA 2001; 285(6):785–95.

41. Alexandru D, So W. Evaluation and management of vertebral compression fractures. Perm J 2012;16(4):46–51.

42. Moran C, Kipen E, Chan P, et al. Understanding post-hospital morbidity associated with immobilisation of cervical spine fractures in older people using

geriatric medicine assessment techniques: a pilot study. Injury 2013;44(12): 1838–42.

43. Muller EJ, Wick M, Russe O, et al. Management of odontoid fractures in the elderly. Eur Spine J 1999;8(5):360–5.

44. Hanigan WC, Powell FC, Elwood PW, et al. Odontoid fractures in elderly patients. J Neurosurg 1993;78(1):32–5.

45. Pepin JW, Bourne RB, Hawkins RJ. Odontoid fractures, with special reference to the elderly patient. Clin Orthop Relat Res 1985;(193):178–83.

46. Ersmark H, Kalen R. A consecutive series of 64 halo-vest-treated cervical spine injuries. Arch Orthop Trauma Surg 1986;105(4):243–6.

47. Lieberman IH, Webb JK. Cervical spine injuries in the elderly. J Bone Joint Surg Br 1994;76(6):877–81.

48. Spivak JM, Weiss MA, Cotler JM, et al. Cervical spine injuries in patients 65 and older. Spine (Phila Pa 1976) 1994;19(20):2302–6.

49. Anderson PA, Bohlman HH. Anterior decompression and arthrodesis of the cervical spine: long-term motor improvement. Part II–Improvement in complete traumatic quadriplegia. J Bone Joint Surg Am 1992;74(5):683–92.

50. Damadi AA, Saxe AW, Fath JJ, et al. Cervical spine fractures in patients 65 years or older: a 3-year experience at a level I trauma center. J Trauma 2008;64(3):745–8.

51. Wang H, Coppola M, Robinson RD, et al. Geriatric trauma patients with cervical spine fractures due to ground level fall: five years experience in a level one trauma center. J Clin Med Res 2013;5(2):75–83.

52. Lomoschitz FM, Blackmore CC, Mirza SK, et al. Cervical spine injuries in patients 65 years old and older: epidemiologic analysis regarding the effects of age and injury mechanism on distribution, type, and stability of injuries. AJR Am J Roentgenol 2002;178(3):573–7.

53. Olerud C, Andersson S, Svensson B, et al. Cervical spine fractures in the elderly: factors influencing survival in 65 cases. Acta Orthop Scand 1999;70(5):509–13.

54. Ryan MD, Taylor TK. Odontoid fractures in the elderly. J Spinal Disord 1993;6(5): 397–401.

55. Anderson LD, D'Alonzo RT. Fractures of the odontoid process of the axis. J Bone Joint Surg Am 1974;56(8):1663–74.

56. Garfin SR, Botte MJ, Nickel VL. Complications in the use of the halo fixation device. J Bone Joint Surg Am 1987;69(6):954.

57. Lind B, Nordwall A, Sihlbom H. Odontoid fractures treated with halo-vest. Spine (Phila Pa 1976) 1987;12(2):173–7.

58. Horn EM, Theodore N, Feiz-Erfan I, et al. Complications of halo fixation in the elderly. J Neurosurg Spine 2006;5(1):46–9.

59. Clark CR, White AA 3rd. Fractures of the dens. A multicenter study. J Bone Joint Surg Am 1985;67(9):1340–8.

60. Platzer P, Thalhammer G, Oberleitner G, et al. Surgical treatment of dens fractures in elderly patients. J Bone Joint Surg Am 2007;89(8):1716–22.

61. Jeanneret B, Magerl F. Primary posterior fusion C1/2 in odontoid fractures: indications, technique, and results of transarticular screw fixation. J Spinal Disord 1992;5(4):464–75.

62. Vaccaro AR, Kepler CK, Kopjar B, et al. Functional and quality-of-life outcomes in geriatric patients with type-II dens fracture. J Bone Joint Surg Am 2013;95(8): 729–35.

63. Sinaki M. Exercise for patients with osteoporosis: management of vertebral compression fractures and trunk strengthening for fall prevention. PM R 2012; 4(11):882–8.

64. Kiel D. Assessing vertebral fractures. National Osteoporosis Foundation Working Group on vertebral fractures. J Bone Miner Res 1995;10(4):518–23.
65. Majumdar SR, Kim N, Colman I, et al. Incidental vertebral fractures discovered with chest radiography in the emergency department: prevalence, recognition, and osteoporosis management in a cohort of elderly patients. Arch Intern Med 2005;165(8):905–9.
66. Eastell R, Cedel SL, Wahner HW, et al. Classification of vertebral fractures. J Bone Miner Res 1991;6(3):207–15.
67. Genant HK, Wu CY, van Kuijk C, et al. Vertebral fracture assessment using a semiquantitative technique. J Bone Miner Res 1993;8(9):1137–48.
68. Genant HK, Jergas M, Palermo L, et al. Comparison of semiquantitative visual and quantitative morphometric assessment of prevalent and incident vertebral fractures in osteoporosis the Study of Osteoporotic Fractures Research Group. J Bone Miner Res 1996;11(7):984–96.
69. Longo UG, Loppini M, Denaro L, et al. Conservative management of patients with an osteoporotic vertebral fracture: a review of the literature. J Bone Joint Surg Br 2012;94(2):152–7.
70. Halaszynski T. Influences of the aging process on acute perioperative pain management in elderly and cognitively impaired patients. Ochsner J 2013;13(2): 228–47.
71. Rovetta G, Monteforte P, Balestra V. Intravenous clodronate for acute pain induced by osteoporotic vertebral fracture. Drugs Exp Clin Res 2000;26(1): 25–30.
72. Rovetta G, Maggiani G, Molfetta L, et al. One-month follow-up of patients treated by intravenous clodronate for acute pain induced by osteoporotic vertebral fracture. Drugs Exp Clin Res 2001;27(2):77–81.
73. Armingeat T, Brondino R, Pham T, et al. Intravenous pamidronate for pain relief in recent osteoporotic vertebral compression fracture: a randomized double-blind controlled study. Osteoporos Int 2006;17(11):1659–65.
74. Nevitt MC, Chen P, Dore RK, et al. Reduced risk of back pain following teriparatide treatment: a meta-analysis. Osteoporos Int 2006;17(2):273–80.
75. Nevitt MC, Chen P, Kiel DP, et al. Reduction in the risk of developing back pain persists at least 30 months after discontinuation of teriparatide treatment: a meta-analysis. Osteoporos Int 2006;17(11):1630–7.
76. Lim V, Clarke BL. New therapeutic targets for osteoporosis: beyond denosumab. Maturitas 2012;73(3):269–72.
77. Pfeifer M, Begerow B, Minne HW. Effects of a new spinal orthosis on posture, trunk strength, and quality of life in women with postmenopausal osteoporosis: a randomized trial. Am J Phys Med Rehabil 2004;83(3):177–86.
78. Bennell KL, Matthews B, Greig A, et al. Effects of an exercise and manual therapy program on physical impairments, function and quality-of-life in people with osteoporotic vertebral fracture: a randomised, single-blind controlled pilot trial. BMC Musculoskelet Disord 2010;11:36.
79. Sinaki M, Itoi E, Wahner HW, et al. Stronger back muscles reduce the incidence of vertebral fractures: a prospective 10 year follow-up of postmenopausal women. Bone 2002;30(6):836–41.
80. Sinaki M, Lynn SG. Reducing the risk of falls through proprioceptive dynamic posture training in osteoporotic women with kyphotic posturing: a randomized pilot study. Am J Phys Med Rehabil 2002;81(4):241–6.
81. Itoi E, Sinaki M. Effect of back-strengthening exercise on posture in healthy women 49 to 65 years of age. Mayo Clin Proc 1994;69(11):1054–9.

82. Papaioannou A, Adachi JD, Winegard K, et al. Efficacy of home-based exercise for improving quality of life among elderly women with symptomatic osteoporosis-related vertebral fractures. Osteoporos Int 2003;14(8):677–82.
83. Silverman SL. The clinical consequences of vertebral compression fracture. Bone 1992;13(Suppl 2):S27–31.
84. McGirt MJ, Parker SL, Wolinsky JP, et al. Vertebroplasty and kyphoplasty for the treatment of vertebral compression fractures: an evidenced-based review of the literature. Spine J 2009;9(6):501–8.
85. Galibert P, Deramond H, Rosat P, et al. Preliminary note on the treatment of vertebral angioma by percutaneous acrylic vertebroplasty. Neurochirurgie 1987;33(2):166–8 [in French].
86. Chandra RV, Yoo AJ, Hirsch JA. Vertebral augmentation: update on safety, efficacy, cost effectiveness and increased survival? Pain Physician 2013;16(4): 309–20.
87. Bostrom MP, Lane JM. Future directions. Augmentation of osteoporotic vertebral bodies. Spine (Phila Pa 1976) 1997;22(Suppl 24):38S–42S.
88. McKiernan F, Faciszewski T, Jensen R. Quality of life following vertebroplasty. J Bone Joint Surg Am 2004;86-A(12):2600–6.
89. Garfin SR, Yuan HA, Reiley MA. New technologies in spine: kyphoplasty and vertebroplasty for the treatment of painful osteoporotic compression fractures. Spine (Phila Pa 1976) 2001;26(14):1511–5.
90. Gaitanis IN, Hadjipavlou AG, Katonis PG, et al. Balloon kyphoplasty for the treatment of pathological vertebral compressive fractures. Eur Spine J 2005;14(3): 250–60.
91. Lin WC, Cheng TT, Lee YC, et al. New vertebral osteoporotic compression fractures after percutaneous vertebroplasty. retrospective analysis of risk factors. J Vasc Interv Radiol 2008;19(2 Pt 1):225–31.
92. Taylor RS, Fritzell P, Taylor RJ. Balloon kyphoplasty in the management of vertebral compression fractures: an updated systematic review and meta-analysis. Eur Spine J 2007;16(8):1085–100.
93. Wardlaw D, Cummings SR, Van Meirhaeghe J, et al. Efficacy and safety of balloon kyphoplasty compared with non-surgical care for vertebral compression fracture (FREE): a randomised controlled trial. Lancet 2009;373(9668):1016–24.
94. Klazen CA, Lohle PN, de Vries J, et al. Vertebroplasty versus conservative treatment in acute osteoporotic vertebral compression fractures (Vertos II): an open-label randomised trial. Lancet 2010;376(9746):1085–92.
95. Buchbinder R, Osborne RH, Ebeling PR, et al. A randomized trial of vertebroplasty for painful osteoporotic vertebral fractures. N Engl J Med 2009;361(6): 557–68.
96. Kallmes DF, Comstock BA, Heagerty PJ, et al. A randomized trial of vertebroplasty for osteoporotic spinal fractures. N Engl J Med 2009;361(6):569–79.
97. Kallmes D, Buchbinder R, Jarvik J, et al. Response to "randomized vertebroplasty trials: bad news or sham news?". AJNR Am J Neuroradiol 2009;30(10): 1809–10.
98. Miller FG, Kallmes DF, Buchbinder R. Vertebroplasty and the placebo response. Radiology 2011;259(3):621–5.
99. Krappinger D, Kastenberger TJ, Schmid R. Augmented posterior instrumentation for the treatment of osteoporotic vertebral body fractures. Oper Orthop Traumatol 2012;24(1):4–12 [in German].
100. Patil S, Rawall S, Singh D, et al. Surgical patterns in osteoporotic vertebral compression fractures. Eur Spine J 2013;22(4):883–91.

101. Frankel BM, Jones T, Wang C. Segmental polymethylmethacrylate-augmented pedicle screw fixation in patients with bone softening caused by osteoporosis and metastatic tumor involvement: a clinical evaluation. Neurosurgery 2007; 61(3):531–7 [discussion: 537–8].

102. Moon BJ, Cho BY, Choi EY, et al. Polymethylmethacrylate-augmented screw fixation for stabilization of the osteoporotic spine: a three-year follow-up of 37 patients. J Korean Neurosurg Soc 2009;46(4):305–11.

Fragility Fractures Requiring Special Consideration
Pelvic Insufficiency Fractures

Catherine A. Humphrey, MD[a,b,]*, Michael A. Maceroli, MD[c]

KEYWORDS

• Pelvis • Fragility • Fracture • Acetabulum • Insufficiency • Osteopenia

KEY POINTS

• Pelvis and acetabulum insufficiency fractures carry a significant morbidity and mortality risk.
• Pelvic fragility fractures can typically be managed without surgery but certain unstable patterns may require operative fixation.
• Presence of an insufficiency fracture, especially in the pelvis, can be the first presentation of osteoporosis, and therefore all patients require a full metabolic bone workup.
• Approved pharmacologic agents should be used as adjunctive treatment of any pelvic fragility fracture.

INTRODUCTION

Fractures of the pelvis and acetabulum in osteoporotic bone represent an important subset of fragility fractures. Pelvic fractures in the elderly patient carry a significant 1-year mortality risk, comparable to that of hip fractures.[1,2] Furthermore, the incidence of pelvic fragility fracture is increasing with overall population age, placing a significant burden on patient, provider, and society.[3]

Pelvic insufficiency fractures impart pain and mobility challenges that often result in decreased independence in a previously high-functioning patient. Therefore, the primary treatment goals in the osteoporotic patient are centered in improving mobility and balance to restore preinjury autonomy. Providers must have an understanding of the unique anatomic and biomechanical characteristics of the pelvis/acetabulum as well as the available treatment strategies. This article aims to provide an overview

[a] Orthopaedics, Highland Hospital, University of Rochester Medical Center, 601 Elmwood Avenue, Box 665, Rochester, NY 14642, USA; [b] Trauma Division, Orthopaedics, Strong Memorial Hospital, University of Rochester Medical Center, 601 Elmwood Avenue, Box 665, Rochester, NY 14642, USA; [c] Department of Orthopaedics, University of Rochester Medical Center, 601 Elmwood Avenue, Box 665, Rochester, NY 14642, USA
* Corresponding author. School of Medicine and Dentistry, University of Rochester Medical Center, 601 Elmwood Avenue, Box 665, Rochester, NY 14642.
E-mail address: Catherine_Humphrey@URMC.Rochester.edu

Clin Geriatr Med 30 (2014) 373–386
http://dx.doi.org/10.1016/j.cger.2014.01.012
0749-0690/14/$ – see front matter © 2014 Elsevier Inc. All rights reserved.

geriatric.theclinics.com

of pelvic insufficiency fractures, demonstrate the anatomic relationships in the pelvis, outline necessary diagnostic techniques, and review operative and nonoperative treatment strategies.

Epidemiology

Pelvis fracture epidemiology

Pelvic fractures account for 7% of all fragility fractures and incur 5% of the total cost for care of osteoporotic fractures in patients older than or equal to 50 years.[4] Most of these fractures occur through a low energy mechanism and, of these, 81% to 95% represent a stable fracture pattern.[5,6]

As one would expect with any fragility fracture, the incidence of pelvic insufficiency fractures is age related. Melton and colleagues[5] reported on the incidence of pelvic fractures during a 10-year period in Rochester, Minnesota. The investigators noted an overall incidence of 37/100,000 person years; however, in men aged between 75 and 84 years the incidence was 63.9/100,000 and in women the incidence was 249.5/100,000. In men and women aged 85 years or greater, the incidence was 220.3/100,000 person years and 446.3/100,000 person years, respectively. The incidence of pelvic fractures continues to rise with the aging of our world population as a whole. Parkkari and colleagues[3] reported on osteoporotic pelvic fractures in Finland from 1970 to 1991 citing an increase from 18% of all pelvic fractures in 1970 to 52% in 1991. They also noted a rise in the proportion of patients older than 60 years from 28% in 1970 to 62% in 1991. Kannus and colleagues[7] noted that incidence of pelvic fractures in patients aged 60 years or older increased by an average of 23% per year from 1970 to 1997. Using these data, the investigators projected the number of pelvic insufficiency fractures per year would triple by year 2030.

Acetabulum fracture epidemiology

Acetabulum insufficiency fractures represent a significant subset of pelvic fractures whose incidence is also increasing. Ferguson and colleagues[8] reported on a consecutive series of operative acetabulum fractures from 1980 to 2007 and demonstrated a 30% increase in the proportion of acetabulum fractures in patients older than 60 years. About 49.8% of these fractures were the result of a low energy ground-level fall. In a 10-year analysis of pelvic fractures treated in Skarborg County, Sweden, a 10% incidence of acetabulum fractures occurred in patients older than 60 years.[6] Boufous and colleagues[9] noted a 11% incidence of acetabulum fractures in their series of geriatric pelvis injuries.

Morbidity and mortality statistics

Pelvic insufficiency fractures are associated with decreased mobility, loss of independence, and significant mortality. In a series of 148 patients aged 65 years or older with a closed pelvic fracture (83% due to low energy trauma), 51.1% required personal assistance for mobility and all patients required device assistance for ambulation at time of discharge.[10] The inability to safely ambulate after sustaining a pelvic fracture makes it especially difficult for the geriatric patient to return home from the hospital.

Breuil and colleagues[11] evaluated outcomes of 60 patients hospitalized with a new pelvic insufficiency fracture and noted 52.5% of patients suffered an adverse event during hospitalization, mainly urinary tract infection, pressure ulcer, cognitive alteration, or thromboembolic event. Furthermore, although 82.5% of the cohort was living autonomously before injury, only 31% returned home on discharge, whereas 3.4% were institutionalized and 65.6% discharged to a geriatric in-patient setting. At time of last follow-up almost 50% of the patients in this series had lost autonomy. Taillandier and colleagues[2] reviewed 10 years of pelvic insufficiency fractures at a single institution and noted that 24 of 41 previously self-sufficient patients returned to this status post-discharge and only 39% returned to their preinjury level of function at 1 year.

Pelvic fractures impart dismal mortality statistics. Hill and colleagues[12] reviewed 273 patients with average age of 74.7 years admitted to the hospital with pubic rami fractures and noted survival rates at 1 and 5 years post-injury as 86.7% and 45.6%, respectively. Patients with dementia had a significantly higher mortality with 80% survival rate at 1 year and 27.8% at 5 years. Bible and colleagues[13] reviewed a series of 86 patients whose average age was 71.1 ± 7.1 years with an isolated acetabular fracture and noted mortality as 2.3% at 30 days, 5.8% at 3 months, 8.1% at 6 months, and 8.1% at 1 year. There were no significant differences in mortality between operatively and nonoperatively treated fractures.

Anatomic and Biomechanical Considerations

The musculoskeletal pelvis is the site at which body weight is transferred from the axial skeleton to the pelvic ring and finally to the lower extremities through the hip articulation. Although all are in close anatomic proximity, injuries to each pelvic component should be considered as a separate entity. The pelvic ring, sacrum, and acetabulum each have unique anatomic characteristics, fracture classifications, and biomechanical properties.

Pelvis anatomy

The bony pelvic ring is composed of the sacrum posteriorly as the keystone structure, bordered on each side by the innominate bones, completing the ring anteriorly at the pubic symphysis. The innominate is formed by 3 ossification centers (ilium, ischium, and pubis) that coalesce at the triradiate cartilage. These bony structures have little inherent stability, and therefore the soft tissue envelope and ligamentous structures are the most biomechanically relevant (**Fig. 1**).

Pelvic injuries are classified by the system defined by Young and Burgess.[14] Elderly patients sustaining pelvic insufficiency fractures will most commonly present with a lateral compression (LC) type pattern resulting from the forces on the hemipelvis after

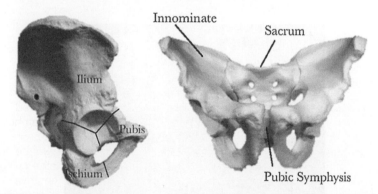

Fig. 1. AP and lateral 3-dimensional representations of the pelvis bony anatomy. The lateral image highlights the 3 ossified centers of the innominate bone: the ilium, the ischium, and the pubis. The dark lines represent the now fused triradiate cartilage. The AP image demonstrates the 3 major structures in the pelvic ring: the innominate bones, the sacrum, and the pubic symphysis. The sacrum is centered between the 2 innominate bones that then converge to complete the ring at the pubic symphysis.

a ground-level fall onto one's side.[15] LC patterns consist of lateral directed force resulting in an anterior internal rotation injury typically in the form of rami fractures and a posterior injury classified as LC-1 (sacral impaction), LC-2 (iliac wing fracture), or LC-3 ("windswept pelvis" LC pattern with contralateral hemipelvis external rotation). In their pelvic fragility fracture series, Melton and colleagues[5] reported LC type 1 or type 2 pattern was present in 95% of all pelvis fractures (**Fig. 2**).

Acetabulum anatomy

The acetabulum, located within the innominate bone, is formed by the articular surface of the hip joint and supported by 2 columns of bone connected to the sacroiliac joint via the sciatic buttress. As described by Letournel,[16] the columns of bone can be separated into the anterior/iliopectineal column and posterior/ilioischial column.

Fractures of the acetabulum are classified via plain radiographs as described by Letournel.[16] The classification consists of 5 elementary types and 5 associated types based on involvement of one or more key structures: anterior column, anterior wall, posterior column, and posterior wall (**Fig. 3**).

Elderly patients can present with any of the 10 fracture types mentioned earlier; however, the pattern most commonly resulting from a ground-level fall onto osteoporotic bone is a comminuted anterior column fracture with disruption of the medial wall of the acetabulum more commonly known as the quadrilateral plate.[17] In their series of acetabulum fractures Ferguson and colleagues[8] noted that comminuted anterior column fractures were significantly more common in the elderly group as compared to a young cohort. Of these acetabular fragility fractures, 50% demonstrated a separate quadrilateral plate component and 40% demonstrated roof impaction; radiologic factors that have been previously established are predictors of poor outcome after reduction and fixation.

EVALUATION
History and Physical Examination

Evaluation of pelvic fragility fractures requires careful history and physical examination coupled with osteoporosis laboratory tests and specific imaging studies. Patients will typically present complaining of hip or groin pain but may also describe buttock or

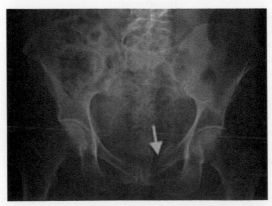

Fig. 2. An AP view of the pelvis demonstrating the classic presentation of the patient with pelvic fragility fracture. There are left-sided superior and inferior rami fractures in the setting of very osteoporotic bone. The sacrum and posterior pelvic elements are difficult to visualize secondary to overlying bowel gas. The arrow is indicating the superior ramus fracture.

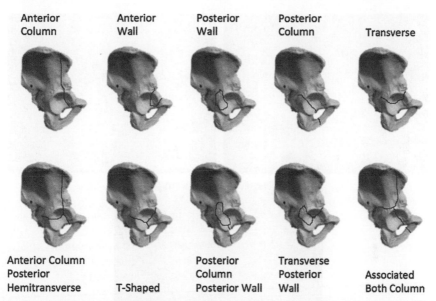

| Anterior Column | Anterior Wall | Posterior Wall | Posterior Column | Transverse |

| Anterior Column Posterior Hemitransverse | T-Shaped | Posterior Column Posterior Wall | Transverse Posterior Wall | Associated Both Column |

Fig. 3. The classification of acetabulum fractures as described by Judet and colleagues.[21] The 5 elementary types consist of the anterior wall, anterior column, posterior column, posterior wall, and transverse. The 5 associated types include the anterior column with posterior hemitransverse, posterior column and posterior wall, transverse posterior wall, T-shaped, and associated both column. Acetabulum fractures in elderly patients commonly involve the anterior column.

lower lumbar pain in the case of sacral fracture.[18] Mechanism of injury is often a low-energy ground-level fall; however, these injuries can also occur without any specific trauma.[10,19,20] Patients will describe pain with ambulation manifesting as either an immediate refusal to bear weight after a fall or a consistent decline in mobility over the course of days to weeks. Because an inciting event may be difficult to identify, physical examination is of the utmost importance.

Patients will be tender to palpation over the groin, pubic symphysis, and occasionally the sacrum. They complain of difficulty initiating hip flexion on the affected side. Often they will describe that the leg feels "heavy". They may also have pain with log rolling (internal and external rotation of the affected extremity) or axial load applied through the heel but this is less common. A full neuromotor examination of the lower extremities including strength, reflexes, and differentiation between light and sharp sensation should always be performed. Most patients will be intact neurologically but any signs of deficit should be met with extreme concern. Furthermore, one must document any signs of spinal cord or nerve root compression including urinary retention, poor rectal tone, and saddle anesthesia, as acute cauda equina syndrome can occur with displaced sacral insufficiency fracture.

Imaging

Plain radiographs
All patients with concern for pelvic or acetabular insufficiency fracture should receive initial evaluation with plain radiographs consisting of anteroposterior (AP), pelvic inlet, pelvic outlet, and Judet radiographs (**Fig. 4**).

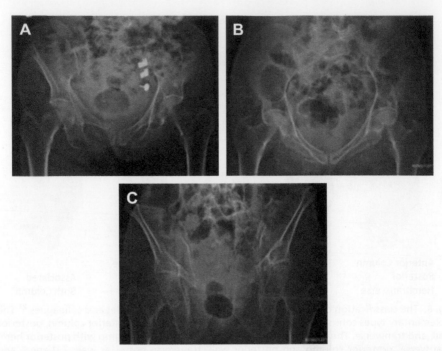

Fig. 4. Radiographic series for pelvic fracture including AP, inlet, and outlet projections. (*A*) AP view of the pelvis in a patient who sustained a ground-level fall onto the right side. Superior and inferior pubic rami fractures are noted on the right side. (*B*) Inlet projection of the pelvis demonstrating the rami fractures, minimal disruption of the ring contour, and a sacral buckle fracture noted on the right. (*C*) Outlet projection of the pelvis demonstrating an "en face" view of the sacrum. The sacral buckle fracture is once again noted on the right. There is no vertical displacement through the sacral fracture. This series demonstrates a stable LC type pelvic fracture.

The 3-view Judet series as described by Judet and colleagues[21] consisting of an AP pelvis, obturator oblique, and iliac oblique projections is used to identify and classify acetabulum fractures (**Fig. 5**).

Advanced imaging

Plain radiographs are the primary screening tool for diagnosis of pelvic insufficiency fractures; however, overlying bowel gas and demineralized bone make these images difficult to interpret. Pubic rami fractures are often identified on plain films while the posterior element injury is missed. In this case, advanced imaging studies such as bone scintigraphy, computed tomography (CT), and magnetic resonance imaging (MRI) can be used (**Fig. 6**).[18,22]

Laboratory Analysis

In addition to imaging studies, an initial osteoporosis screening is performed for all patients who present with fragility fracture. Providers should evaluate for both primary osteoporosis as well as secondary causes of decreased bone mineral density.[23,24] Rapid identification of primary or secondary causes for decreased bone mineral density is vital in formulating an appropriate treatment plan. Further discussion on osteoporosis diagnostic testing and surveillance can be found in Chapter 14.

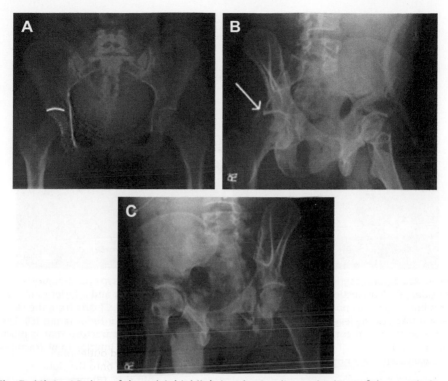

Fig. 5. (A) An AP view of the pelvis highlighting the 6 radiographic lines of the acetabulum: Solid White – acetabular roof; Solid Green – ilioischial line corresponding to the posterior column; Solid Red – illopectineal line corresponding to the anterior column; Blue – radiographic teardrop formed by the quadrilateral plate and anterior wall; Dotted Blue – anterior wall; Dotted Purple – posterior wall. (B) Obturator oblique projection used to highlight the anterior column and posterior wall; the *arrow* is indicating a large, displaced posterior wall fracture. (C) Iliac oblique projection used to highlight the posterior column and anterior wall; the posterior column and anterior wall are intact demonstrating that this fracture pattern is an elementary posterior wall fracture.

Author's Preferred Management

At the authors' institution, any patient with suspected pelvic insufficiency fracture receives an initial radiographic series of AP, inlet, and outlet views. If there is presumed acetabular injury a Judet series is obtained. All patients are examined by a Geriatrician and undergo a full set of laboratory studies as outlined in the prior section. There is controversy in the literature as to whether a CT or MRI is indicated as a diagnostic screening tool for pelvic insufficiency fracture.[20,25,26] At this institution a CT pelvis with coronal and sagittal reconstructions is obtained if there is a neuromotor deficit, concern for instability on physical examination, signs of displacement on radiographs, or high suspicion of fracture that is unseen on plain radiographic studies. CT is also used for preoperative planning in any acetabular or pelvic surgery.

MANAGEMENT GOALS

The ultimate management goal in pelvic and acetabular fragility fractures is a return to preoperative functional status. Unfortunately, pelvic injuries cause severe pain, gait

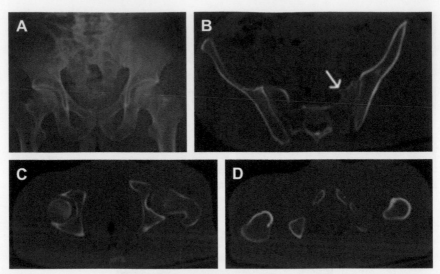

Fig. 6. Radiographic series of an elderly patient who sustained an LC type pelvis injury to the left side. (*A*) AP projection of the pelvis clearly illustrates left superior and inferior rami fractures but no obvious posterior pelvic injury is identified. (*B–D*) Axial CT cuts from the same patient taken at the level of the sacrum (*B*), superior ramus (*C*), and inferior ramus (*D*). The *arrow* on the sacral cut image demonstrates the left sacral buckle fracture that is much better identified on CT than plain radiographs. The superior and inferior rami fractures are again seen. Take note of the detailed comminution in the inferior ramus.

instability, and imbalance resulting in loss of autonomy.[2,11] In the elderly patient, prolonged immobility is met with severe complications.

Ideally all fractures could be managed without weight-bearing restrictions; however, some injuries are simply too unstable to safely allow weight bearing. In these instances, nonimpact joint range of motion and contralateral weight bearing for transfers are used.

The management goals for pelvis and acetabulum fragility fracture treatment as defined by our Geriatric Fracture Center are as follows:

1. Early mobilization: as soon as the fracture is deemed stable the patient can be weight bearing as tolerated and begin to mobilize.
2. Personal independence: similar to physical therapy, patients can begin occupational therapy on post-injury day zero. Therapists can help patients perform their activities of daily living and provide strategies to modify activities without sacrificing autonomy.
3. Fracture union
4. Pain control: pelvic and acetabulum fractures are painful and often worse with movement. Careful titration of pain medicines is required to alleviate pain such that the patient can participate in therapy but should not overly sedate him or her.
5. Osteoporosis treatment

NONPHARMACOLOGIC STRATEGIES

Nonpharmacologic treatment strategies for pelvic and acetabular insufficiency fractures consist of nonoperative and operative management. Nonoperative treatment is preferable in all cases in which the patient is expected to have an acceptable result without incurring the risks of surgery. There are specific criteria that the orthopedic surgeon will use to determine if a patient is a candidate for operative treatment; however, these indications are mutually exclusive pertaining to pelvis or acetabulum fractures. Orthopedic surgeons, for the purpose of surgical decision making, consider pelvic ring injuries and acetabulum fractures as separate entities. The following section separates pelvis and acetabulum fragility fractures and outlines the indications, strategies, and available options for both operative and nonoperative treatment.

Nonoperative Considerations

Pelvis

Most pelvic fragility fractures can be managed nonoperatively with progressive mobilization and serial radiographs. Surgical decision making is based on an assessment of stability. Thorough assessment of the anterior ring and the posterior ring, including the sacrum, is required to determine if a fracture pattern is stable and amenable to nonoperative treatment.

Patients with stable pelvic fractures can be mobilized on post-injury day zero. Repeat radiographs with AP/inlet/outlet projections are taken 1 week after the initial injury and are repeated at 4 to 6 weeks, 3 months, 6 months, and 1 year. Patients will begin formal inpatient physical and occupational therapy while in the hospital. Depending on progression in therapy, many patients will require home or inpatient rehabilitation services after leaving the hospital.

Acetabulum

Acetabulum insufficiency fractures present a unique challenge to the orthopedic surgeon. Any acetabulum fracture with minimal displacement, hip joint stability, and concentric reduction can be managed without surgery (**Fig. 7**); however, in the case of fragility fractures, there is often significant displacement and comminution. Goals for surgical treatment are often simply to restore the relationship between the femoral head and the weight-bearing dome. Injuries that do not disrupt this relationship can be managed without surgery as post-traumatic arthritis is often much less of a consideration in this population.

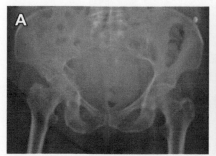 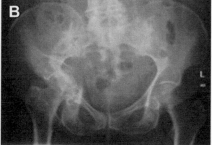

Fig. 7. Radiographic series of an elderly patient who sustained a displaced, associated both column acetabulum fracture after a ground-level fall. (*A*) Post-injury pelvis AP projection demonstrating fracture through both the anterior and posterior acetabulum columns. Note the medial displacement of the femoral head through the quadrilateral plate. Despite the displacement, the fragments maintain congruity to the femoral head effectively retaining a concentric joint space. (*B*) AP projection taken 8 weeks post-injury. There are signs of osseous healing and, although the medial displacement remains, the "secondary congruence" of the joint space is unchanged from initial post-injury alignment.

If nonoperative management is chosen, the patient must undergo an initial period of non–weight bearing with bed rest for pain control only. Once symptoms resolve, the patient may begin toe-touch weight bearing, which allows the patient to control balance using the injured side but prevents further fracture displacement or joint subluxation that could occur with full weight bearing. Toe-touch weight bearing can be difficult to perform in the elderly population and most, if not all, will require use of a rolling walker. Patients are followed with AP and Judet radiographs weekly for the first 4 weeks, then again at 6 weeks, 3 months, 6 months, and 1 year. It is important for the physical therapist to continually work on hip range of motion, starting at post-injury day 1, to prevent stiffness. Development of severe post-traumatic arthritis could alter the plan to an arthroplasty surgery but only after the fracture demonstrates radiographic healing.

Operative Considerations

Pelvis
The absolute operative indications for pelvic insufficiency fractures include open fractures, displaced H- or U-type sacral fractures (vertical fractures through the bilateral sacral foramen with a connecting transverse fracture line) with cauda equina syndrome, and the rare case of locked pubic symphysis. In addition, if a patient is unable to mobilize secondary to pain or altered gait, operative fixation can stabilize the fracture enough to relieve pain and enhance ambulation (**Fig. 8**).[27] In the case of symptomatic nonunion or malunion, operative manipulation and fixation are used to correct the deformity.

Acetabulum
The absolute operative indications in acetabular fragility fractures or acetabulum fractures in osteopenic bone include open fractures, hip joint instability, and intra-articular loose bodies. Hip joint incongruity and intra-articular displacement greater than 2 to 3 mm, particularly in the weight-bearing dome, are associated with risk of early post-traumatic arthritis and therefore are also considered surgical indications. Surgical options include traditional open reduction and internal fixation, percutaneous

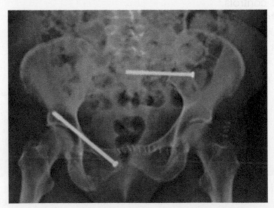

Fig. 8. AP view of the pelvis in a patient who underwent operative stabilization of a right-sided superior and inferior rami fractures and a left-sided sacroiliac joint injury. A sacroiliac screw was placed percutaneously on the left from the iliac wing into the S1 body. A partially threaded screw was placed from the right superior ramus into the supra-acetabular region. This case is an example of percutaneous techniques used to stabilize both posterior and anterior pelvic ring injuries.

minimally invasive fixation, and early total hip arthroplasty. Additionally, it should be noted that any fracture treated nonoperatively or operatively with internal fixation has the potential to progress into post-traumatic arthritis. These patients may become candidates for delayed total hip arthroplasty.

Post-operative care

Post-operative care in elderly acetabulum fractures consists of early hip range of motion exercises with weight bearing limited to toe touch only with walker or crutches. After 6 weeks patients can begin progressive weight bearing as tolerated. Patients are prescribed an accepted form of chemical deep venous thrombosis prophylaxis for 6 weeks total treatment period. Prophylaxis against heterotopic ossification is not routinely performed. Otherwise, AP/Judet projections are obtained at regularly scheduled follow-up to assess for osseous union and fracture alignment.

PHARMACOLOGIC STRATEGIES

In addition to the aforementioned nonoperative and operative management strategies, there are a variety of pharmacologic treatment options available for fragility fracture care. These medicines are designed for a variety of purposes including increasing bone mineral density, decreasing fracture healing times, preventing future fragility fractures, or a combination of these purposes. Patients presenting with an osteoporotic fragility fracture have a 1.8 to 2.0 relative risk of incurring a second fragility fracture in the future.[28] Patients with pelvic insufficiency fractures could be considered a higher risk population due to potential alterations in gait and balance mechanics. Careful consideration should be given to starting the patient on a pharmacologic osteoporosis treatment regimen. Further discussion of the management of osteoporosis in fragility fracture patients can be found in Chapter 14.

Vitamin D/Calcium

Vitamin D and calcium supplementation is a common mainstay of an osteoporosis treatment regimen. Population-based series have demonstrated a decreased risk of fragility fracture in patients receiving Vitamin D and calcium supplements as compared to nonmedicated controls.[29] After a pelvic insufficiency fracture, vitamin D and calcium supplementation should be initiated alone or as an adjunct to other pharmaceuticals to help reduce the risk of future fracture. Current National Osteoporosis Foundation recommended Vitamin D dosing for patients aged 50 years or older is 800 to 1000 IU per day.[24] Current recommended calcium dosing for men aged between 51 and 71 years is 1000 mg/d and that for men older than 71 years and women aged 51 years or older is 1200 mg/d.[24] Patients with Vitamin D deficiency are treated with higher doses. In the authors' Geriatric Fracture Center all patients presenting with fragility fracture are placed on a vitamin D and calcium regimen as outlined earlier.

Bisphosphonates

Bisphosphonates are a class of antiresorptive medications that are approved for treatment and prevention of osteoporosis in both men and women. Bisphosphonates target and inhibit the osteoclast cell type thereby decreasing bone resorption and turnover.[30] Through this mechanism of action bisphosphonates can slow the progression of osteoporosis.

Daily use of bisphosphonates is associated with reduced risk for insufficiency fracture, and a significant risk reduction can be appreciated within 6 months of therapy initiation.[31] In a randomized, placebo controlled trial, patients taking 5 mg of risedronate daily experienced a 39% to 59% overall reduction of nonverbral fractures over the 3-year study arc.[31,32] Patients receiving 10 mg of alendronate daily compared to placebo demonstrated significant bone mineral density increases in the spine, femoral neck, trochanter and total body.[33]

Bisphosphonates have been shown to significantly reduce fracture rates and increase bone mineral density; however, they are not without risk. The most common adverse reaction to bisphosphonates is gastrointestinal distress including dyspepsia, nausea, and ulcer formation.[33] Other less common side effects include renal damage, osteonecrosis of the jaw, and atypical subtrochanteric femur fracture.[24]

Calcitonin also inhibits osteoclast activity but has not been shown to prevent non-vertebral fragility fractures.[24]

Human Recombinant Parathyroid Hormone

Recombinant human parathyroid hormone (PTH 1-34) is in a class of anabolic medications approved by Food and Drug Administration for osteoporosis treatment in men and women at high risk for fracture.[24] Rh-PTH is administered through daily subcutaneous injections. The medication is designed to increase bone formation on trabecular, endosteal, and periosteal surfaces.[34]

In a randomized controlled trial, Piechl[35] reported that patients with pelvic fragility fractures treated with human recombinant PTH 1-84 demonstrated decreased healing times and improved functional scores as compared to untreated controls. Patients were evaluated with CT scans, Visual Analog Scale, and the Up and Go functional test. Patients in the PTH 1-84 group demonstrated a 7.8 weeks mean time to radiographic healing compared to 12.6 weeks for controls. Furthermore, the experimental group demonstrated significantly lower VAS pain scores and at 8 weeks the average Up and Go test was 22.9 ± 7.7 seconds compared to 54.3 ± 19.9 seconds in the control group. The improved functional scores in the PTH 1-84–treated group are likely due to earlier fracture union and reduced pain allowing for greater mobility.

Administration of rh-PTH has also been associated with decreased rates of fragility fracture occurrence. Rajzbaum and colleagues[36] evaluated 290 osteoporotic patients treated with PTH 1-34 over a period of 36 months. Of these patients, approximately 20% had experienced a pelvic fracture before initiation of therapy. By the end of the treatment period patients had significantly reduced risk of fracture. Of note, no pelvis fractures occurred during the course of the study.

Human recombinant PTH therapy should be initiated with caution. PTH 1-34 has been linked with osteosarcoma and is not recommended for patients with a prior history of osteosarcoma or conditions associated with skeletal malignancy such as Paget disease of bone.[24] Furthermore, all safety and efficacy data are based on 2 years of therapy, and adverse events for longer durations are unknown.[24]

SUMMARY

Fragility fracture of the pelvis and acetabulum are a growing concern. As the population ages, the incidence is rising dramatically. Pelvic ring injuries are painful and restrict mobility. Patients often lose their ability to function independently in the community that has immeasurable psychological impact in addition to a financial and social impact. Although much of the world is familiar with the concept of a hip fracture, the pelvis is not nearly as well understood creating concern and confusion for patients, their families, and General Practitioners.

Operative strategies are fraught with complications even in the most skilled of hands. Fortunately, most injuries to the pelvis and acetabulum can be well managed without a surgical intervention. A thorough discussion of the likely course of recovery, the prolonged need for pain medications, and the risks and benefits of intervention can help patients and their families cope with the disability. For many patients their pelvic fracture may be the first indicator of osteoporosis. In this group, treatment of their bone density is essential to reducing their risk of further fractures. A complete bone health evaluation is an essential component of pelvic fracture management.

REFERENCES

1. Browner WS, Pressman AR, Nevitt MC, et al. Mortality following fractures in older women: the study of osteoporotic fractures. Arch Intern Med 1996;156(14): 1521–5.
2. Taillandier J, Langue F, Alemanni M, et al. Mortality and functional outcomes of pelvic insufficiency fractures in older patients. Joint Bone Spine 2003;70:287–9.
3. Parkkari J, Kannus P, Niemi S, et al. Secular trends in osteoporotic pelvic fractures in Finland: number and incidence of fractures in 1970-1991 andprediction for the future. Calcif Tissue Int 1996;59(2):79–83.
4. Burge R, Dawson-Hughes B, Solomon DH, et al. Incidence and economic burden of osteoporosis-related fractures in the United States, 2005–2025. J Bone Miner Res 2006;22(3):465–75.
5. Melton LJ, Sampson JM, Morrey BF, et al. Epidemiologic features of pelvic fractures. Clin Orthop Relat Res 1981;155:43–7.
6. Ragnarsson B, Jacobsson B. Epidemiology of pelvic fractures in a Swedish county. Acta Orthop Scand 1992;63:297–300.
7. Kannus PP, Palvanen MM, Niemi SS, et al. Epidemiology of osteoporotic pelvic fractures in elderly people in Finland: sharp increase in 1970–1997 and alarming projections for the new millennium. Osteoporos Int 2000;11(5):443–8.
8. Ferguson TA, Patel R, Bhandari M, et al. Fractures of the acetabulum in patients aged 60 years and older: an epidemiological and radiological study. J Bone Joint Surg Br 2010;92(2):250–7.
9. Boufous S, Finch C, Lord S, et al. The increasing burden of pelvic fractures in older people, New South Wales, Australia. Injury 2005;36:1323–9.
10. Morris RO, Sonibare A, Green DJ, et al. Closed pelvic fractures: characteristics and outcomes in older patients admitted to medical and geriatric wards. Postgrad Med J 2000;76:646–50.
11. Breuil V, Roux CH, Testa J, et al. Outcome of osteoporotic pelvic fractures: an underestimated severity. Survey of 60 cases. Joint Bone Spine 2008;75:585–8.
12. Hill RM, Robinson CM, Keating JF. Fractures of the pubic rami: epidemiology and 5 year survival. J Bone Joint Surg Br 2001;83-B:1141–4.
13. Bible JE, Wegner A, McClure JM, et al. One-year mortality after acetabular fractures in elderly patients presenting to a level-one trauma center. J Orthop Trauma 2014;28(3):154–9.
14. Young JW, Burgess AR, Brumback RJ, et al. Pelvic fractures: value of plain radiography in early assessment and management. Radiology 1986;160(2):445–51.
15. Krappinger D, Kammerlander C, Hak DJ, et al. Low-energy osteoporotic pelvic fractures. Arch Orthop Trauma Surg 2010;130(9):1167–75.
16. Letournel E. Acetabular fractures: classification and management. Clin Orthop 1980;151:81–106.
17. Mears DC. Surgical treatment of acetabular fractures in elderly patients with osteoporotic bone. J Am Acad Orthop Surg 1999;7:128–41.
18. Gotis-Graham I, McGuigan L, Diamond T, et al. Sacral insufficiency fractures in the elderly. J Bone Joint Surg Br 1994;76:882–6.

19. Linstrom NJ, Heiserman JE, Kortman KE, et al. Anatomical and biomechanical analyses of the unique and consistent locations of sacral insufficiency fractures. Spine 2009;34(4):309–15.
20. Sembler-Soles GL, Ferguson TA. Fragility fractures of the pelvis. Curr Rev Musculoskelet Med 2012;5:222–8.
21. Judet R, Judet J, Letournel E. Fractures of the acetabulum. Classification and surgical approaches for open reduction. J Bone Joint Surg Am 1964;46A:1615–38.
22. Lyders EM, Whitlow CT, Baker MD, et al. Imaging and treatment of sacral insufficiency fractures. AJNR Am J Neuroradiol 2010;31(2):201–10.
23. Kanis JA, Melton LJ 3rd, Christiansen C, et al. The diagnosis of osteoporosis. J Bone Miner Res 1994;9(8):1137–41.
24. National Osteoporosis Foundation. Clinician's guide to the prevention and treatment of osteoporosis. Washington, DC: National Osteoporosis Foundation; 2013.
25. Scheyerer MJ, Osterhoff G, Wehrle S, et al. Detection of posterior pelvic injuries in fractures of the pubic rami. Injury 2012;43(8):1326–9.
26. Schädel-Höpfner M, Celik I, Stiletto R, et al. Computed tomography for the assessment of posterior pelvic injuries in patients with isolated fractures of the pubic rami in conventional radiography. Chirurg 2002;73(10):1013–8.
27. Barei DP, Shafer BL, Beingessner DM, et al. The impact of open reduction internal fixation on acute pain management in unstable pelvic ring injuries. J Trauma 2010;68:949–53.
28. Klotzbuecher CM, Ross PD, Landsman PB, et al. Patients with prior fractures have an increased risk of future fractures: a summary of the literature and statistical synthesis. J Bone Miner Res 2000;15(4):721–39.
29. Larsen ER, Mosekilde L, Foldspang A. Vitamin D and calcium supplementation prevents osteoporotic fractures in elderly community dwelling residents: a pragmatic population-based 3-year intervention study. J Bone Miner Res 2004;19(3):370–8.
30. Rodan GA, Fleisch HA. Bisphosphonates: mechanism of action. J Clin Invest 1996;97(12):2692–6.
31. Harrington JT, Ste-Marie LG, Brandi ML, et al. Risedronate rapidly reduces the risk for nonvertebral fractures in women with postmenopausal osteoporosis. Calcif Tissue Int 2004;74(2):129–35.
32. Harris ST, Watts NB, Genant HK, et al. Effects of risedronate treatment on vertebral and nonvertebral fractures in women with postmenopausal osteoporosis: a randomized controlled trial. Vertebral Efficacy with Risedronate Therapy (VERT) Study Group. JAMA 1999;282(14):1344–52.
33. Liberman UA, Weiss SR, Broll J, et al. Effect of oral alendronate on bone mineral density and the incidence of fractures in postmenopausal osteoporosis. The alendronate phase III osteoporosis treatment study group. N Engl J Med 1995;333(22):1437–43.
34. Bukata SV. Systemic administration of pharmacological agents and bone repair: what can we expect. Injury 2011;42:605–8.
35. Peichl P. Parathyroid hormone 1–84 accelerates fracture- healing in pubic bones of elderly osteoporotic women. J Bone Joint Surg Am 2011;93(17):1583.
36. Rajzbaum G, Grados F, Evans D, et al. Treatment persistence and changes in fracture risk, back pain, and quality of life amongst patients treated withteriparatide in routine clinical care in France: results from the European Forsteo Observational Study. Joint Bone Spine 2013. http://dx.doi.org/10.1016/j.jbspin.2013.05.001. pii:S1297–319X(13)00120-6.

Index

Note: Page numbers of article titles are in **boldface** type.

Clin Geriatr Med 30 (2014) 387–393
http://dx.doi.org/10.1016/S0749-0690(14)00028-7
0749-0690/14/$ – see front matter © 2014 Elsevier Inc. All rights reserved.

geriatric.theclinics.com

Moving?

Make sure your subscription moves with you!

To notify us of your new address, find your **Clinics Account Number** (located on your mailing label above your name), and contact customer service at:

Email: journalscustomerservice-usa@elsevier.com

800-654-2452 (subscribers in the U.S. & Canada)
314-447-8871 (subscribers outside of the U.S. & Canada)

Fax number: 314-447-8029

Elsevier Health Sciences Division
Subscription Customer Service
3251 Riverport Lane
Maryland Heights, MO 63043

*To ensure uninterrupted delivery of your subscription, please notify us at least 4 weeks in advance of move.

Printed and bound by CPI Group (UK) Ltd, Croydon, CR0 4YY

03/10/2024

01040493-0005